Applied Animal
Reproduction

Applied Animal Reproduction

Sixth Edition

H. Joe Bearden
John W. Fuquay
Scott T. Willard
Mississippi State University

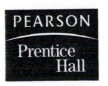

Upper Saddle River, New Jersey 07458

Library of Congress Cataloging-in-Publication Data

Bearden, H. Joe (Henry Joe)

    Applied animal reproduction / H. Joe Bearden, John W. Fuquay, Scott T. Willard.— 6th ed.
       p. cm.

Includes bibliographical references and index.

ISBN 0-13-112831-0

  1. Livestock—Reproduction. 2. Livestock—Breeding. 3. Veterinary obstetrics.
4. Artificial insemination. I. Fuquay, John W. II. Willard, Scott T. III. Title.

SF871.B4 2004

636.08′ 2—dc21

2003046013

Editor-in-Chief: Stephen Helba
Executive Editor: Debbie Yarnell
Editorial Assistant: Jonathan Tenthoff
Managing Editor: Mary Carnis
Production Editor: Amy Hackett/Carlisle Communications
Production Liaison: Janice Stangel
Director of Manufacturing and Production: Bruce Johnson
Manufacturing Buyer: Cathleen Petersen
Creative Director: Cheryl Asherman
Cover Design Coordinator: Miguel Ortiz
Marketing Manager: Jimmy Stephens
Cover Illustration: Courtesy © Joe McDonald/Corbis

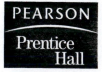

10 9 8 7 6 5 4 3 2 1
ISBN 0-13-112831-0

Contents

Preface xv

Chapter 1   ***Introduction and Early History***   ***1***
Suggested Reading   4

PART 1   **Anatomy, Function, and Regulation**

Chapter 2   ***The Female Reproductive System***   ***7***
2–1   Ovaries   7
2–2   Oviducts   13
2–3   Uterus   13
2–4   Cervix   17
2–5   Vagina   19
2–6   Vulva   19
2–7   Support Structures, Nerves, and Blood Supply   19
          Suggested Reading   21

Chapter 3   ***The Male Reproductive System***   ***22***
3–1   Testes   22
3–2   Scrotum and Spermatic Cord   27
3–3   Epididymis   29
3–4   Vasa Deferentia and Urethra   31
3–5   Accessory Glands   31
3–6   Penis   33
3–7   Prepuce   33
          Suggested Reading   35

Chapter 4   ***Neuroendocrine and Endocrine Regulators of Reproduction***   ***36***
4–1   Primary Reproductive Hormones of the Pituitary Gland   38
4–2   Neuroendocrine Control of the Pituitary Gland   40
4–3   Hormones of the Gonads   44

4–4   Primary Reproductive Hormones of the Adrenal Cortex   48
4–5   Endocrine Function of the Uterine/Placental Unit   49
4–6   Reproductive Role of Prostaglandins   49
4–7   Hormone-like Factors and Other Hormonal Mediators   50
4–8   Regulation of Hormonal Receptor Sites   52
4–9   Intracellular Mechanisms of Hormone Actions   53
4–10   Methods of Hormone Detection and Measurement   55
4–11   Summary   57
        Suggested Reading   57

PART 2   **Reproductive Processes**

Chapter 5   *The Estrous Cycle   61*

5–1   Puberty   61
5–2   Periods of the Estrous Cycle   63
5–3   Hormonal Control of the Estrous Cycle   64
5–4   Follicular Dynamics   67
5–5   Seasonal Breeders   70
        Suggested Reading   73

Chapter 6   *Spermatogenesis and Maturation of Spermatozoa   75*

6–1   Puberty   75
6–2   The Process of Spermatogenesis   77
6–3   The Seminiferous Epithelial Cycle and Spermatogenic Wave 82
6–4   Capacitation of Spermatozoa and Acrosome Reaction   84
        Suggested Reading   86

Chapter 7   *Mating Behavior   87*

7–1   Regulation of Mating Behavior   87
7–2   Behavioral Characteristics of Estrus   90
7–3   Mating Behavior in Males   91
        Suggested Reading   95

Chapter 8   *Ovigenesis and Fertilization   96*

8–1   Ovigenesis   96
8–2   Ovulation   98
8–3   Gamete Transport   99
8–4   Fertilization   103
8–5   Polyspermy   105
8–6   Aging of Gametes   105
        Suggested Reading   107

Chapter 9   *Gestation   109*

9–1   Cleavage   110
9–2   Differentiation   112
9–3   Fetal Growth   119

9–4   Maintenance of Pregnancy   121
9–5   Twinning   124
      Suggested Reading   126

Chapter 10   *Parturition and Postpartum Recovery*   128

10–1   Overview of the Parturition Process   128
10–2   Approaching Parturition   128
10–3   Parturition   131
10–4   Dystocia   135
10–5   Care of the Newborn   135
10–6   Retained Placentae   136
10–7   Postpartum Recovery   137
       Suggested Reading   140

Chapter 11   *Lactation*   142

11–1   Structure of Mammary Glands   142
11–2   Hormonal Regulation of the Development and Function
       of the Mammary Gland   146
11–3   Composition of Milk   150
       Suggested Reading   152

PART 3   Artificial Insemination

Chapter 12   *Introduction and History of Artificial Insemination*   155

12–1   Introduction   155
12–2   History   156
12–3   Advantages and Disadvantages   159
       Suggested Reading   159

Chapter 13   *Semen Collection*   160

13–1   Facilities Needed for Semen Collection   160
13–2   Methods of Semen Collection   160
       Suggested Reading   172

Chapter 14   *Semen and Its Components*   173

14–1   Spermatozoa   173
14–2   Seminal Plasma   177
14–3   Energy Metabolism by Spermatozoa   178
14–4   Factors Affecting Rate of Metabolism   179
       Suggested Reading   182

Chapter 15   *Semen Evaluation*   183

15–1   Gross Examination   183
15–2   Progressive Motility   184
15–3   Concentration of Sperm Cells   186

15–4   Sperm Cell Morphology   190

15–5   Differential Staining of Live and Dead Sperm   192

15–6   Speed of Sperm   192

15–7   Evaluating Frozen Semen   193

15–8   Computer Automated Semen Analyzer   195

15–9   Other Tests   196

        Suggested Reading   197

Chapter 16   **Semen Processing, Storage, and Handling**   **198**

16–1   Importance and Properties of Semen Diluters   199

16–2   Buffer Solutions Used in Semen Diluters   200

16–3   Antimicrobial Agents for Semen Diluters   201

16–4   Effective Diluters for Bull Semen   202

16–5   Processing Bull Semen   204

16–6   Storage and Handling of Bull Semen   211

16–7   What Does the Future Hold for Liquid Bull Semen?   212

16–8   Processing Boar Semen   214

16–9   Processing Ram Semen   217

16–10   Processing Stallion Semen   218

16–11   Processing Buck Semen   221

        Suggested Reading   221

Chapter 17   **Insemination Techniques**   **223**

17–1   Insemination of the Cow   223

17–2   Insemination of the Ewe and Doe   230

17–3   Insemination of the Sow   231

17–4   Insemination of the Mare   233

        Suggested Reading   234

PART 4   **Management for Improved Reproduction**

Chapter 18   **Synchronization of Estrus and Superovulation with Embryo Transfer**   **237**

18–1   Synchronization of Estrus   237

18–2   Superovulation and Embryo Transfer   249

        Suggested Reading   259

Chapter 19   **Reproductive Biotechnology**   **261**

19–1   Assisted Reproductive Technologies   261

19–2   Sex Determination and Control   269

19–3   Cloning   276

19–4   Genetic Engineering (Transgenics)   278

19–5   Gene Discovery—Markers for Reproduction   282

19–6   Technologies for the Future—Definitions   286

        Suggested Reading   289

Chapter 20   *Reproductive Management*   *291*

20–1   Measurements of Reproductive Efficiency   291
20–2   Management Related to the Female   292
20–3   Management Related to the Male   309
20–4   Altering Male Reproduction   313
Suggested Reading   317

Chapter 21   *Pregnancy Diagnosis*   *318*

21–1   Cow   318
21–2   Ewe and Doe   329
21–3   Mare   331
21–4   Sow   334
Suggested Reading   337

Chapter 22   *Environmental Management*   *338*

22–1   Environmental Stressors   338
22–2   Physiological Relationship of Environmental Stress to
         Reproduction   341
22–3   Thermoregulation   343
22–4   Modification of Summer Environments
         to Reduce Stress   343
22–5   Other Management Considerations in Hot Environments   345
Suggested Reading   346

Chapter 23   *Nutritional Management*   *348*

23–1   Nutritive Components   348
23–2   Growing Animals   354
23–3   Maintaining Reproductive Efficiency   355
Suggested Reading   357

PART 5   **Causes of Reproductive Failure**

Chapter 24   *Anatomical and Inherited Causes of Reproductive*
               Failure   *361*

24–1   Freemartin   361
24–2   Infantile Reproductive System   363
24–3   Incomplete Structures—Oviduct, Uterus, Cervix,
         or Vagina   363
24–4   Hermaphrodite   364
24–5   Cryptorchid   365
24–6   Injuries   366
24–7   Prolapse of Vagina and Uterus   368
24–8   Genetic Abnormalities   369
Suggested Reading   369

Chapter 25   *Physiological, Toxicological, and Psychological Causes of Reproductive Failure*   *370*

     25–1   Cystic Ovaries   370
     25–2   Retained Corpus Luteum   373
     25–3   Anestrus   374
     25–4   Irregular Estrous Cycles   375
     25–5   Quiet Ovulation   376
     25–6   Age   377
     25–7   Reproductive Toxicology   378
     25–8   Psychological Disturbances   385
     Suggested Reading   387

Chapter 26   *Infectious Diseases That Cause Reproductive Failure*   *389*

     26–1   Bacterial Diseases   389
     26–2   Protozoan Diseases   403
     26–3   Viral Diseases   406
     Suggested Reading   411

Index   *413*

List of Tables

Table 1–1   Accuracy of sire proofs for predicting milk yield   3

Table 2–1   Reproductive organs of the female with their major functions   9

Table 3–1   Reproductive organs of the male with their major functions   25

Table 4–1   Molecular size of peptide and protein hormones that regulate reproduction   37

Table 4–2   Hormones that regulate reproduction   39

Table 4–3   Major steroid hormones produced by the gonads   44

Table 5–1   Species differences in various characteristics of the estrous cycle   62

Table 5–2   Species and breed differences in age and weight at puberty   62

Table 5–3   Primary characteristics of the periods of the estrous cycle in the cow   63

Table 6–1   Effect of time of insemination on ovulation and fertility in cows   85

Table 7–1   Characteristics of average ejaculate of semen for different species   93

Table 8–1   Transport time of oocytes in the oviduct of farm animals   100

Table 8–2   Estimated fertile life of sperm and ova in farm animals   106

Table 8–3   Effect of age of the ovum on fertility in cattle   106

Table 8–4   Effect of the length of time of storage of extended semen on its fertility level and the difference between 1-month and 5-month nonreturns   106

Table 9–1   Species and breed differences in gestation length   110

Table 9–2   Time comparisons during early embryonic development for different farm
species   112

Table 9–3   Certain organs that have been identified as forming from specific
germ layers   114

Table 9–4   Developmental features in cattle and swine during differentiation   118

Table 9–5   Weight changes of the bovine uterus and its contents during pregnancy   120

Table 9–6   Average daily growth rates and relative growth rates for single and twin
fetal sheep at different stages of gestation   120

Table 10–1   Average time required for the three stages of parturition for different
species of farm animals   129

Table 10–2   Interaction of energy level and suckling on postpartum anestrus in
beef cows   139

Table 11–1   Comparison of the mammary glands of various species   143

Table 11–2   Species and breed differences in milk composition   150

Table 11–3   Comparison of the composition of colostrum with that of normal
milk   151

Table 13–1   Common characteristics of ejaculates for farm species   161

Table 13–2   Characteristics of ejaculates from bulls with and without sexual
stimulation   163

Table 14–1   Sources and relative contribution (volume %) to semen   174

Table 14–2   Average chemical composition of semen from different species
(mg/100 ml)   174

Table 14–3   Characteristics of semen from farm animals   174

Table 16–1   Fertility with antibacterial agents in 50% yolk-citrate: High and low
fertility bulls   201

Table 16–2   Commonly used diluters for processing bull semen   203

Table 16–3   Freeze rates of semen in straws C/minute   210

Table 16–4   Composition of Beltsville F5 diluter and thawing solution
for boar semen   214

Table 16–5   Number of motile ram sperm ($\times 10^6$) per breeding unit as affected by
deposit site and processing   217

Table 16–6   Sample diluters for liquid ram semen   218

Table 16–7   Sample diluters for liquid stallion semen   219

Table 16–8   Sample diluters used in freezing stallion semen   220

Table 18–1   Plasma progesterone levels, response rate, and conception rate of dairy
heifers injected with $PGF_{2\alpha}$ in early, middle, and late diestrus   240

Table 18–2   Distribution of estrus following 25 mg $PGF_{2\alpha}$ injected intramuscularly to
Holstein heifers that had been observed for estrus for 5 days   241

Table 18–3   Effect of timing of insemination on the pregnancy rate of heifers treated with Norgestomet ear implants for 9 days   243

Table 18–4   Summary of events in superovulation and embryo transfer in the cow using unpurified FSH extracts   251

Table 18–5   Modified Dulbecco's phosphate-buffered medium   255

Table 19–1   Defined medium (DM) for *in vitro* fertilization   262

Table 19–2   Time of *in vitro* fertilization events and embryo development   268

Table 19–3   The effect of sample size on sex determination rate by amplification of a bovine Y chromosome–specific sequence   272

Table 19–4   Confirmation of sex prediction of embryos by amplification of Y chromosome–specific sequences by birth of live calves or ultrasound pregnancy diagnosis   272

Table 19–5   Comparative flow cytometric reanalysis for DNA of sorted nuclei and sorted, intact sperm from three different species   276

Table 19–6   Selected listing of milk gene promoters and expressed proteins   281

Table 19–7   Logistic regression analysis of the presence or absence of AFLP markers with classifications of good or bad freezability and semen quality assessments   286

Table 20–1   Recommended body weight and size of heifers at puberty, first breeding, and first calving for the dairy breeds and selected beef breeds   292

Table 20–2   Cows detected in estrus when checked three or four times daily, compared with twice daily   293

Table 20–3   Cows detected in estrus during A.M. versus P.M.   294

Table 20–4   Time of insemination and 150- to 180-day percentage of nonreturns   300

Table 20–5   Recommended time for breeding cows and sows in relation to onset of estrus   300

Table 20–6   Effect of winter turn-out management on nonreturn rate in cows   300

Table 20–7   Relationship of postpartum breeding interval to percent nonreturns and interval to conception   302

Table 20–8   Incidence of retained placenta in the Mississippi State University dairy herd by breed (Jan. 1971–Dec. 1977)   308

Table 20–9   Semen characteristics of a Holstein bull ejaculated three times per week, 4 consecutive years following puberty   309

Table 21–1   Diameter of pregnant bovine uterine horn at different stages of pregnancy   321

Table 21–2   Average size of bovine conceptus at different ages: variation occurs between breeds and within breeds   322

Table 21–3   Fertilization, embryonic survival, and embryonic mortality rates of bulls with histories of either low or high fertility in artificial breeding   327

Table 22–1   Options available to animal managers to reduce heat stress and that are likely to be economically feasible during the summer   344

Table 23–1   Nutrient-related abnormalities in reproduction   349

Table 23–2   Influence of plane of nutrition on reproductive performance of Holsteins   350

Table 23–3   Effect of dietary energy on ovulation rate in cycling gilts   355

Table 25–1   Number and percentage of normal and abnormal intervals between heats, as determined from ovarian examination of 200 cows through 500 cycles   376

Table 25–2   Conception rates in cows bred during and following various ovarian conditions   377

Table 25–3   Percent conception for cows by age groups, compared with cows more than 36 months of age   378

Table 25–4   Breeding efficiency of inexperienced inseminators in areas where AI was new and in areas where AI had previously been established   386

Table 26–1   Summary of diseases affecting reproduction in farm species   390

Preface

We are pleased to present the sixth edition of *Applied Animal Reproduction.* Some significant changes will be apparent in this edition, as compared with earlier editions. Dr. Scott T. Willard is now a part of the author team. Dr. Willard is an emerging reproductive physiologist with an interest in and a philosophy for teaching undergraduate students that is compatable with that of the other two authors of this text. There is some reorganization of chapters in this edition and three new chapters have been included. A new chapter, "Mating Behavior," has combined elements from Chapter 5, "The Estrous Cycle," and old Chapter 11, "Male Mating Behavior." This is the new Chapter 7 and is located in front of the chapter entitled "Ovigenesis and Fertilization." Chapter 18 from earlier editions is now two chapters, Chapter 18, "Synchronization of Estrus and Superovulation with Embryo Transfer," and Chapter 19, "Reproductive Biotechnology." The information in these chapters has been updated and expanded considerably. Several tables and figures have been added to the text, and color plates that are representative of material covered in the book are grouped at two locations.

There has been substantial revision of several other chapters. Two new sections, "Hormone-like Factors and Other Hormonal Mediators" and "Methods of Hormone Detection and Measurement," are found in Chapter 4, "Neuroendocrine and Endocrine Regulators of Reproduction." A section on immunological considerations has been added to Chapter 9, "Gestation," and a section on reproductive toxicology has been added to Chapter 25, "Physiological, Toxicological, and Psychological Causes of Reproductive Failure." Further, Chapter 11, "Lactation," has been expanded to include new information on the biosynthesis of milk. Updated information can be found throughout the text.

Even though there is considerable revision in this edition, the writing style has not changed. Also, the reorganization has been minor and should not affect the lecture format of instructors who have been using this text. This text is intended to give the undergraduate student majoring in animal or dairy science a complete overview of the reproductive processes. It is assumed that these students have a limited background in physiology. Therefore, a major effort has been made to maintain clarity. It is hoped that this style of writing will also encourage use of this text in 2-year agricultural curricula and in short courses where participants have a more limited educational background. Sixty combined years of experience in teaching a course in physiology of reproduction to students with a wide divergence of backgrounds have influenced the level of writing and the organization of the book. Comments and suggestions from students were given careful consideration during the preparation of the text.

Parts 1 and 2 are designed to help students develop both the terminology needed to discuss problems associated with physiology of reproduction and an understanding of the physiological processes controlling reproduction. These parts have been updated to provide students with recent information. Chapter 4 will be difficult because the concept of endocrine regulation will be new to most undergraduate students. When this information is reinforced in later chapters on reproductive processes in the female and the male, these concepts will seem less troublesome. Early introduction permits development of a more profound understanding of the neuroendocrine and endocrine regulation of reproduction.

Parts 3, 4, and 5 emphasize the application of basic concepts to the management of reproduction in livestock. This text is unique in the emphasis that is given to the applied aspects of reproduction. Five chapters are devoted to artificial insemination. These include collection, evaluation, storage, and utilization of semen through artificial insemination. Five chapters are written on reproductive management with specific chapters on environmental management, nutritional management, pregnancy diagnosis, and diseases affecting reproduction. The goal of these chapters goes beyond description of simple techniques for good reproductive management. They are designed to help students understand the rationale and principles used in developing guidelines for good reproductive management.

Several steps have been taken to make this text more readable. Important terms are italicized and defined when first introduced. Only the most prevalent theories are presented, and these have been simplified rather than presented in lengthy discussions on the pros and cons of these concepts. A consensus is presented where disagreement exists in the literature. Also, reference citations are not listed in the text. A carefully selected reading list has been included at the end of each chapter. It is intended to provide the student with references to classical as well as more recent literature pertaining to reproduction. These lists of suggested reading are not intended as a complete and up-to-date bibliography used in the development of each chapter. The references have been limited to encourage additional reading, rather than overwhelming students with the vast number of publications available on each topic. The writing style used in this book may be troublesome to instructors who are accustomed to delving into scientific literature. Referenced texts are currently available, while few have been written specifically for undergraduates. The selected readings after each chapter include both reviews and publications of original research, which will be useful for documentation.

H. Joe Bearden
John W. Fuquay
Scott T. Willard

Introduction and Early History

Reproduction is a complex science, so much so that Dr. William Hansel of Cornell University told his classes, "It is not a wonder that reproduction sometimes fails, but rather a miracle that so many pregnancies terminate successfully." This is obviously an overstatement. However, it does indicate the complexity of the subject. In order to understand the science of reproduction, it is necessary to include anatomy, physiology, endocrinology, embryology, histology, cytology, microbiology, and some nutrition. Reproduction involves a series of physiological and psychological events that must be properly timed. The endocrine system, through the production of several hormones, is responsible for this timing.

Much of the existing knowledge pertaining to reproduction has been generated during the past 60 years. However, Hippocrates (460–377 B.C.), the "Father of Modern Medicine," makes reference to the differences between castrates and intact males and wrote about the relationship between promiscuous behavior and the spread of disease. He erroneously credited the observed physical differences between castrates and intact males and the higher incidence of disease in prominicuis as compared to chaste men to the "power of semen which was retained in intact and chaste men." Hippocrates also believed that illness had a physical and rational explanation, rejecting views that considered illnesses to be caused by superstitions such as possession of evil spirits and disfavor of the gods. These views were supported by Aristotle (384–322 B.C.), whose greatest contribution was to turn the human mind away from superstition, replacing it with observation. Aristotle also wrote the first scientific papers on embryology. His great work was so far ahead of the age in which he lived it was nearly 2,000 years before anything of significance was added. Working without a microscope, Aristotle had to speculate on some things and here he fell into error. He formulated two theories for embryonic development: (1) the embryo was preformed and grew or enlarged during development, or (2) it was the result of differentiation from a formless being. He decided on the latter, crediting the popular belief that slime and decaying matter were capable of producing living animals. He described the human embryo as being organized out of the mother's menstrual blood. New developments awaited the invention of the microscope.

In 1562, Fallopius, an Italian anatomist and botanist, discovered and described the oviduct (hence, the term "fallopian" tubes in human anatomy) and was an early authority on the sexual transmission of syphilis. Coiter described the corpus luteum in 1573, and in 1668 Redi published papers which tended to disprove Aristotle's theory that the human embryo developed from menstrual blood. De Graaf described the ovarian follicle in 1672, while Hamm and Leewenhoek, with the aid of the early microscope, observed and described human spermatozoa in 1677. During the period from 1759 to 1769, Wolf observed parts of the chick embryo take shape and virtually destroyed the preformation theory. However, he was not able to show that development began with a single cell. He set forth the theory of *epigenesis*—development of an embryo by progressive growth and differentiation. Some individuals tended to hang onto the preformation theory until about 1860. Some believed that the pre-formed animal existed in the ovum and that growth was stimulated by seminal fluid from the male. Others believed that the preformed animal existed in the sperm cell, which grew after entering the egg. Dumas in 1825 discovered that follicles contained ova and that when sperm united with the ova it produced an embryo, which proved that sperm were fertilizing agents. The first recorded *endocrine* experiment (i.e., hormonal integration of the body) was con-ducted in 1849 by Berthold, who castrated roosters and then transplanted testes back into the castrated birds. The castrated roosters exhibited small combs and wattles, no interest in hens, weak crowing abilities, and listless fighting behavior. When one or both testes were replaced, combs and wattles developed normally, and the roosters showed interest in hens, exhibited strong crowing abilities, and aggressive fighting behavior. Through these studies, Berthold identified the testis as important for normal sexual development and for the development of secondary sex characteristics in the male. Pasteur in 1864 demonstrated that bacteria repro-duced themselves through cell division, thus destroying the theory of spontaneous generation. Driesh in 1900 provided the final proof that life came from single cells by separating daugh-ter cells of a fertilized egg and showed that they could each develop into an embryo.

A tremendous amount of knowledge pertaining to reproduction has been generated since 1900, but the subject remains very dynamic. Reproductive efficiency has been greatly enhanced as improved practices based on new scientific information have been put into use. Greater use of these practices by those who use this book will result in further improvements.

Recent research has resulted in major advances in *in vitro* fertilization as well as cloning using stem cells of embryos and adult animals. Some of these techniques will no doubt rank with the discovery of the microscope in helping us to understand reproductive processes. The student must keep in mind that the concepts presented in this book are as current as our present knowledge will allow but that future research will change some of them. It will be only through continued basic research that major improvements in repro-ductive efficiency will be accomplished.

Reproduction has at least three purposes:

1. *Perpetuation of the species.* The strongest desire of an individual in any species, including humans, is to maintain itself. The strongest impulse in an individual is saving its own life. Reproduction is nature's second strongest impulse, thus, the maintenance of the species.

2. *To provide food.* Humans have learned to manage both domestic and wild species so that surplus animals may be harvested to supply meat. Through selection, they have developed the milk-producing capabilities of a few species, so that milk, too, has become an important link in the human food chain. Reproduction is essential for the maintenance and continuity of nature's food chain as well.

3. *Genetic improvement.* The management and alteration of natural reproductive processes have been utilized as genetic tools.

Genetic improvement of any species is accomplished by selecting males and females with superior transmitting ability as parents of succeeding generations. Selection pressures have been applied for thousands of years, but more genetic progress has been made during the past 50 years than in any previous 100-year period. Some of this progress has been made through genetic knowledge and techniques; however, a large part of it has been accomplished by manipulating, or harnessing, the reproductive process.

The rate of genetic improvement through selection depends on several factors. *Variation,* that difference in production level for individual animals for characteristics such as milk production, rate of gain, weaning weight, and so on, must exist. Otherwise, there would be no basis for selection. *Heritability* is the percentage of total variation that is controlled by the genetic makeup of the individual. This portion of the variation is also referred to as *genetic variation.* If all of the difference in the records made by different individuals were due to genetic variation, heritability would be 1 or 100%; thus, an animal's production records or appearance would perfectly measure its genetic value. Heritability for most economic traits in farm animals ranges from 0% to 60%; milk production 25%; number of pigs per litter 5% to 10%; yearling body weight in sheep 20% to 59%; feedlot gain in beef cattle 50% to 55%; and fertility in cattle 5%. *Environmental variation* is the difference between total variation and genetic variation. In order to measure genetic gain, it is necessary to either control or account for environmental variation. *Selection intensity* is a factor that affects the rate of genetic improvement by determining the ratio of offspring utilized for extensive breeding versus the number culled after adequate sampling. The higher the culling rate, the faster genetic progress should be. *Generation interval* is the average interval between the birth of an animal and the birth of its offspring. The shorter the generation interval, the faster progress can be made. Selection intensity can be changed at will, but only minor changes can be made in generation interval. From these accurately measured factors, one can estimate the rate of genetic progress per generation or per year.

Artificial insemination (AI) is an example of reproductive processes being used as a genetic tool. The true transmitting ability for milk production and overall type score in dairy bulls was virtually impossible to obtain prior to the introduction of AI. The wide variation that exists, plus a relatively low heritability of the traits, requires a large number of offspring with production records or type scores. These records also need to be made in many different herds to account for environmental variation. Table 1–1 shows the accuracy of sire proofs for predicting milk yields, assuming heritability of 25% and an environmental correlation of

Table 1–1   *Accuracy of sire proofs for predicting milk yield*

Number of daughters	Accuracy when all cows are in different herds	Accuracy when all cows are in one herd
1	25%	25%
5	50	46
10	63	53
20	76	60
40	85	65
50	88	66
70	91	67
100	93	68
200	96	69
1,000	99	70

From Schmidt and Van Vleck, *Principles of Dairy Science*, W. H. Freeman and Co., copyright © 1974.

6% among daughters in the same herd. An *environmental correlation* exists when daughters of a sire are treated more alike than unrelated cows. Note that when all daughters are in different herds the accuracy reaches 99% only when there are 1,000 daughters with records. When all daughters are in one herd, the accuracy is only 70% with records on 1,000 daughters. Before AI, a bull seldom had more than 20 daughters and usually these were in one or possibly two herds. The example given here is for milk yield, but the general principle applies to essentially all economic traits of all species of farm animals. Traits with higher heritability will require fewer numbers. For traits with extremely low heritability, such as fertility in cattle, little progress can be expected through selection.

Other reproductive processes that have been or may be used as genetic tools are

1. Frozen semen
2. Separation of male- and female-producing sperm
3. Synchronization of estrus
4. Superovulation
5. Embryo transfer
6. Storing of embryos
7. *In vitro* fertilization
8. Environmental influence on puberty
9. Cloning of embryos and adult animals
10. Transfer of genetic material

These processes will be discussed in detail in later chapters as they relate to genetic improvement and enhancement of reproductive efficiency in livestock.

SUGGESTED READING

ASDELL, S. A. 1977. Historical introduction. *Reproduction in Domestic Animals.* (3rd ed.) eds. H. H. Cole and P. T. Cupps. Academic Press.

HADLEY, M. E. 1988. *Endocrinology.* Prentice Hall.

SALISBURY, G. W., N. L. VANDEMARK, and J. R. LODGE. 1978. *Physiology of Reproduction and Artificial Insemination of Cattle.* (2nd ed.) W. H. Freeman and Co.

SCHMIDT, G. H. and L. D. VAN VLECK. 1974. *Principles of Dairy Science.* W. H. Freeman and Co.

Part 1

Anatomy, Function, and Regulation

The chapters in Part 1 are intended to acquaint students with the nomenclature as well as the physiological control systems that are necessary for their comprehension of later chapters on the physiological processes involved in reproduction and how sound physiological principles are used in management of reproduction. Chapters 2 and 3 detail functional anatomy in the female and the male. There may be questions as to why the female and male chapters are not grouped by gender. Given the fact that viable gametes from both females and males are necessary for fertilization, information on females and males needs to be presented somewhat concurrently up to completion of the fertilization process. Chapter 4 presents concepts that will be new and therefore difficult for many undergraduate students. However, a comprehension of these basic concepts is important for developing an understanding of how these reproductive processes are controlled and how they can be manipulated.

The Female Reproductive System

The female reproductive system, as illustrated for the cow in Figure 2–1, consists of two ovaries and the female duct system. The duct system includes the oviducts, uterus, cervix, vagina, and vulva. The embryonic origin of the ovaries is the *secondary sex cords* of the genital ridges. The *genital ridges* are first seen in the embryo as a slight thickening near the kidneys. The duct system originates from the *Müllerian ducts*, a pair of ducts that appear during early embryonic development (Chapter 9). An overview of the organs of reproduction for the female and the major functions of these organs is shown in Table 2–1. Color plates of the cow (Plates 1 and 2) and sow/gilt (Plates 3 and 4) reproductive tracts are provided as a supplement to the text and accompanying figures.

2–1 OVARIES

The *ovaries* are considered the primary reproductive organs in the female. They are primary because they produce the female gamete (the *ovum*) and the female sex hormones (estrogens and progestins). The cow, mare, and ewe are *monotocous,* normally giving birth to one young each *gestation period.* Therefore, one ovum is produced each estrous cycle. The sow is *polytocous,* producing 10 to 25 ova each estrous cycle and giving birth to several young each gestation period.

The ovary of the cow is described as almond-shaped, but the shape is altered by growing follicles or corpora lutea. The average size is about 35 mm × 25 mm × 15 mm. The size will vary among cows, and active ovaries are larger than inactive ovaries. Therefore, one ovary is frequently larger than the other in a given cow. The ovaries of the ewe and doe (goat) are almond-shaped and less than half the size of those of a cow. The ovaries in the mare are kidney-shaped and are two or three times larger than ovaries of a cow. The ovaries in the sow are slightly larger than those found in the ewe and appear as a "cluster of grapes" because of the extensive follicle growth and associated corpora lutea.

The ovary is composed of an inner *medulla* and its outer shell, the *cortex.* The medulla is composed primarily of blood vessels, nerves, and connective tissue. The cortex contains those cell and tissue layers associated with ovum and hormone production. The outermost layer of the cortex of the ovary is the *surface epithelium.* The surface epithelium, a single layer of cuboidal cells, was originally called the germinal epithelium because it was believed to be the origin of female germ cells (oogonia). It is now known that germ cells do

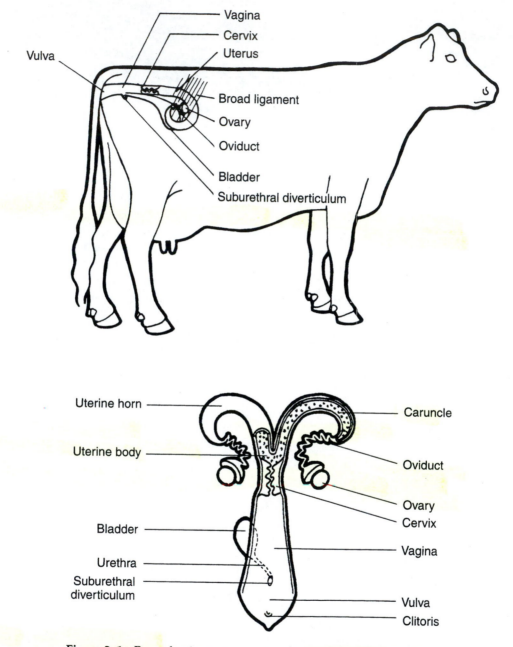

Figure 2–1 Reproductive system and associated parts of the urinary system of the cow as it appears in the natural state *(top)* and excised *(bottom)*.

Table 2–1 *Reproductive organs of the female with their major functions*

Organ	Function(s)
Ovary	Production of oocytes
	Production of estrogens (Graafian follicle)
	Production of progestins (corpus luteum)
Oviduct	Gamete transport (spermatozoa and oocytes)
	Site of fertilization
Uterus	Retains and nourishes the embryo and fetus
Cervix	Prevents microbial contamination of uterus
	Reservoir for semen and transport of spermatozoa
	Site of semen deposit during natural mating in sows and mares
Vagina	Organ of copulation
	Site of semen deposit during natural mating in cows, does, and ewes
	Birth canal
Vulva	External opening to reproductive tract

not arise from this epithelial layer. They arise from embryonic gut tissue and then migrate to the cortex of the embryonic gonad. Just beneath the surface epithelium is a thin, dense layer of connective tissue, the *tunica albuginea ovarii*. Below the tunica albuginea ovarii is the *parenchyma,* known as the functional layer because it contains ovarian follicles and the cells that produce ovarian hormones.

It is accepted that all primary follicles are formed during the prenatal period of the female. The greatest number are found in the fetal gilt 50 to 90 days postconception; the fetal calf 110 to 130 days postconception. A *primary follicle* is a germ cell surrounded by a single layer of follicular (granulosa) cells. They are located in the parenchyma and are frequently seen in groups called *egg nests*. It is estimated that approximately 75,000 primary follicles are found in the ovaries of a young calf. With continual follicular growth and maturation throughout her reproductive life, an old cow may have only 2,500 potential ova. Some potential ova reach full maturity and are released into the duct system for possible fertilization and development of offspring. Most start development and become *atretic* (i.e., they degenerate). Therefore, the potential harvest of ova that could produce offspring is far greater than is actually realized.

Follicles are in a constant state of growth and maturation. A histological section of the cortex of a reproductively active female will reveal these maturation stages (Figure 2–2), which can also be viewed by ultrasonography (Figure 2–3). The primary follicle has been described. This stage is followed by a proliferation of granulosa cells surrounding the potential ovum. A potential ovum surrounded by two or more layers of granulosa cells is a *secondary follicle.* Later in the development, an *antrum* (cavity) will form by fluid collecting between the granulosa cells and separating them. When the antrum has formed, the follicle is classified as a *tertiary follicle.* The mature tertiary follicle, which appears as a fluid-filled blister on the surface of the ovary, is also called a *Graafian follicle.* The fluid in the antrum of a tertiary follicle is called *liquor folliculi.* It is a viscous fluid that is rich in steroid reproductive hormones. A number of other reproductive hormones as well as nonhormonal factors that help regulate the function of the ovary have been identified in follicular fluid (Chapter 4).

Several cell layers in the Graafian follicle have been identified and are of functional importance (Figure 2–4, and 2–5). The outer, more fibrous cell layer is the *theca externa.*

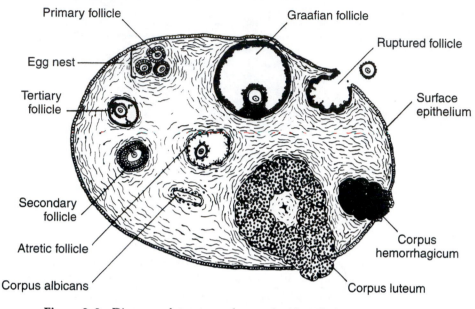

Figure 2–2   Diagram of structures that can be identified in a cross section of an ovary of a reproductively active female. Different maturation stages for follicles and the corpus luteum can be observed. (Adapted from Patten. 1964. *Foundations of Embryology.* (2nd ed.) McGraw-Hill.)

Inside this layer is the *theca interna.* These two cell layers are supplied with blood by a capillary network and can be differentiated microscopically with special histological staining techniques. Thecal cells and the capillary network are acquired as the follicle enlarges and pushes into the medulla. A basement membrane separates the theca interna from the innermost cell layer, the *granulosa cells,* and prevents entry of the vascular system into these cells (Figure 2–5). The granulosa cells surround the antrum. In addition, the *cumulus oophorus,* a hillock (mound) of granulosa cells, is located at one side of the antrum. The potential ovum rests upon the cumulus oophorus with other granulosa cells extending around the potential ovum in a loose matrix. The granulosa cells surrounding and in immediate contact with the potential ovum are termed the *corona radiata.* Both theca interna and granulosa cells are involved in the production of estrogen. The accepted theory is that the theca interna cells produce androgens, which diffuse through the basement membrane for conversion to estrogen by the aromatase enzyme in the granulosa cells. In addition, granulosa cells are the principal progesterone producing cells in the corpus luteum. They also secrete other compounds that have been identified in follicular fluid, which help regulate the function of the ovary. When ovulation occurs, the follicle ruptures, expelling the liquor folliculi, some granulosa cells, and the potential ovum (oocyte) into the body cavity near the opening to the oviduct. At the time of expulsion, the oocyte is surrounded by the corona radiata and a sticky mass containing other granulosa (*cumulus*) cells which aid the oviduct in picking up the oocyte and moving it down the oviduct. In some species, the corona radiata is present at the time of fertilization. In other species, these cells are shed quickly and are not present when fertilization occurs.

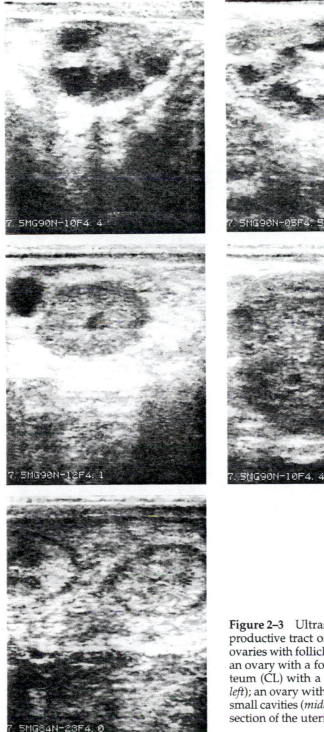

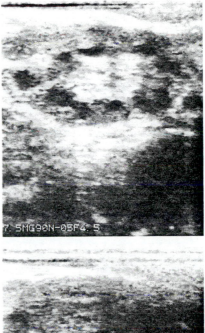

Figure 2–3 Ultrasonograms of the reproductive tract of the bovine female: ovaries with follicles (*top left and right*); an ovary with a follicle and corpus luteum (CL) with a small cavity (*middle left*); an ovary with two CLs, both with small cavities (*middle right*); and a cross section of the uterine horns (*left*).

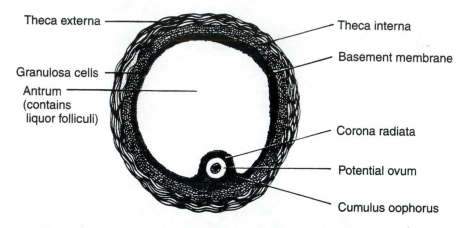

Figure 2–4 Functionally important features of a Graafian follicle. (Redrawn from Hafez. 1974. *Reproduction in Farm Animals.* (3rd ed.) Lea and Febiger.)

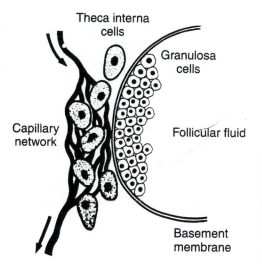

Figure 2–5 Structure of the wall of the Graafian follicle showing how the granulosa cells are deprived of a blood supply by the basement membrane. (Austin and Short. 1972. *Reproduction in Mammals. 3. Hormones of Reproduction.* Cambridge University Press.)

With rupture of the follicle, bleeding occurs and a blood clot forms at the ovulation site. The ruptured follicle with its blood-filled cavity is called a *corpus hemorrhagicum.* The corpus hemorrhagicum is replaced by the *corpus luteum* (*corpora lutea,* pl.), a solid body that forms rapidly from a mixture of thecal and granulosa cells (Figure 2–2). The corpus luteum has a yellowish color in cows and mares but is grayish white in sows and ewes. Two distinct cell types are found in the corpus luteum. They are small luteal cells of thecal origin and large luteal cells of granulosa origin. While enlarging, granulosa cells acquire additional mitochondria and other intracellular structures involved in synthesis of progesterone. The corpus luteum is well supplied with blood vessels and is the only ovarian source of progesterone and other progestins. In a Holstein heifer between 1 and 4 days of the cycle, the average diameter of the corpus luteum is 8 mm. Between 5 and 9 days, it has grown to an average of 15 mm. The average maximum size of 20.5 mm is reached in 15 or

16 days in a heifer that is not pregnant. This increased size is primarily due to enlargement of cells. The corpus luteum then regresses in size, with an average diameter of 12.5 mm at 18 to 21 days. When the corpus luteum regresses, it no longer produces progestins. It loses its color, eventually appearing as a small white scar on the surface of the ovary, which is called a *corpus albicans* (*corpora albicantia*, pl.). If the animal is pregnant, the corpus luteum will not regress until late pregnancy for most species, but species differences do exist (Section 9–5).

2–2　OVIDUCTS

The *oviducts* (also called *fallopian tubes*) are a pair of convoluted tubes extending from near the ovaries to and becoming continuous with the tips of the uterine horns. Their functions include transport of ova and spermatozoa, which must be conveyed in opposite directions. In addition, they are the site of fertilization and the early cell divisions of the embryo. His-tologically, they contain three distinct cell layers. The outer layer, basically connective tis-sue, is the *tunica serosa*. The middle layer, composed of both circular and longitudinal smooth muscle fibers, is the *tunica muscularis*. The innermost layer, which contains both ciliated and secretory epithelial cells, is the *tunica mucosa*. The same basic histological arrangement is found in the remainder of the female duct system, with some differences in the inner two layers, which will be noted when we discuss specific organs.

An oviduct, which is from 20 cm to 30 cm long for most farm species, is divided into three segments (Figure 2–6). The funnel-shaped opening near the ovaries is the *infundibulum*, with its lacelike edging, the *fimbria*, which serves to capture the ovum after ovulation. In some species (cat, rabbit, mink, and others), the infundibulum forms a bursa around the ovary. In the cow, doe, ewe, sow, and mare, the infundibulum is separate from the ovary. There are numerous folds in the mucosa, and most mucosal cells in the infundibulum are ciliated. The *ampulla*, the middle segment, is from 3 mm to 5 mm in diameter and ac-counts for about half of the total length of the oviduct. The mucosal lining of the ampulla has from 20 to 40 longitudinal folds, which greatly increase the surface area of the lumen. The majority of the cells in the mucosa of the ampulla are ciliated, but some secretory cells are present. Action of the cilia aids movement of the ovum down the ampulla. The ampulla joins the *isthmus*, the third segment, at the *ampullary-isthmic junction*. This junction is dif-ficult to locate anatomically and has been described as a physiological stricture that delays the ovum several hours during transport. Fertilization occurs at this junction. The isthmus is smaller than the ampulla, being 0.5 mm to 1 mm in diameter. It is further distinguished by having a thicker smooth muscle layer than the ampulla and from 4 to 8 mucosal folds. A higher ratio of secretory to ciliated cells is characteristic of the isthmus. The isthmus is in-volved in transport of motile sperm to the site of fertilization while filtering out dead sperm. The isthmus joins the tip of the uterine horn at the *uterotubal junction*. In general, contrac-tile activity of the oviduct is stimulated by estrogens and inhibited by progestins.

2–3　UTERUS

The *uterus* (*uteri*, pl.) extends from the uterotubal junctions to the cervix. For the cow, sow, and mare, the overall length may range from 35 cm to 60 cm. For the sow, doe, ewe, and cow, the uterine horns account for 80% to 90% of the total length, while in the mare the

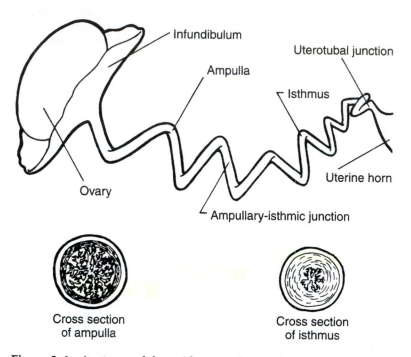

Figure 2–6   Anatomy of the oviduct: *top,* longitudinal view illustrating the macroscopic features of the oviduct; *bottom,* cross section of the ampulla and isthmus comparing the thickness of the musculature of the wall and the complexity of the mucosal folds.

uterine horns account for about 50% of the total length. The uteri of the ewe and doe are less than half the size of the other mentioned species. The major function of the uterus is to retain and nourish the embryo and fetus. Before the embryo becomes attached to the uterus, the nourishment comes from *yolk* within the embryo or from *uterine milk,* which is secreted by glands in the mucosal layer of the uterus. After attachment to the uterus, nutrients and waste products are conveyed between maternal and embryonic and fetal blood by way of the placenta (Chapter 9).

Four basic types of uteri are found in animals (Figure 2–7). Only two of these types are found in farm animals. The *bicornuate uterus* is found in the sow, cow, doe, and ewe. It is characterized by a small uterine body just anterior to the cervical canal and two long uterine horns (Figure 2–1). Fusion of the uterine horns of the cow and ewe near the uterine body gives the impression of a larger uterine body than actually exists and has sometimes resulted in their uteri being classified bipartite. The sow has longer uterine horns than the cow, and they may be slightly convoluted. The mare has a *bipartite uterus.* There is a prominent uterine body anterior to the cervical canal and two uterine horns that are not as long and distinct as in the bicornuate type. During pregnancy in mares, the fetal body extends into both horns, whereas the fetuses do not occupy the uterine body in monotocous species with bicornuate-type uteri. The *duplex uterus,* which consists of two uterine horns, each with a separate cervical canal that opens into the vagina, is found in the rat, rabbit, guinea pig, and

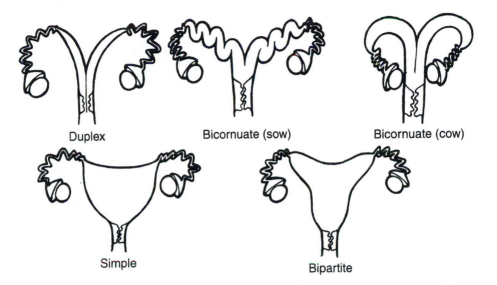

Duplex　　　　　Bicornuate (sow)　　　　Bicornuate (cow)

Simple　　　　　　　Bipartite

Figure 2–7　Basic types of uteri found in mammals.

other small animals. The *simple uterus,* a pear-shaped body with no uterine horns, is characteristic of humans and other primates.

As in the oviduct, the tunica serosa is the outer layer of the uterus. The *myometrium,* the middle layer, is composed of two thin longitudinal layers of smooth muscle, with a thicker, circular layer sandwiched between. Estrogens increase the tone of the myometrium, giving the uterus a firm, turgid feel. Progestins decrease the tone of the myometrium, causing the uterus to feel more flaccid. The *endometrium,* the mucosal lining of the uterus, is more complex than the rest of the duct system and has simple glands. Estrogens increase the vascularity and cause a thickening of the endometrium. In addition, estrogens stimulate growth of the endometrial glands. Progestins cause the endometrial glands to coil, to branch, and to secrete uterine milk. The synergistic actions of estrogens and progestins on the endometrium are for preparation of the uterus for pregnancy.

The endometrium provides a mechanism for attachment of the extraembryonic membranes. This union forms the placenta, and the process is called *placentation.* With formation of the placenta, nutrients from maternal blood can be transferred to embryonic and fetal blood, and waste products from embryonic and fetal blood can be eliminated through the maternal systems. The nature of the placental attachment differs among species (Figures 2–8 and 2–9). Cows, does, and ewes have *cotyledonary* placental attachments. *Chorionic villi* from the extraembryonic membranes penetrate into *caruncles,* which are buttonlike projections on the endometrium. This union, chorionic villi and caruncle, forms the *placentome* (also called the cotyledon). There are 70 to 120 such cotyledonary attachments in a cow in late pregnancy. There are 88 to 96 in ewes and does, and these are smaller than in cows. The sow and mare have a *diffuse* (surface) placental attachment. Their extraembryonic membranes lie in folds on the endometrium, with chorionic villi extending into the endometrium in a more fragile attachment than is found in the cow, doe, or ewe. The placenta

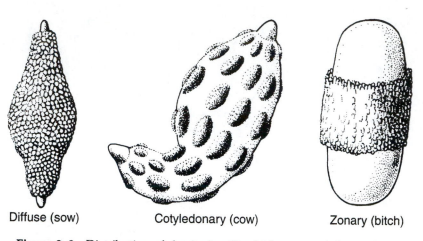

Diffuse (sow)   Cotyledonary (cow)   Zonary (bitch)

Figure 2–8   Distribution of chorionic villi which serve as a basis of placental shape in several species. (Redrawn from Arey. 1974. *Developmental Anatomy.* (7th ed.) W.B. Saunders Co.)

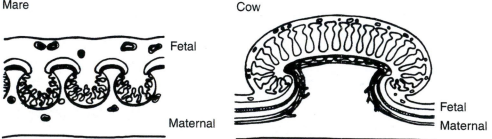

Figure 2–9   Diffuse attachment found in the mare and cotyledonary attachment found in the cow.

of the mare is further distinguished by development of *endometrial cups* that form a semicircular ring around the pregnant horn between the 6th and 20th week of the gestation (Figure 2–9). These endometrial cups are of fetal origin and are associated with secretion of pregnant mare serum gonadotropin (PMSG). Both the bitch and female cat have a *zonary* attachment with chorionic villi arranged in an equatorial belt (Figure 2–8). A *discoidal* attachment with chorionic villi arranged in a circular plate is found in many rodents and in primate species that include the human.

      Placental attachments are classified by degree of attachment also, with up to six tissue layers separating maternal and fetal blood after placentation. These layers are the maternal uterine vascular endothelium, connective tissue, and epithelium along with the fetal allanto-chorionic epithelium, connective tissue, and vascular endothelium. The placental attachments of the mare, sow, cow, ewe, and doe are *epitheliochorial,* with all six layers remaining after placentation. The uterine epithelium rests against the epithelium of the allanto-chorion

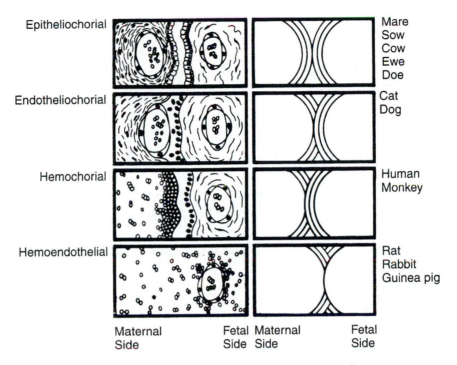

Epitheliochorial — Mare, Sow, Cow, Ewe, Doe

Endotheliochorial — Cat, Dog

Hemochorial — Human, Monkey

Hemoendothelial — Rat, Rabbit, Guinea pig

Maternal Side   Fetal Side   Maternal Side   Fetal Side

Figure 2–10 Placental types showing the cellular barriers between maternal and fetal blood for several species. (Adapted from Arey. 1974. *Developmental Anatomy.* (7th ed.) W.B. Saunders Co.)

(Figure 2–10). There is no erosion of either the maternal or the fetal layers. Formation of the placenta in primates results in extensive erosion of the endometrium. Classified as *hemochorial,* nutrients from maternal blood must pass only through the three fetal tissue layers to reach fetal blood. The placental attachments of the rat, rabbit, and guinea pig are classified *hemoendothelial,* with only the fetal vascular endothelium separating maternal and fetal blood. There is erosion of both maternal and fetal tissue layers. Erosion is not extensive enough to permit direct mixing of maternal and fetal blood in any mammalian species.

The epitheliochorial arrangement does not permit large molecules such as immunoglobulins to diffuse from the maternal to the fetal systems. Therefore, offspring from these species do not have circulating maternal immunoglobulins at birth. This is not the case for offspring from species with hemochorial attachments, as maternal immunoglobulins do diffuse into the fetal systems.

2–4   CERVIX

While technically a part of the uterus, the *cervix* will be discussed as a distinct organ. It is thick-walled and inelastic, the anterior end being continuous with the body of the uterus while the posterior end protrudes into the vagina. For most farm species, the length will range from 5 cm

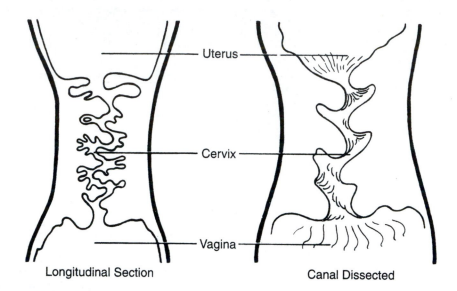

Uterus

Cervix

Vagina

Longitudinal Section   Canal Dissected

Figure 2–11   The cervix of the cow demonstrating the relationship of the annular rings. (Redrawn from Hafez. 1974. *Reproduction in Farm Animals.* (3rd ed.) Lea and Febiger.)

to 10 cm with an outside diameter of 2 cm to 5 cm. It contains a canal, which is the opening into the uterus. A major function of the cervix is to prevent microbial contamination of the uterus. In cows, ewes, and does, it serves as a sperm reservoir after mating and functions to filter out dead sperm as motile sperm channel through the cervical mucus into the uterus (Section 8–3.2). Semen is deposited into the cervix during natural mating in sows and mares.

The cervical canals in the cow, doe, and ewe have transverse interlocking ridges known as *annular rings* (Figure 2–11), which help seal the uterus from contaminants. The cervical canal in the sow is funnel-shaped, with ridges in the canal having a corkscrew configuration, which conforms to that of the glans penis in the boar (Chapter 3). The cervical canal of the mare is more open than in other farm species, but mucosal folds in the canal which project into the vagina help prevent contamination.

Histologically, the outer layer of the cervix is the tunica serosa. The middle layer is connective tissue interspersed with smooth muscle fibers, which gives the cervix its firm and inelastic properties. The inner layer, the mucosa, is composed mainly of secretory epithelial cells, but some ciliated epithelial cells are present. High levels of estrogens cause the cervical canal to dilate during estrus (standing heat). Synergism between high levels of estrogens and relaxin causes greater dilation just before parturition. This dilation of the canal would appear to make the uterus more vulnerable to invading organisms. However, estrogens cause the epithelial cells of the cervix to secrete mucus that has antibacterial properties, therefore protecting the uterus.

If cervical mucus is obtained at estrus and allowed to dry on a glass slide, it will form a fernlike pattern. This ferning pattern does not form from cervical mucus obtained at other stages of the cycle when estrogens are low. During pregnancy, the mucus thickens into a gel-like plug, which seals and protects the uterus during the pregnancy. Removal of the *mucous plug* will increase the chance of abortion.

2–5   VAGINA

The *vagina* is tubular in shape, thin-walled, and quite elastic. It is from 25 cm to 30 cm in length in the cow and mare, and 10 cm to 15 cm in length in the sow, doe, and ewe. In the cow, doe, and ewe, semen is deposited into the anterior end of the vagina, near the opening to the cervix, during natural mating. The vagina is the female organ of copulation.

The outer layer, the tunica serosa, overlays a smooth muscle layer containing both circular and longitudinal fibers. In most species, the mucosal layer is composed of stratified squamous epithelial cells (the cow a possible exception). These epithelial cells cornify (become cells without nuclei) under the influence of estrogens. Vaginal smears can be used as an aid in detecting estrus but are most useful in laboratory animals. This layer of cornified cells at the time of estrus may serve as a lubricating or protective mechanism which prevents abrasions during copulation. Under the influence of progestins, the epithelial lining regenerates.

2–6   VULVA

The *vulva,* or external genitalia, consists of the vestibule with related parts and the labia. The *vestibule* is that portion of the female duct system that is common to both the reproductive and urinary systems. It is from 10 cm to 12 cm in length in the cow and mare, half that length in the sow, and one-quarter that length in the ewe and doe. The vestibule joins the vagina at the *external urethral orifice.* A *hymen* (ridge) at that point is well defined in the ewe and mare but less prominent in the cow and sow. A *suburethral diverticulum* (blind-pocket) is located just posterior to the external urethral orifice. The labia consists of the *labia minora,* inner folds or lips of the vulva, and *labia majora,* outer folds or lips of the vulva. The labia minora is homologous to the prepuce (sheath) in the male and is not prominent in farm animals. The labia majora, homologous to the scrotum in the male, is that portion of the female system that is visible externally. In the cow, the labia majora is covered with fine hair up to the mucosa. The *clitoris,* homologous to the glans penis in the male, is located ventrally and about 1 cm inside the labia. It contains erectile tissue and is well supplied with sensory nerves. It is erect during estrus. While not prominent enough to be used in estrus detection in most species, the clitoris of the mare is an exception. In the mare during estrus, frequent contractions of the labia (winking) expose the erected clitoris. *Vestibular glands,* located in the posterior part of the vestibule, are active during estrus and secrete a lubricating mucus. The activity of these glands accounts for the moist appearance of the vulva of the cow during estrus.

2–7   SUPPORT STRUCTURES, NERVES, AND BLOOD SUPPLY

Even though the female reproductive tract may be partially resting on the floor of the pelvis, the *broad ligament* is considered the principal supporting structure. This ligament suspends the ovaries, oviducts, and uterus from either side of the dorsal wall of the pelvis. Blood vessels and nerves pass through the broad ligament to the female reproductive system. The female reproductive system is supplied primarily with autonomic nerves. However, sensory nerves are found in the region of the vulva, especially the clitoral region.

The *ovarian arteries,* also called utero-ovarian arteries, branch and supply blood to the ovaries, the oviducts, and a portion of the uterine horns. These arteries are larger on the side of the ovary containing an active corpus luteum in cows and other species where one active corpus luteum is the rule. The *middle uterine artery* supplies blood to the rest of the uterine horns and the body of the uterus. It enlarges during middle and late pregnancy and can be palpated as an aid in pregnancy diagnosis in cows and mares (Chapter 21). The hypogastric artery branches to supply the cervix, vagina, and vulva, while the *hypogastric vein* is the return route for blood from these organs.

Interest in the circulatory patterns of the reproductive tract has increased with the discovery that the uterus, by release of prostaglandin $F_{2\alpha}$ ($PGF_{2\alpha}$), controls the life of the corpus luteum. *Prostaglandin* $F_{2\alpha}$ is luteolytic (causes the regression of the corpus luteum) but is readily oxidized, and about 90% is destroyed during one passage through the pulmonary circulation. It did not seem likely that $PGF_{2\alpha}$, if released into the systemic circulation (uterus→veins→heart and lungs→arteries→ovaries), could be responsible for luteolysis (regression of the corpus luteum). Now there is evidence of a countercurrent circulation pattern, whereby $PGF_{2\alpha}$ diffuses from the *utero-ovarian vein* into the ovarian artery, thereby reaching the ovary by a local rather than a systemic route. A common utero-ovarian vein drains blood from the ovary, the oviduct, and a large portion of the uterine horn. In the sow, ewe, and cow, the ovarian artery is in close apposition to the utero-ovarian vein (Figure 2–12). In the ewe and cow, it is very tortuous, increasing the area of contact with the utero-ovarian vein. The arterial walls are thinnest where they are in contact with this vein. Therefore, it seems likely that

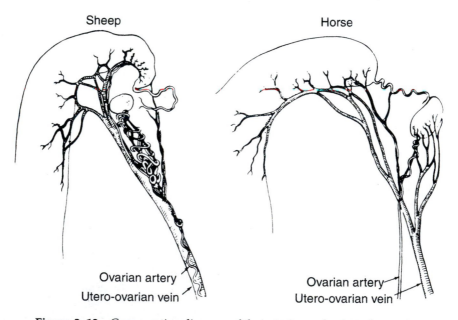

Figure 2–12   Comparative diagram of the arteries and veins of a uterine horn and adjacent ovary in the ewe and the mare. (Del Campo and Ginther. 1973. *Amer. J. Vet. Res.,* 34:305.)

sufficient $PGF_{2\alpha}$ can diffuse from the utero-ovarian vein into the ovarian artery to cause luteolysis in the sow, ewe, and cow. During synchronization of estrus, the effective dose of $PGF_{2\alpha}$ is much smaller when infused into the uterus as compared with a systemic injection (5 mg versus 25 mg).

The ovarian artery of the mare is straight and caudal to the utero-ovarian vein (Figure 2–12). They are in contact in a limited area where the ovarian artery crosses the utero-ovarian vein. While a local route for $PGF_{2\alpha}$ from the uterus to the ovary seems less likely in mares than in other species, uterine prostaglandins have been identified as the natural luteolysin in mares.

SUGGESTED READING

AREY, L. B. 1974. *Developmental Anatomy.* (7th ed.) W. B. Saunders Co.

ASDELL, S. A. 1946. *Patterns of Mammalian Reproduction.* Comstock Pub. Assoc.

COLE, H. H. 1930. A study of the genital tract of the cow with special reference to the cyclic changes. *Amer. J. Anat.,* 46:261.

DEL CAMPO, C. H. and O. J. GINTHER. 1973. Vascular anatomy of the uterus and ovaries: Horse, sheep and swine. *Amer. J. Vet. Res.,* 34:305.

GETTY, R., ed. 1975. *Sisson and Grossman—the Anatomy of Domestic Animals.* W. B. Saunders Co.

GINTHER, O. J. and C. H. DEL CAMPO. 1974. Vascular anatomy of the uterus and ovaries and the unilateral luteolytic effect of the uterus: Cattle. *Amer. J. Vet. Res.,* 35:193.

HAFEZ, E. S. E. 1974. Functional anatomy of the female. *Reproduction in Farm Animals.* (3rd ed.) Lea and Febiger.

PARKES, A. S., ed. 1956. *Marshall's Physiology of Reproduction.* Vol. 1. Part 1. Longmans, Green and Co.

The Male Reproductive System

The male reproductive system (Figure 3–1) consists of the scrotum, spermatic cords, testes, accessory glands, penis, prepuce, and male duct system. The duct system includes vasa efferentia located within the testis along with the epididymis, vas deferens, and urethra external to the testis. The embryonic origin of the testes is the primary sex cords of the genital ridge, whereas the male duct system originates from the Wolffian ducts (Chapter 9). A summary of the reproductive organs of the male and their major functions is given in Table 3–1.

3–1 TESTES

The *testes* (*testis,* sing.) are the primary organs of reproduction in males, just as ovaries are the primary organs of reproduction in females. Testes are considered primary because they produce male gametes (*spermatozoa*) and male sex hormones (androgens). Testes differ from ovaries in that not all potential gametes are present at birth. Germ cells, located in the seminiferous tubules, undergo continual cell divisions, forming new spermatozoa throughout the normal reproductive life of the male.

Testes also differ from ovaries in that they do not remain in the body cavity. They descend from their site of origin, near the kidneys, down through the inguinal canals into the scrotum. Descent of the testes occurs because of an apparent shortening of the gubernaculum, a ligament extending from the inguinal region and attaching to the tail of the epididymis. This apparent shortening occurs because the gubernaculum does not grow as rapidly as the body wall. The testes are drawn closer to the inguinal canals and intraabdominal pressure aids passage of the testes through the inguinal canals into the scrotum. Androgens or other testicular factors help regulate descent of the testes. This descent is completed by midpregnancy in bulls and rams, late pregnancy in boars, and just before or just after birth in stallions. In some cases, one or both testes fail to descend due to a defect in development. This is fairly common in stallions but occurs in all farm species. If neither testis descends, the animal is termed a *bilateral cryptorchid.* Bilateral cryptorchids are sterile (Section 3–2). If only one testis descends, he is a *unilateral cryptorchid.* The unilateral cryptorchid is usually fertile due to the descended testis. The cryptorchid condition can be corrected by surgery, but this is not recommended for farm animals (Chapter 24). The condition can be inherited; therefore, surgical correction would result in the perpetuation of an undesirable trait.

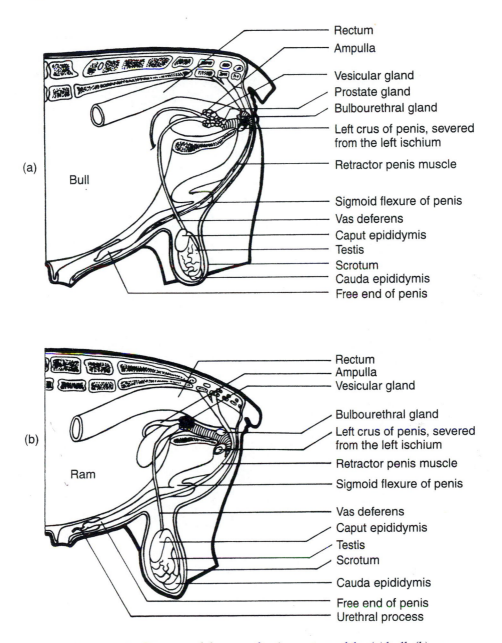

Figure 3–1 Diagram of the reproductive system of the *(a)* bull; *(b)* ram. (Redrawn from Sorenson. 1979. *Animal Reproduction: Principles and Practices.* McGraw-Hill.)

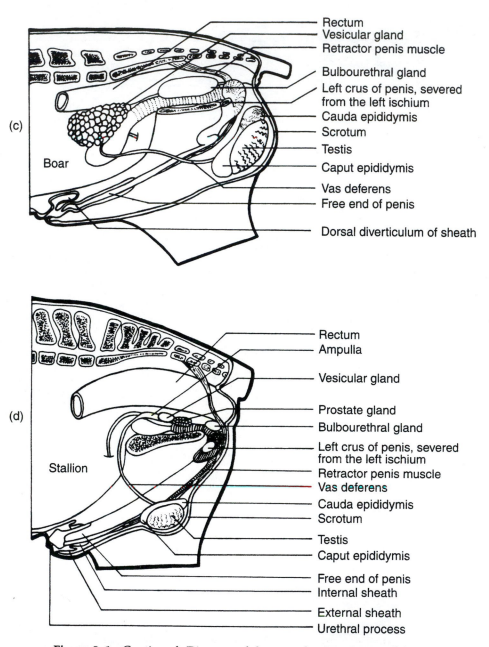

Figure 3–1 Continued. Diagram of the reproductive system of the *(c)* boar; and *(d)* stallion. (Redrawn from Sorenson. 1979. *Animal Reproduction: Principles and Practices.* McGraw-Hill.)

Table 3–1 *Reproductive organs of the male with their major functions*

Organ	Function(s)
Testis	Production of spermatozoa
	Production of androgens
Scrotum	Support of the testes
	Temperature control of the testes
	Protection of the testes
Spermatic cord	Support of the testes
	Temperature control of the testes
Epididymis	Concentration of spermatozoa
	Storage of spermatozoa
	Maturation of spermatozoa
	Transport of spermatozoa
Vas deferens	Transport of spermatozoa
Urethra	Transport of semen
Vesicular gland	Contributes fluid, energy substrates, and buffers to semen
Prostate gland	Contributes fluid and inorganic ions to semen
Bulbourethral gland	Flushes urine residue from urethra
Penis	Male organ of copulation
Prepuce	Encloses free end of penis

3–1.1 *Functional Morphology*

The testis of the bull is 10 cm to 13 cm long, is 5 cm to 6.5 cm wide, and weighs 300 g to 400 g. The testis is of similar size in boars but is smaller in rams, bucks (goats), and stallions.

In all species, testes are covered with the *tunica vaginalis,* a serous tissue, which is an extension of the peritoneum. This serous coat is obtained as the testes descend into the scrotum and is attached along the line of the epididymis. The outer layer of the testes, the *tunica albuginea testis,* is a thin white membrane of elastic connective tissue. Numerous blood vessels are visible just under its surface (Color Plate 7). Beneath the tunica albuginea testis is the *parenchyma,* the functional layer of the testes. The parenchyma has a yellowish color and is divided into segments by incomplete septa of connective tissue (Figure 3–2). Located within these segments of parenchymal tissue are the *seminiferous tubules.* Seminiferous tubules are formed from primary sex cords. They contain germ cells (*spermatogonia*) and nurse cells (Sertoli cells) (Figure 3–3). *Sertoli cells* are larger and less numerous than spermatogonia. Their tight junction at the basement membrane forms the blood-testis barrier. With stimulation by FSH, Sertoli cells produce both androgen-binding protein and inhibin (Chapter 4). Seminiferous tubules are the site of spermatozoa production. They are small, convoluted tubules approximately 200 μ in diameter. It has been estimated that the seminiferous tubules from a pair of bull testes, stretched out and laid end to end, are approximately 3 km to 5 km in length. They make up 85% of the weight of the testes in bulls and rams and somewhat less in stallions and boars. Seminiferous tubules join a network of tubules, the *rete testis,* which connects to 12 to 15 small ducts, the *vasa efferentia,* which converge into the head of the epididymis. Production of spermatozoa will be discussed in Chapter 6.

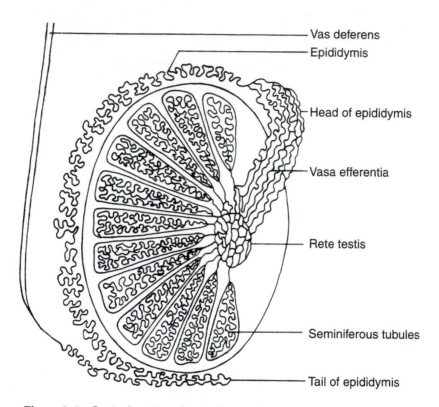

Figure 3–2 Sagittal section of testis illustrating segments of parenchymal tissue, which contain the seminiferous tubules, rete testis, vasa efferentia, epididymis, and scrotal portion of the vas deferens.

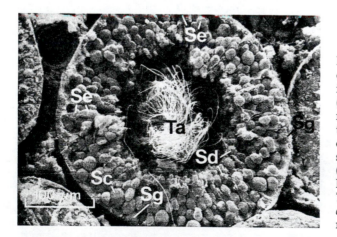

Figure 3–3 Scanning electron micrograph of a cross section of a seminiferous tubule. A tangle of tails (Ta) in the lumen represents spermatozoa that have been released through spermiation. Se = Sertoli cell; Sg = spermatogonium; Sc = spermatocyte; Sd = spermatid. (Copyright by R. G. Kessel and R. H. Kardon, *Tissues and Organs: A Text-Atlas of Scanning Electron Microscopy,* W. H. Freeman, 1979, all rights reserved.)

Leydig (interstitial) *cells* are found in the parenchyma of the testes between the seminiferous tubules (Figure 6–2). When stimulated by LH, Leydig cells produce testosterone and small quantities of other androgens.

Testosterone is needed for development of secondary sex characteristics and for normal mating behavior. In addition, it is necessary for the function of the accessory glands, production of spermatozoa, and maintenance of the male duct system. Through its effects on the male, testosterone aids in maintenance of optimum conditions for spermatogenesis, transport of spermatozoa, and deposition of spermatozoa into the female tract. Normal body temperature will not affect the function of the Leydig cells. For example, bilateral cryptorchids develop secondary sex characteristics, have normal sexual vigor, and can do all things associated with reproduction except production of spermatozoa.

3–2 SCROTUM AND SPERMATIC CORD

The *scrotum* is a two-lobed sac which encloses the testes (Color Plate 8). It is located in the inguinal region between the rear legs of most species. The scrotum has the same embryonic origin as the labia majora in the female. It is composed of an outer layer of thick skin, with numerous large sweat and sebaceous glands. This outer layer is lined with a layer of smooth muscle fibers, the *tunica dartos,* which is interspersed with connective tissue. The tunica dartos divides the scrotum into two pouches and is attached to the tunica vaginalis at the bottom of each pouch.

The *spermatic cord* connects the testis to its life support mechanisms, the convoluted testicular arteries and surrounding venous plexus, and nerve trunks. In addition, the spermatic cord is composed of muscle fibers, connective tissue, and a portion of the vas deferens. Both the spermatic cords and scrotum contribute to the physical support of the testes. Also, they have a joint function in regulating the temperature of the testes.

3–2.1 *Temperature Control*

Several examples can be given to illustrate the importance of temperature control of the testes. If a ram's scrotum is insulated, or the testes are tied against the abdomen, sterility results. The higher temperature causes degeneration of the cells lining the wall of the seminiferous tubules. Fertility will be restored if the testes and scrotum are returned to their natural state before total degeneration occurs. However, a few weeks will be required before fertile semen is again produced. (Sometimes men with high fevers are sterile for short periods after recovery.) The bilateral cryptorchid is sterile, again illustrating that production of spermatozoa stops when the temperature inside the testes is as high as normal body temperature (Section 24–5).

Low fertility semen produced by several species of farm animals during the summer has been attributed to the inability of the body's cooling mechanisms to keep the testes cool enough (Section 22–1.1). In cattle, when ambient temperatures range from 5°C to 21°C, the temperature inside the testes will be about 4°C below body temperature (38.6°C). As the ambient temperature increases to approximately 38°C, the temperature of both the body and the testes will be elevated, and the difference between the two will be reduced by about one-half (2°C). The elevation in temperature inside the testes will be sufficient to stop spermatogenesis. There is no evidence that low ambient temperature will lower fertility.

The role of the scrotum and spermatic cord in temperature control of the testes involves drawing the testes closer to the body as ambient temperature falls and letting the testes swing farther away from the body as ambient temperature rises. Two muscles are involved. The tunica dartos, the smooth muscle lining the scrotum, and the *external cremaster*, a striated muscle around the spermatic cord, are sensitive to temperature. During cold weather, the tunica dartos contracts causing the skin to pucker and draw the testes closer to the body. By reflexly contracting, the external cremaster can shorten the spermatic cord to assist in drawing the testes closer to the body. During hot weather, these muscles relax, permitting the scrotum to stretch and the spermatic cord to lengthen. Thus, the testes swing down, away from the body. The tunica dartos does not respond to changes in ambient temperature until near the age of puberty, when testosterone increases and sensitizes this smooth muscle.

Actual cooling of the testes occurs by two mechanisms. The skin of the scrotum has both sweat and sebaceous glands, which are more active during hot weather. Evaporation of the excretions of these glands cools the scrotum and thus the testes. The external scrotum has been observed to be 2°C to 5°C cooler than the temperature inside the testes. As the scrotum stretches during hot weather, more surface area is provided for cooling by evaporation. In addition to cooling by evaporation, significant cooling occurs through heat exchange in the circulatory system (Figure 3–4). As arteries transporting blood at internal

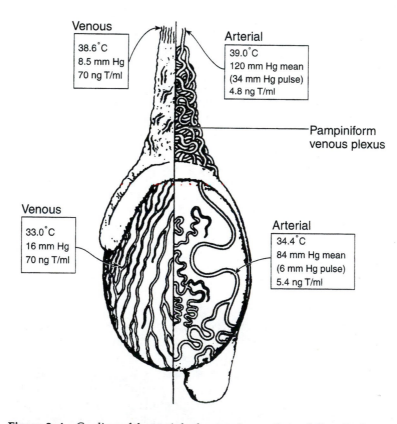

Venous

38.6°C
8.5 mm Hg
70 ng T/ml

Arterial

39.0°C
120 mm Hg mean
(34 mm Hg pulse)
4.8 ng T/ml

Pampiniform
venous plexus

Venous

33.0°C
16 mm Hg
70 ng T/ml

Arterial

34.4°C
84 mm Hg mean
(6 mm Hg pulse)
5.4 ng T/ml

Figure 3–4   Cooling of the testis by heat exchange through the circulatory system. (Setchell. 1977. *Reproduction in Domestic Animals*. (3rd ed.) eds. Cole and Cupps. Academic Press.)

body temperature descend along the spermatic cord, their convoluted folds pass through a network of veins, the *pampiniform venous plexus,* transporting cooler blood back toward the heart. With this countercurrent mechanism, some cooling of arterial blood then occurs before it reaches the testes. The lengthening of the cord during hot weather provides more surface area for this heat exchange.

3–3 EPIDIDYMIS

The *epididymis* (*epididymides,* pl.), the first external duct leading from the testis, is fused longitudinally to the surface of the testis and is encased in the tunica vaginalis with the testis (Color Plate 7). The single convoluted duct is covered with an extension of the tunica albuginea testis (Figure 3–5). The *caput* (head) of the epididymis is a flattened area at the apex of the testis, where 12 to 15 small ducts, the vasa efferentia, merge into a single duct. The *corpus* (body) extending along the longitudinal axis of the testis is a single duct, which becomes continuous with the *cauda* (tail). The total length of this convoluted duct is about 34 meters in the bull and is longer in the ram, boar, and stallion. The lumen of the cauda is wider than the lumen of the corpus. The structure of the epididymis and other external ducts (vas deferens and urethra) is similar to that of the tubular portion of the female tract. The tunica serosa (outer layer) is followed by a smooth muscle layer (middle) and an epithelial layer (innermost).

3–3.1 *Transport*

As a duct leading from the testis, the epididymis serves to transport spermatozoa. In sexually active males, the time involved in transport is 9 to 14 days in boars, 13 to 15 days in rams, and 9 to 11 days in bulls. Frequent ejaculation has been reported to speed transport by 10% to 20%.

Several factors contribute to movement of spermatozoa through the epididymis. One factor is pressure from the production of new spermatozoa. As spermatozoa are produced in the seminiferous tubules, they are forced out through the rete testis and vasa efferentia into the epididymis. In a sexually inactive male, they are eventually forced through the epididymis. Such movement of spermatozoa is aided by external pressure created by the massaging effect on the testes and epididymis that occurs during normal exercise. The lining of

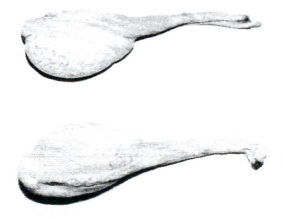

Figure 3–5 View of the epididymis as it is fused to the surface of the testis. Note the tunica albuginea testis, which covers the testis.

the epididymis contains some ciliated epithelial cells, but the role of these cilia in facilitating movement of spermatozoa is not clear. As mentioned previously, movement of spermatozoa is aided by ejaculation. During ejaculation, peristaltic contractions involving the smooth muscle layer of the epididymis and a slight negative pressure (sucking action) created by peristaltic contractions of the vas deferens and urethra actively move spermatozoa from the epididymis into the vas deferens and urethra.

3–3.2 *Concentration*

A second function of the epididymis is concentration of spermatozoa. Spermatozoa entering the epididymis from the testis of the bull, ram, and boar are relatively dilute (approximately 100 million spermatozoa/ml). In the epididymis, they concentrate to about 4×10^9 (4 billion) spermatozoa per ml. Concentration occurs as the fluids, which suspend spermatozoa in the testes, are absorbed by the epithelial cells of the epididymis. Absorption of these fluids occurs principally in the caput and proximal end of the corpus.

3–3.3 *Storage*

A third function of the epididymis is storage of spermatozoa. Most are stored in the cauda of the epididymides, where concentrated spermatozoa are packed into the wide lumen. The epididymis of a mature bull may contain 50 to 74 billion sperm. Capacities of other species are not reported. Conditions are optimum in the cauda for preserving the viability of spermatozoa for an extended period. The low pH, high viscosity, high carbon dioxide concentration, high potassium-to-sodium ratio, the influence of testosterone, and probably other factors combine to contribute to a lower metabolic rate and extended life. These conditions have not been duplicated outside the epididymis. If the epididymis is ligated to prevent entry of new spermatozoa and removal of old, spermatozoa have remained alive and fertile for about 60 days. On the other hand, after a long period of sexual rest, the first few ejaculates may contain a high percentage of nonfertile spermatozoa.

3–3.4 *Maturation*

A fourth function of the epididymis is that of maturation of spermatozoa. When recently formed spermatozoa enter the caput from the vasa efferentia, they have the ability for neither motility nor fertility. As they pass through the epididymis, they gain the ability to be both motile and fertile. If the cauda is ligated at each end, those spermatozoa closest to the corpus increase in ability to be fertile for up to 25 days, but those closest to the vas deferens lose the ability. Therefore, it appears that spermatozoa gain ability to be fertile in the cauda and then start to age and deteriorate if they are not removed. Actual fertility is gained when spermatozoa undergo a second maturation process after deposition into the female tract (Section 6–4).

While in the epididymis, spermatozoa lose the cytoplasmic droplet that forms on the neck of each spermatozoa during spermatogenesis (Chapter 6). The physiological significance of the cytoplasmic droplet is not known, but it has been used as an indicator of sufficient maturation of spermatozoa in the epididymis. If a high percentage of spermatozoa in freshly ejaculated semen has cytoplasmic droplets, they are considered immature and have low fertilizing capacity.

3–4   VASA DEFERENTIA AND URETHRA

The *vasa deferentia* (*vas deferens,* sing.) are a pair of ducts with one leading from the distal end of the cauda of each epididymis. Initially supported by folds of the peritoneum, they pass along the spermatic cord, through the inguinal canal to the pelvic region, where they merge with the urethra at its origin near the opening to the bladder. The enlarged end of the vas deferens near the urethra is the *ampulla.* The vasa deferentia have a thick layer of smooth muscles in their walls and appear to have the single function of transport of spermatozoa. Some have suggested that ampullae serve as a short-term storage depot for semen. However, spermatozoa age quickly in the ampullae. It seems more likely that spermatozoa may pool in the ampullae during ejaculation before being expelled into the urethra.

The urethra is a single duct that extends from the junction of the ampullae to the end of the penis. It serves as an excretory duct for both urine and semen. During ejaculation in the bull and ram, there is a complete mixing of spermatozoa concentrate from the vasa deferentia and epididymides with fluids from the accessory glands in the pelvic part of the urethra to form semen. In stallions and boars, mixing is not as complete, with the ejaculate containing sperm-free and sperm-rich fractions (Chapter 7).

3–5   ACCESSORY GLANDS

The *accessory glands* (Figure 3–6) are located along the pelvic portion of the urethra, with ducts that empty their secretions into the urethra. They include the *vesicular glands,* the *prostate gland,* and the *bulbourethral glands.* They contribute greatly to the fluid volume of semen. In addition, their secretions are a solution of buffers, nutrients, and other substances needed to assure optimum motility and fertility of semen.

3–5.1   *Vesicular Glands*

The vesicular glands (sometimes called seminal vesicles) are a pair of lobular glands that are easily identified because of their knobby appearance. They have been described as having the appearance of a "cluster of grapes." They are of similar length in the bull, boar, and stallion (13 cm to 15 cm), but the width and thickness of the vesicular glands of the bull are approximately half that of the boar and stallion. The vesicular glands of the ram and buck are much smaller, being about 4 cm in length. The excretory ducts of the vesicular glands open near the bifurcation where the ampullae merge with the urethra. In bulls, they contribute well over half of the total fluid volume of semen and appear to make a substantial contribution in other species. Several organic compounds found in secretions of the vesicular glands are unique in that they are not found in substantial quantities elsewhere in the body. Two of these compounds, fructose and sorbitol, are major sources of energy for bull and ram spermatozoa but are found in lower concentration in boar and stallion semen. Both phosphate and carbonate buffers are found in these secretions and are important in that they protect against shifts in the pH of semen. Such shifts in pH would be detrimental to spermatozoa.

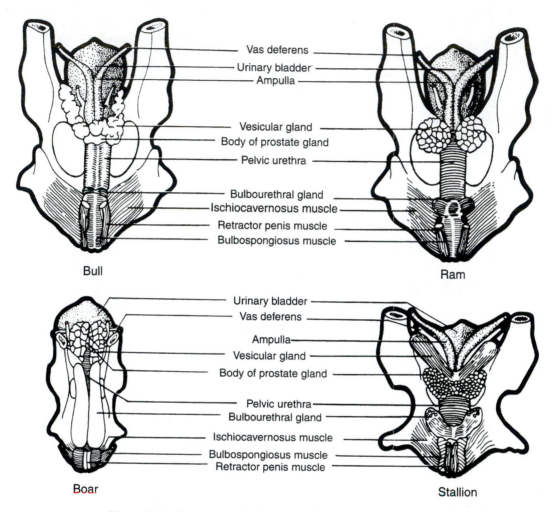

Vas deferens
Urinary bladder
Ampulla

Vesicular gland
Body of prostate gland
Pelvic urethra

Bulbourethral gland
Ischiocavernosus muscle
Retractor penis muscle
Bulbospongiosus muscle

Bull

Ram

Urinary bladder
Vas deferens

Ampulla
Vesicular gland
Body of prostate gland

Pelvic urethra
Bulbourethral gland

Ischiocavernosus muscle

Bulbospongiosus muscle
Retractor penis muscle

Boar

Stallion

Figure 3–6   Accessory glands of the bull, boar, ram, and stallion showing their relationship to the ampulla and urethra. (Redrawn from Ashdown and Hancock. 1974. *Reproduction in Farm Animals.* (3rd ed.) ed. Hafez. Lea and Febiger.)

3–5.2 *Prostate Gland*

The prostate is a single gland located around and along the urethra just posterior to the excretory ducts of the vesicular glands. A prostate body is visible in excised tracts and can be palpated in bulls and stallions. In rams, all of the prostate is embedded in urethral muscles, as is part of this glandular tissue in bulls and boars. It makes a small contribution to the fluid volume of semen in most species studied. However, the contribution of the prostate gland is more substantial than that of the vesicular glands in boars. The prostate of the boar is larger than that of the bull. The secretions of the prostate are high in inorganic ions with sodium, chlorine, calcium, and magnesium all in solution.

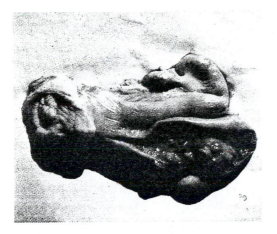

Plate 1 Gross examination of the cow reproductive tract—I. The os cervix is clearly visible where the anterior portion of the vagina has been retracted. The two uterine horns can be seen, with maternal caruncles evident in the incised horn. The brown fluid within this horn is evidence of pyometria (a uterine infection). The corpus luteum is prominent on the left ovary.

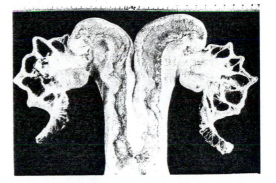

Plate 2 Gross examination of the cow reproductive tract—II. Both uterine horns have been incised to reveal the lumen and maternal caruncles. The oviduct is prominently displayed between the uterine horns and the ovaries. A corpus luteum is evident on the left ovary.

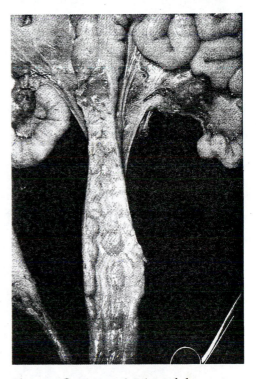

Plate 4 Gross examination of the sow reproductive tract—II. The cervix has been incised to reveal the prominent interdigitating folds. This configuration facilitates the corkscrew-like shape of the boar's penis to lock into the cervix. Note the presence of corpora lutea on both the right and left ovaries.

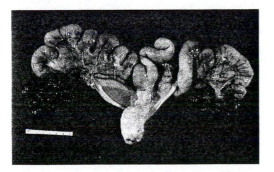

Plate 3 Gross examination of the gilt reproductive tract.—I. The prominent cervix and long uterine horns of a gilt are presented. Note the large number of corpora lutea on both the right and left ovaries.

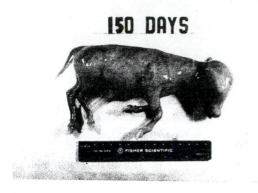

Plate 5 A bovine fetus at 150 days of gestation.

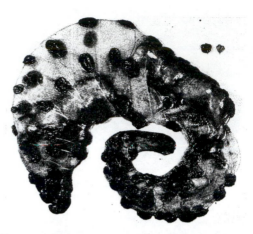

Plate 6 A bovine placenta containing twin fetuses. Cotyledons are evident across the entire placenta. (Photo courtesy of D. Porter, Ontario College of Veterinary Medicine, University of Guelph, and P. Ryan, Department of Animal and Dairy Science, Mississippi State University).

(A)

(B)

(C)

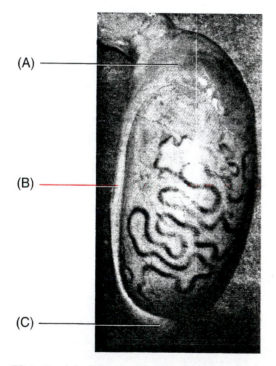

Plate 7 A bull testis. The outer layer of the testis is referred to as the tunica albuginea. The caput (A), corpus (B), and cauda (C) epididymis are prominent. (Photo courtesy of R. Godfrey, University of the Virgin Islands–St. Croix, USVI).

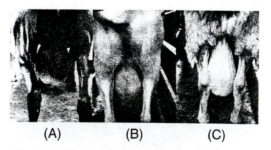

(A) (B) (C)

Plate 8 The pendulous scrotum of the ram which houses the testes. Three breeds of rams are represented in the plate: the Barbados Blackbelly (A), St. Croix White (B) and Dorper (C). (Photo courtesy of R. Godfrey, University of the Virgin Islands–St. Croix, USVI).

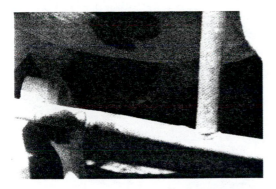

Plate 9 Extension of the penis of the bull from the prepuce. An electroejaculator was used to stimulate extension of the penis for ejaculation and semen collection. Note the semen collection cone (left side of the plate) being brought forth for collection of the ejaculate. (Photo courtesy of R. Godfrey, University of the Virgin Islands–St. Croix, USVI).

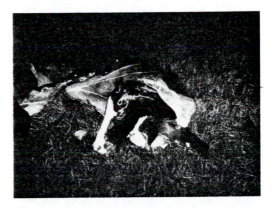

Plate 10 Parturition in the mare. The foal has been expelled and the fetal membranes ruptured and peeled back from the head of the newborn foal. (Photo courtesy of P. Ryan, Department of Animal and Dairy Science, Mississippi State University).

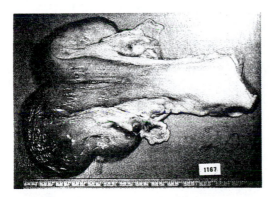

Plate 11 Recovery of the bovine uterus after calving–I. The exterior of the reproductive tract shows that there is still some enlargement at 20 days after normal calving (Note also the prominent corpus luteum on the left ovary, this cow had been in heat since calving which is uncommon within 20 days after calving). (Photo courtesy of N. L. VanDemark and University of Illinois, Urbana, IL).

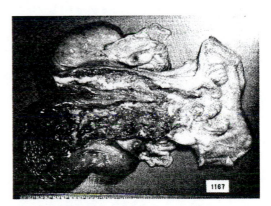

Plate 12 Recovery of the bovine uterus after calving—II. The interior of the uterus shown in Plate 11 is presented. Note the pus that is present within the tract, and that the lining of the uterus is far from being the healthy pink color found in a fully recovered uteri. (Photo courtesy of N. L. VanDemark and University of Illinois, Urbana, IL).

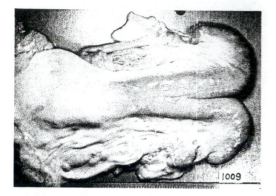

Plate 13 Recovery of the bovine uterus after calving–III. The exterior of the reproductive tract at 35 days after normal calving. Note that this uterus has returned to normal size, shape and tone. (Photo courtesy of N. L. VanDemark and University Illinois, Urbana, IL).

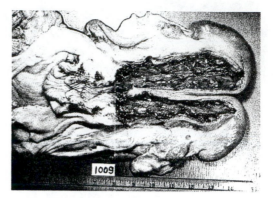

Plate 14 Recovery of the bovine uterus after calving–IV. The interior of the uterus shown in Plate 13 is presented. While the exterior of the tract indicates near return to normal size, the interior reflects a tract that has not yet recovered completely. The lining of the uterus is still red and inflamed, and the caruncles are still somewhat enlarged. (Photo courtesy of N. L. VanDemark and University of Illinois, Urbana, IL).

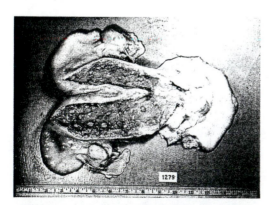

Plate 15 Recovery of the bovine uterus after calving–V. The interior of the uterus at 46 days after calving. The lining of the uterus is still not fully recovered, with still a slight enlargement of the caruncles and reddening of the uterine lining. (Photo courtesy of N. L. VanDemark and University of Illinois, Urbana, IL).

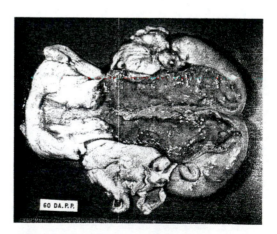

Plate 16 Recovery of the bovine uterus after calving–VI. The interior of the uterus at 60 days after calving. It is apparent that the uterine size, shape and tone are good and the uterine lining is a healthy pink color indicating that full recovery has taken place. (Photo courtesy of N. L. VanDemark and University of Illinois, Urbana, IL).

3–5.3 *Bulbourethral Glands*

The bulbourethral (Cowper's) glands are a pair of glands located along the urethra near the point where it exits from the pelvis. They are about the size and shape of walnuts in bulls but are much larger in boars. In bulls, they are embedded in the bulbospongiosus muscle. They contribute very little to the fluid volume of semen. In bulls, their secretions flush urine residue from the urethra before ejaculation. These secretions are seen as dribblings from the prepuce just before copulation. In boars, their secretions account for the gel-like portion of boar semen. This is strained from boar semen before it is used for artificial insemination. During natural service, the white coagulated lumps may prevent semen from flowing back through the cervix into the vagina of sows.

3–6   PENIS

The *penis* is the organ of copulation in males (Figure 3–1). It forms dorsally around the urethra from the point where the urethra leaves the pelvis, with the external urethral orifice at the free end of the penis. Bulls, boars, and rams have a *sigmoid flexure*, an S-shaped bend in the penis, which permits it to be retracted completely into the body. These three species and the stallion have *retractor penis muscles*, a pair of smooth muscles which will relax to permit extension of the penis and contract to draw the penis back into the prepuce. These retractor penis muscles arise from the vertebrae in the coccygeal region and are fused to the ventral penis just anterior to the sigmoid flexure. The *glans penis* (Figure 3–7 and Color Plate 9), which is the free end of the penis, is well supplied with sensory nerves and is homologous to the clitoris in the female (Chapter 2). There is considerable variation in the glans penis across species. The urethra opens into a twisted groove in the glans penis of the bull. The ram has a urethral process known as a filiform appendage extending beyond the glans penis. The glans penis of the boar spirals in a corkscrew manner. The glans penis of the stallion is flattened, with a small urethral process extending beyond the flattened end. In most species, the penis is fibroelastic, containing small amounts of erectile tissue. The penis of a stallion is vascular, containing more erectile tissue than is found in bulls, boars, bucks, or rams.

Erectile tissue is cavernous (spongy) tissue located in two regions of the penis (Figure 3–8). The *corpus spongiosum penis* is the cavernous tissue around the urethra. It enlarges into the penile bulb, which is covered with *bulbospongiosus muscle* at the base of the penis. The *corpus cavernosum penis* is a larger area of cavernous tissue located dorsally to the corpus spongiosum penis. It arises as two cavernous rods from the *ischiocavernosus muscle*, eventually fusing to form one cavernous area as it proceeds toward the glans penis. These cavernous areas engorge with blood during sexual excitement, causing extension of the penis (erection) and facilitation of the final ejection of semen during ejaculation (Chapter 7). Both the bulbospongiosus muscle and ischiocavernosus muscle are striated muscles rather than the smooth muscle associated with most of the male and female tracts.

3–7   PREPUCE

The *prepuce* (sheath) is an invagination of skin that completely encloses the free end of the penis. It has the same embryonic origin as the labia minora in the female. It can be divided into a prepenile portion, which is the outer fold, and the penile portion, or inner folds. The

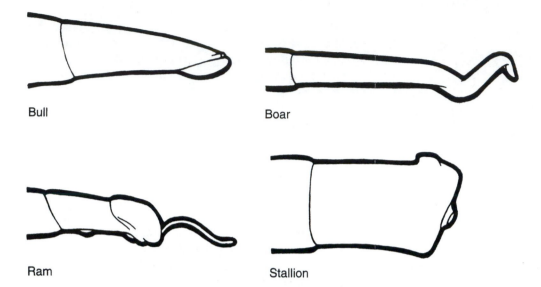

Bull

Boar

Ram

Stallion

Figure 3–7   Comparative diagram showing the shape of the glans penis of the bull, boar, ram, and stallion. Note the twisted groove containing the external urethral orifice in the bull, the urethral process (filiform appendage) extending beyond the glans penis in the ram, the corkscrew spiral in the boar, and the flattened glans penis in the stallion, with the small urethral process extending beyond. (Redrawn from Ashdown and Hancock. 1974. *Reproduction in Farm Animals.* (3rd ed.) ed. Hafez. Lea and Febiger.)

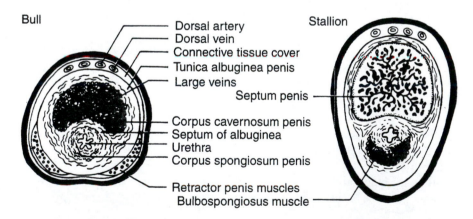

Figure 3–8   Cross section of penis showing corpus cavernosum penis and corpus spongiosum penis. (Redrawn from Sorensen. 1979. *Animal Reproduction: Principles and Practices.* McGraw-Hill.)

prepuce of the boar has a pouch dorsal to the orifice. Secretions that accumulate here contribute to the boar odor. The orifice of the prepuce is surrounded by long and tough preputial hairs.

SUGGESTED READING

AREY, L. B. 1947. *Developmental Anatomy.* (5th ed.) W. B. Saunders Co.

ASHDOWN, R. R. and J. L. HANCOCK. 1974. Functional anatomy of male reproduction. *Reproduction in Farm Animals.* (3rd ed.) ed. E. S. E. Hafez. Lea and Febiger.

GETTY, R., ed. 1975. *Sisson and Grossman—the Anatomy of Domestic Animals.* W. B. Saunders Co.

JOHNSON, A. D., W. R. GOMES, and N. L. VANDEMARK. 1970. *The Testes.* Vol. 1. Academic Press.

PARKES, A. S. 1956. *Marshall's Physiology of Reproduction.* Vol. 1. Part 1. Longmans, Green and Co.

SALISBURY, G. W., N. L. VANDEMARK, and J. R. LODGE. 1978. The reproductive tract of the bull. *Physiology of Reproduction and Artificial Insemination of Cattle.* (2nd ed.) W. H. Freeman and Co.

SETCHELL, B. P. 1977. Male reproductive organs and semen. *Reproduction in Domestic Animals.* (3rd ed.) eds. H. H. Cole and P. T. Cupps. Academic Press.

4

Neuroendocrine and Endocrine Regulators of Reproduction

Before undertaking a study of reproduction, it is important to become familiar with the physiological system most responsible for regulating the natural reproductive processes. The neuroendocrine system (Figure 4–1), through the hormones that it produces, is responsible for much of this regulation. Even reproductive reflexes that are considered neural reflexes (e.g., copulation) have a hormonal requirement.

Endocrine glands are ductless glands and secrete internally. They secrete directly into the bloodstream, as opposed to exocrine glands, which have ducts and secrete externally, not into the bloodstream. Endocrine glands secrete hormones—chemical agents—which are carried by the blood to cells within a target organ or to other target cells where they regulate a specific physiological activity. Thus, by the classic definition, hormones exert their influence through cells at a site away from the glands that produce them. However, some hormones also exert these effects locally. These effects may be *autocrine* (affecting the cells that secrete them) or *paracrine* (affecting other cells in the same organ). These effects differ from endocrine effects in that movement to the sites of action involves local diffusion rather than the circulatory system.

Cells that respond to a specific hormone do so because they have *receptor sites* which bind that hormone. Receptor sites can be defined as recognition units in cells that have a high affinity for a particular hormone. When a hormone binds to a receptor site, it initiates reactions within that cell, which bring about the specific physiological response associated with the bound hormone. The concentration of receptor sites in a target organ will increase or decrease depending on the endocrine status of the animal. Regulation of hormonal receptor sites in organs of reproduction will be discussed in Section 4–8. Knowledge of how receptor sites are regulated has added a new realm of understanding to the endocrine control of reproduction.

Chemically, hormones of reproduction can be divided into two major classes. One class includes the peptide and protein hormones (Table 4–1). These hormones are formed by the bonding of a series of amino acids, with molecular size being the determinant of whether they are called peptide or protein. Peptide and protein hormones are soluble in water. They are denatured by strong acids, strong bases, or heat which makes them physiologically inactive. To be physiologically effective, they must be administered systemically (i.v., i.m., or s.c.) rather than orally.

The second class of hormones of reproduction are steroids. Steroids are a special class of lipids having a tetracyclic configuration (Figure 4–2). All steroid hormones have cholesterol as a common precursor. They are not soluble in water but are soluble in ether

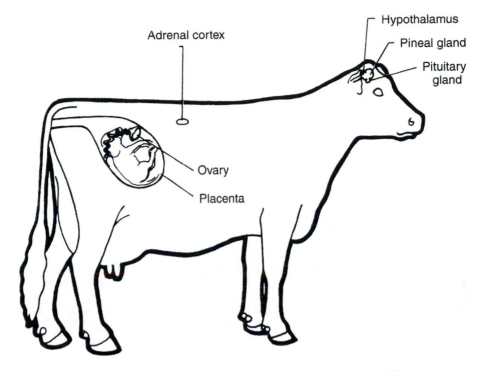

Figure 4–1 Approximate location of the endocrine glands of the cow which secrete hormones that regulate reproduction. (Redrawn from Foley et al. 1972. *Dairy Cattle: Principles, Practices, Problems, Profits.* Lea and Febiger.)

Table 4–1 *Molecular size of peptide and protein hormones that regulate reproduction*

Hormone	Molecular weight
Follicle-stimulating hormone (FSH)	30,000–37,000
Luteinizing hormone (LH)	26,000–32,000
Prolactin	23,000–25,000
Adrenocorticotropic hormone (ACTH)	4,500
Inhibin	32,000
Oxytocin	1,007
Gonadotropin-releasing hormone (GnRH)	1,200
Human chorionic gonadotropin (hCG)	37,700
Pregnant mare serum gonadotropin (PMSG)	28,000
Relaxin	6,500

and other solvents, which can be used to extract lipids from tissue or blood. Some steroids can be effectively absorbed through the gastrointestinal tract but are usually less effective with oral administration than with systemic administration. Natural estrogens are usually more effective than natural progestins or androgens when given orally. Synthetic progestins have been developed for oral administration.

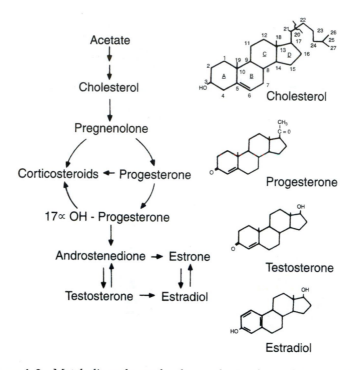

Figure 4–2   Metabolic pathway for the synthesis of gonadal steroid hormones and the chemical structure of the three most important sex steroids. (Niswender et al. 1974. *Reproduction in Farm Animals.* (3rd ed.) ed. Hafez. Lea and Febiger.)

Functionally, hormones can be classified as either *primary hormones of reproduction* or *secondary hormones of reproduction*. The primary hormones of reproduction are those that directly regulate a reproductive activity. Most other hormones are classified as secondary hormones of reproduction. These hormones regulate other physiological systems which directly or indirectly influence the reproductive processes. The discussion in this chapter will be limited to the primary hormones of reproduction (Table 4–2). The functions of the hormones which are mentioned briefly in this chapter will be discussed in greater detail in later chapters.

4–1 PRIMARY REPRODUCTIVE HORMONES OF THE PITUITARY GLAND

The pituitary, a gland located in a bony depression (the sella turcica) at the base of the brain, is embryologically and functionally two separate glands in the adult animal. The anterior lobe or *anterior pituitary* (also called adenohypophysis) arises from embryonic gut tissues of the roof of the mouth. The posterior lobe or *posterior pituitary* (also called neurohypophysis) forms from embryonic brain tissue. Thus, the posterior pituitary is a neural structure that serves an endocrine function and should be called a neuroendocrine gland.

Table 4–2 *Hormones that regulate reproduction*

Gland	Hormone	Chemical class	Principal functions
Hypothalamus	Gonadotropin-releasing hormone (GnRH)	Peptide	(1) FSH and LH release
	Prolactin-inhibiting factor (PIF)	"	(1) Prolactin retention
	Prolactin-releasing factor (PRF)	"	(1) Prolactin release
	Corticotropin-releasing hormone (CRH)	"	(1) ACTH release
Anterior pituitary	Follicle-stimulating hormone (FSH)	Protein	(1) Follicle growth (2) Estrogen release (3) Spermatogenesis
	Luteinizing hormone (LH)	"	(1) Ovulation (2) Corpus luteum formation and function (3) Testosterone release
	Prolactin	"	(1) Milk synthesis
	Adrenocorticotropin (ACTH)	Polypeptide	(1) Release of glucocorticoid
Posterior pituitary	Oxytocin	Peptide	(1) Parturition (2) Milk ejection
Ovary	Estrogens (estradiol)	Steroid	(1) Mating behavior (2) Secondary sex characteristics (3) Maintenance of female duct system (4) Mammary growth
	Progestins (progesterone)	Steroid	(1) Maintenance of pregnancy (2) Mammary growth
Relaxin	Relaxin	Polypeptide	(1) Expansion of pelvis (2) Dilation of cervix
	Inhibin	Protein	(1) Prevention of release of FSH
Testis	Androgens (testosterone)	Steroid	(1) Male mating behavior (2) Spermatogenesis (3) Maintenance of male duct system (4) Function of accessory glands
	Inhibin	Protein	(1) Prevention of release of FSH
Adrenal cortex	Glucocorticoids (cortisol)	Steroid	(1) Parturition (2) Milk synthesis
Placenta	Human chorionic gonadotropin (hCG)	Protein	(1) LH-like
	Pregnant mare serum gonadotropin (PMSG)	Protein	(1) FSH-like (2) Supplementary corpora lutea in mare
	Estrogens Progestins Relaxin	(See ovary)	
Uterus	Prostaglandin $F_{2\alpha}$ ($PGF_{2\alpha}$)	Lipid	(1) Regression of corpus luteum (2) Parturition

The anterior pituitary produces three primary hormones of reproduction. These protein hormones of the anterior pituitary are *follicle-stimulating hormone (FSH), luteinizing hormone (LH),* and *prolactin.* Collectively, FSH and LH are known as *gonadotropins* because they stimulate the gonads. In the male, LH was originally called *interstitial cell stimulating hormone (ICSH).*

In the female, FSH promotes follicle growth and estrogen production by granulosa cells in the ovarian follicle. Also, *inhibin* is secreted by granulosa cells, with its production being enhanced by FSH. Inhibin, a protein hormone, was first identified in males, where it is secreted by Sertoli cells, but follicular fluid is a richer source than are the testes. Other protein hormones secreted by granulosa cells are *activin* and *follistatin.* Secretion of follistatin is regulated by FSH. Little is known about the regulation of activin at this time. Stimulation of the theca interna cells by LH causes production of testosterone, which then diffuses across the basement membrane, where it is converted to estrogens by granulosa cells under the influence of FSH. Also, LH causes maturation of the oocyte and ovulation (rupture of follicle with release of oocyte), and it is *luteotropic.* That is, it stimulates formation of the corpus luteum and production of progesterone. Prolactin synergizes with LH by increasing LH receptor sites in the corpus luteum in some species. Also, prolactin has a stimulating effect on development of the mammary gland and the synthesis of milk. *Adrenocorticotropic hormone (ACTH),* a small protein hormone of the anterior pituitary, stimulates the release of *glucocorticoids* from the adrenal cortex. Glucocorticoids play a role in parturition and in the synthesis of milk.

In the male, FSH is needed for quantitative production of spermatozoa in the seminiferous tubules with specific action on Sertoli cells. Sertoli cells secrete inhibin and *androgen-binding protein* when stimulated by FSH. Androgen-binding protein is secreted into the lumen of the seminiferous tubules and serves as a carrier for testosterone. The cells of Leydig, located in the interstitial tissue of the testes, produce testosterone and other androgens when stimulated by LH. Prolactin appears to synergize with LH by increasing hormone receptor sites for LH in the testes.

Oxytocin, a peptide hormone released from the posterior pituitary, stimulates the contraction of smooth muscle in the oviduct and uterus. Because of this activity, it has been postulated that oxytocin aids both sperm and ovum transport in the female tract and stimulates uterine contractions during parturition. Also, oxytocin stimulates the myoepithelial cells of the mammary gland, causing the ejection of milk.

4–2 Neuroendocrine Control of the Pituitary Gland

Release of hormones from the anterior pituitary is controlled by neurosecretory substances produced in the brain. These include releasing hormones (called releasing factors if not well characterized) and inhibiting factors from the hypothalamus, endogenous opioids from the hypothalamus and adjacent tissues, and melatonin from the pineal gland.

4–2.1 *Hypothalamus*

The *hypothalamus* is a neuroendocrine gland that forms along the floor and lateral wall of the third ventricle of the brain. It is closely linked with the pituitary. The hypophyseal por-

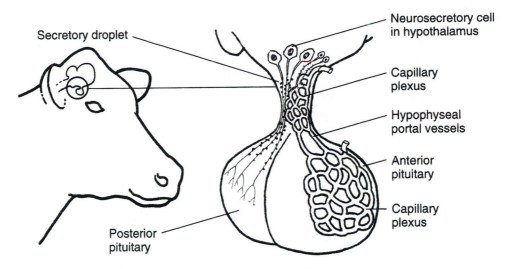

Figure 4–3 Relationship between the hypothalamus and the pituitary gland. (The pituitary-hypothalamic area is enlarged to permit a more detailed illustration.)

a. The hypophyseal portal blood system is the route by which GnRH and other releasing hormones of the hypothalamus are transported to the anterior pituitary.

b. Neurosecretory cells in the hypothalamus secrete oxytocin, which is transported by carrier proteins as secretory droplets along nerve fibers to the posterior pituitary.

tal blood system connects the hypothalamus with the anterior pituitary and is the route by which hormones of the hypothalamus reach the anterior pituitary. The hypothalamic hormones are released from terminals of axons (nerve fibers) into blood vessels that serve the anterior pituitary. The area of the hypothalamus where this exchange takes place is the *median eminence,* and the pituitary vessels that receive releasing hormones or releasing factors are the *hypophyseal portal vessels*. Also, a portion of the venous return from the anterior pituitary is by way of the hypothalamus. This permits a direct, short-loop feedback system whereby hormones of the anterior pituitary may help regulate release of hormones from the hypothalamus. The posterior pituitary is an extension of the hypothalamus. Axons from neurosecretory cells in the hypothalamus extend down into the posterior pituitary (Figure 4–3).

Secretion of gonadotropic hormones from the anterior pituitary is controlled by a peptide-releasing hormone which is produced by neurosecretory cells in the hypothalamus. This peptide, *gonadotropin-releasing hormone (GnRH),* was first isolated and characterized by Guillemin and Schally, who, working independently of one another, purified GnRH from the hypothalamus of sheep and pigs, respectively. Guillemin and Schally shared the Nobel Prize for Physiology and Medicine in 1977 for their discovery of both GnRH and *thyrotropin-releasing hormone (TRH)*. GnRH causes the release of both FSH and LH. At one time, it was postulated that separate releasing agents (FSH-releasing hormone and LH-releasing hormone) regulated the release of FSH and LH from the anterior pituitary. While physiological evidence for separate releasing hormones still exists, a specific FSH-releasing hormone has not been isolated. In a clinical situation, GnRH can be used instead of LH for treatment of cystic ovaries in cows. There is evidence that both a *prolactin-releasing factor (PRF)* and *prolactin-inhibiting factor (PIF)* control the release and retention of prolactin in the anterior pituitary. *Corticotropin-releasing hormone (CRH)* stimulates the release of ACTH, *growth hormone–releasing hormone (GHRH)* stimulates the release of *growth hormone (GH),* and TRH stimulates the release of *thyroid-stimulating hormone (TSH).*

Oxytocin, which is released from the posterior pituitary, is produced by the supraoptic and paraventricular nuclei (neurosecretory cells) in the hypothalamus. After synthesis, oxytocin is transported by carrier proteins (neurophysins) as secretory droplets along nerve fibers extending into the posterior pituitary. Stimulation of sensory nerves in the teats or the cervix will cause oxytocin to be released from nerve endings in the posterior pituitary.

4–2.2 *Endogenous Opioids*

After discovery of specific binding sites in brain tissue for synthetic opiate drugs such as morphine, a number of *endogenous opioid peptides* were identified in brain tissue. One of these, β-*endorphin,* is found in high concentration in the hypothalamus and hypophyseal portal blood with its concentration changing during the estrous cycle and during different reproductive states. Injection of opioid peptides inhibits the secretion of FSH and LH but stimulates release of prolactin. Injection of *naloxone,* a specific opioid inhibitor, can cause release of gonadotropic hormones (FSH and LH). There is evidence that opioid peptides have their effect on gonadotropin release by preventing release of GnRH from nerve terminals in the median eminence (stalk of pituitary). Therefore, GnRH is not transferred to hypophyseal portal blood and from there to the anterior pituitary for release of FSH and LH. Similarly, there is experimental evidence that opioid peptides can inhibit release of oxytocin from nerve terminals in the posterior pituitary. Their physiological role seems to be that of a modulator of hormone release from the anterior pituitary and posterior pituitary.

4–2.3 *Pineal Gland*

The *pineal gland* is located posterior to the hypothalamus between the hemispheres of the brain. Its embryonic origin is the brain, but direct connection to the central nervous system is lost during development with innervation thereafter coming from sympathetic nerves. While the pineal gland of the amphibian has photoreceptors, they are not found in the pineal gland of mammals. However, the pineal gland responds to environmental lighting and senses changes in photoperiod (day length).

The sensor of photoperiod change in mammals is the eye (Figure 4–4). Nerve impulses from these photic signals are transmitted from the retina along the retinohypothalamic tract to the suprachiasmatic nuclei, located anterior to the hypothalamus, and then to the superior cervical ganglia near the base of the brain, from which arise the sympathetic nerves that innervate the pineal gland. The diurnal rhythm of secretory activity of the pineal gland is generated by these suprachiasmatic nuclei. This rhythm is abolished by placement of the animal

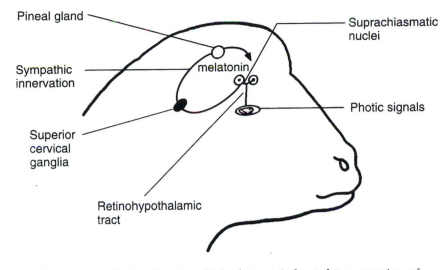

Figure 4–4 Mechanism by which photoperiod regulates secretion of melatonin from the pineal gland. Nerve impulses resulting from photic signals to the eye are transmitted from the retina along the retinohypothalamic tract to the suprachiasmatic nuclei, then to the superior cervical ganglia, and from there to the pineal gland via sympathetic nerve stimulation.

in constant light, by destruction of the suprachiasmatic nuclei, or by destruction of the superior cervical ganglia which prevent the signals generated by the suprachiasmatic nuclei from reaching the pineal gland. Neither constant darkness, removal of the eyes, nor severing of the retinohypothalamic tract will abolish the diurnal secretory rhythm of the pineal gland. However, the retained rhythm will be free-running and not affected by changing photoperiod.

The best characterized hormone of the pineal gland is *melatonin,* a derivative of the amino acid tryptophan. Darkness causes increased sympathetic activity to the pineal gland, which increases the secretion rate of melatonin. Studies indicate there is a diurnal pattern, with higher melatonin secretion at night and lower secretion during the day in seasonal and nonseasonal species. However, it is only in seasonal breeders (animal species that are reproductively active for only a part of each year) that a clear reproductive role for melatonin has been demonstrated. That role is as a regulator of reproductive activity by either stimulating or inhibiting gonadal function. The long duration of high melatonin secretion during short photoperiod (long nights) switches on short-day breeders such as sheep and goats and switches off long-day breeders such as the hamster. A role for melatonin in onset of puberty has also been suggested. The mechanism by which the pattern of melatonin release either turns on or turns off the reproductive system is not clear. The most likely site of action is the hypothalamus through regulation of the release of GnRH. The effects of melatonin could be direct on the hypothalamus or could be indirect by initiating release of other physiologically active compounds. A number of physiologically active peptides, produced by the pineal gland, have been identified, with some having effects on the reproductive system. There is some experimental evidence that melatonin elicits their release, but these peptides have not yet been fully characterized.

4–3   HORMONES OF THE GONADS

Major steroid hormones produced by the gonads are shown in Table 4–3.

4–3.1 *Female*

Two classes of hormones produced by the ovaries are *estrogens* and *progestins*. Chemically, estrogens and progestins are classified as steroids and have cholesterol as a common precursor.

Estrogens, representing a group of steroids with similar physiological activity, are produced by specific cells in the Graafian follicle. The thecal cells of the follicle are stimulated by LH to produce androgens which diffuse across the basement membrane, where they are converted to estrogens by aromatase activity in granulosa cells, which are under the influence of FSH. The estrogen of greatest importance, quantitatively and physiologically, is *estradiol.* Others of importance include estriol and estrone. The principal actions of estrogens are their influence on (1) the manifestation of mating behavior during estrus; (2) cyclic changes in the female tract; (3) duct development in the mammary gland; and (4) development of secondary sex characteristics in females. Estrogens have been called the "female sex hormone." Estrogens are luteolytic (causing lysis of the CL) in cows and ewes but are luteotropic (supportive of CL function) in sows.

Progestins are another group of hormones with similar physiological activity, the most important being *progesterone.* They are secreted by the corpus luteum. The larger luteal cells of granulosa origin are the principal progesterone-secreting cells in the corpus luteum, but small luteal cells of thecal origin secrete progesterone when stimulated by LH. Important functions are (1) inhibition of sexual behavior; (2) maintenance of pregnancy by inhibiting uterine contractions and promoting glandular development in the endometrium; and (3) promotion of alveolar development of the mammary gland. The synergistic actions of estrogens and progestins are notable in preparing the uterus for pregnancy and the mammary gland for lactation.

Estrogens and progestins help regulate the release of gonadotropins, acting through both the hypothalamus and anterior pituitary (Figure 4–5). High concentrations of progestins inhibit the release of GnRH, FSH, and LH—a negative feedback control. Endogenous opioids are likely a part of this negative feedback system. Whereas low concentrations

Table 4–3   *Major steroid hormones produced by the gonads*

Class	Hormone
Estrogens	Estradiol-17 β
	Estriol
	Estrone
Progestins	Progesterone
	17-Hydroxyprogesterone
	20 β-dihydroprogesterone
Androgens	Testosterone
	Androstenedione
	Dihydrotestosterone

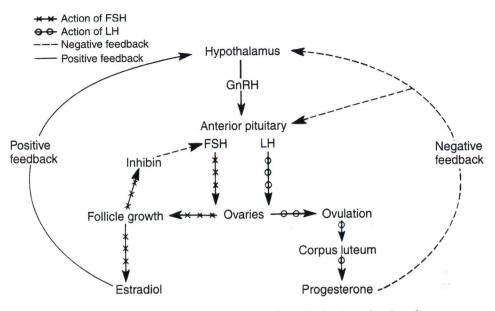

Figure 4–5 Relationship among the hypothalamic releasing hormones, gonadotropins, and ovarian hormones in regulating reproductive function.

a. GnRH from the hypothalamus stimulates the release of FSH and LH from the anterior pituitary.

b. FSH stimulates production of estradiol and inhibin by granulosa cells in the ovarian follicle.

c. Inhibin selectively inhibits release of FSH.

d. When progesterone is low, high concentrations of estradiol stimulate a greater surge of GnRH, FSH, and LH, a positive feedback control.

e. LH stimulates production and release of progesterone by granulosa cells in the corpus luteum.

f. High concentrations of progesterone inhibit the release of GnRH, FSH, and LH, a negative feedback control.

of estrogens are inhibitory and important in regulation of tonic release of gonadotropins, high concentrations stimulate the release of GnRH, LH, FSH, and prolactin—a positive feedback control. This positive feedback effect is seen near the time of ovulation when progesterone is low. The influence of the gonadotropins on estrogen and progestin release has been mentioned previously. Therefore, it can be seen that reciprocal action between the gonadotropins and the steroid hormones of the ovaries is necessary for maintenance of the hormone balance essential for normal reproduction.

Both inhibin and follistatin, protein hormones secreted by granulosa cells in ovarian follicles, suppress release of FSH from the anterior pituitary, without apparent effect on release of LH. The effects of follistatin on FSH release are weaker than for inhibin but the effects of the two are additive. These actions may account for some of the reported differences in the release patterns of FSH and LH that appear inconsistent with a single gonadotropin-releasing hormone. Activin, another protein hormone produced by granulosa cells, increases the secretion of FSH but is found in lower concentrations in follicular fluid than is inhibin.

Relaxin is a polypeptide hormone produced by the corpus luteum and placenta. Little is known about the mechanisms controlling its production, but higher concentrations are seen during pregnancy. It causes a relaxation of pelvic ligaments and softening of the connective tissue of the uterine muscles to allow the expansion necessary to accommodate the growing fetus. Synergizing with estrogen, it causes further expansion of the pelvis and softening of the connective tissue of the cervix to permit the fetus to be expelled during parturition.

Oxytocin is secreted by the corpus luteum, also. In some species, the concentration in the corpus luteum is almost as high as that found in the posterior pituitary. Injection of prostaglandin $F_{2\alpha}$ ($PGF_{2\alpha}$), a luteolytic agent (Section 2–7), causes release of luteal oxytocin. Therefore, luteal oxytocin may either mediate or enhance the effects of $PGF_{2\alpha}$ during regression of the corpus luteum.

4–3.1a Follicular Fluid

Follicular fluid (liquor folliculi) is the fluid that fills the antrum of a tertiary follicle bathing the granulosa cells. There is free exchange of fluids and many compounds between blood and follicular fluid across the basement membrane. However, large plasma proteins (> 1,000,000 MW) do not cross the basement membrane and are not in follicular fluid. Follicular fluid is rich in steroid reproductive hormones, including testosterone, estradiol, and progesterone. Concentrations of these steroids are much higher in follicular fluid than in blood. This is not surprising, since testosterone produced by theca cells is converted to estradiol in granulosa cells. As the follicle matures, the increasing number of granulosa cells is reflected by the decreased concentration of testosterone while estradiol concentration increases.

The pituitary hormones, FSH, LH, and prolactin, are found in follicular fluid. The lower concentrations of LH as compared with FSH may in part be due to binding of LH to theca cells outside the basement membrane, whereas granulosa cells have receptor sites for both FSH and LH. The conversion of testosterone to estradiol by granulosa cells is stimulated by FSH, whereas LH stimulates progesterone production by granulosa cells. Prolactin inhibits progesterone synthesis by granulosa cells (*in vitro*), and higher progesterone is seen in follicular fluid when prolactin is low. Prostaglandins ($PGF_{2\alpha}$ and PGE_2) are found in the follicular fluid of Graafian follicles as the time of ovulation approaches (Section 8–2).

A number of other peptide ovarian factors have been identified in follicular fluid in recent years. These include inhibin, activin, and follistatin. Inhibin has an apparent molecular weight of about 32,000 and is composed of two subunits linked by a disulfide bond. Activin is of similar structure and size to inhibin, but follistatin does not exhibit the same subunit structure. These hormones have both endocrine and local effects. Endocrine effects are demonstrated by their effect on the secretion of FSH from the anterior pituitary. Local effects of inhibin include inhibition of production of estradiol by granulosa cells (autocrine action) and a stimulatory effect on LH-induced androgen secretion by thecal cells (paracrine action). An autocrine function of activin is its enhancing effect on FSH-induced progesterone secretion by granulosa cells. A paracrine effect of activin is its inhibitory effect on LH-induced androgen production by thecal cells. Follistatin has autocrine effects by inhibiting FSH-induced inhibin secretion and aromatase activity. Further, follistatin may serve as an activin-binding protein in follicular fluid.

GnRH or a similar substance has been identified in follicular fluid. The concentrations in follicular fluid are thought to be too high for it to be of hypothalamic origin, but cells in the ovary that secrete GnRH have not been identified. Production of estradiol and progesterone is suppressed by GnRH, thus interfering with ovulation and corpus luteum formation. The concentration of GnRH that originates from the hypothalamus is not high enough in peripheral blood to have these depressing effects on ovarian function.

Insulin, a pancreatic hormone, and insulin-like growth factor, secreted by granulosa cells, are found in follicular fluid. Although it has been suggested that many actions of insulin are mediated through insulin-like growth factor receptors, granulosa cells have separate receptors for both insulin and insulin-like growth factor. Endocrine actions of insulin are reduced atresia in tertiary follicles and increased ovulation rate in pigs. The negative relationship between insulin-like growth factor and follicular atresia suggests an autocrine role for insulin-like growth factor (Section 4–7).

Oocyte maturation inhibitor, a factor that prevents resumption of meiosis until a few hours before ovulation, may be produced by granulosa cells under the influence of FSH. A peptide with a molecular weight of less than 10,000, its activity declines shortly before ovulation, thereby permitting meiosis to resume. Other peptide factors with either stimulating or inhibiting effects on ovarian function are poorly characterized, but some will likely prove to be important to natural regulation of ovarian function (Section 4–7). Factors that have been reported in research literature include luteinizing stimulator, luteinizing inhibitor, FSH receptor binding inhibitor, gonadostatin, and gonadocrinin, the latter having actions similar to GnRH.

4–3.2 *Male*

Upon stimulation by LH, the Leydig cells of the testes produce *androgens,* which are a class of steroid hormones. The principal androgen in mature males is *testosterone,* which has been labeled the male sex hormone. Functions of testosterone include (1) development of secondary sex characteristics; (2) maintenance of the male duct system; (3) expression of male sexual behavior (libido); (4) function of the accessory glands; (5) function of the tunica dartos muscle in the scrotum; (6) spermatogenesis; and (7) embryonic differentiation of the male duct system and external genitalia. The role of testosterone in regulating the release of hypothalamic and gonadotropic hormones is similar to that described for progesterone in the female (Figure 4–6). High concentrations of testosterone inhibit the release of GnRH, FSH, and LH, a negative feedback control. Conversely, when testosterone concentrations are low, higher concentrations of GnRH, FSH, and LH are released. Thus, reciprocal action of testosterone with the hypothalamic and gonadotropic hormones is necessary for regulation of normal reproduction in the male. Inhibin and androgen-binding protein are produced by Sertoli cells under the influence of FSH. As in the female, inhibin selectively inhibits the release of FSH while not affecting the release of LH. Androgen-binding protein binds testosterone, making it available for its function in spermatozoa production. Under the influence of FSH, Sertoli cells convert testosterone to estradiol, but a role for estradiol in regulation of reproduction in the male has not been clearly established. Activin and other proteins are secreted by Sertoli cells, also.

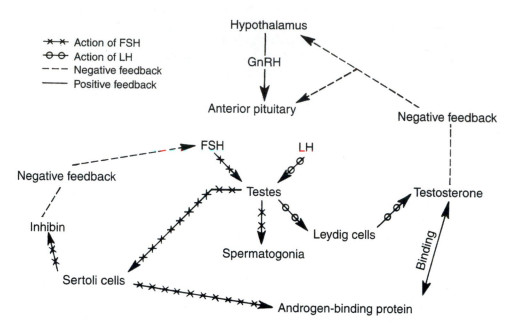

Figure 4–6   Interrelationship of the hormones regulating reproduction in the male.

a. GnRH from the hypothalamus stimulates the release of FSH and LH from the anterior pituitary.

b. LH stimulates the Leydig cells to produce testosterone.

c. High concentrations of testosterone inhibit the release of GnRH, FSH, and LH, whereas low levels of testosterone permit these hormones to be released, a negative feedback control.

d. FSH stimulates the Sertoli cells to produce inhibin and androgen-binding protein.

e. Inhibin inhibits the release of FSH.

f. Androgen-binding protein binds testosterone in the seminiferous tubules, assuring a supply for continuance of spermatogenesis.

4–4   PRIMARY REPRODUCTIVE HORMONES OF THE ADRENAL CORTEX

The adrenal cortex produces two classes of steroid hormones that have been associated with mineral metabolism (mineralocorticoids) and carbohydrate metabolism (glucocorticoids). Glucocorticoids, the principal one being *cortisol,* have been classified as antistress hormones, also. While progestins, estrogens, and androgens have been isolated from the adrenal cortex, they have not been seen in quantities high enough to affect the reproductive processes. It is believed that glucocorticoids, when released at high levels during periods of stress, may alter (suppress) normal reproductive function in livestock (Section 23–2).

A role for glucocorticoids in the initiation of parturition in sheep has been demonstrated. Furthermore, the glucocorticoids involved in this process are of fetal rather than maternal origin (Section 10–3.1). In addition, a role for glucocorticoids in milk synthesis has been advanced (Chapter 11).

4–5 ENDOCRINE FUNCTION OF THE UTERINE/PLACENTAL UNIT

The placenta does not fit the classical definition of an endocrine gland but does assume an endocrine function during pregnancy. Estrogens, progestins, prostaglandins, and relaxin are produced by the placenta in certain species and supplement production of these hormones by the ovaries. In addition, placental hormone(s) with luteotropic and/or lactogenic activity have been identified in some species and may be present in others. *Human chorionic gonadotropin (hCG)* has been isolated from the urine of pregnant women. Its principal action is LH-like and it maintains the function of the corpus luteum during pregnancy. *Pregnant mare serum gonadotropin (PMSG)*, which is sometimes called equine chorionic gonadotropin (eCG), is produced by endometrial cups that form when specialized cells in the chorion invade the endometrium of the pregnant uterus of the mare. Principally, PMSG has FSH-like action but it has some LH-like activity, also. It has been isolated from the serum of mares during early pregnancy. PMSG stimulates the formation of accessory corpora lutea in the mare during pregnancy. Both hCG and PMSG are proteins.

Placental lactogen has been isolated from a number of species, including goats, sheep, and cows. It is a polypeptide and is extracted from the placenta of these species. Its properties are similar to both prolactin and growth hormone. Possible functions include development of the mammary gland for postpartum milk production, regulation of fetal growth through altered maternal or fetal metabolism, and stimulation of progesterone synthesis by the ovary or placenta. Concentrations are higher during late gestation than during early gestation. Higher concentrations have also been reported for cows with high milk production than for low milk producers.

Pregnancy specific proteins of placental origin have been identified in cattle and sheep. One pregnancy-specific protein is produced for only a few days during early pregnancy in cattle and sheep. It is known as bovine (or ovine) *interferon-τ*. In sheep, its concentrations increase from day 13 to day 17 of the gestation period and then decline to undetectable levels by day 23. Another protein, identified as *protein B,* has been detected in the blood of pregnant cows as early as 24 days after conception. Production of protein B continues for the rest of the gestation period, with higher concentrations present in late gestation. It has not been detected in urine or milk. The assay used to detect protein B in the blood of pregnant cows has detected this protein in the blood of pregnant sheep.

A role for *interferon-τ* in maternal recognition and maintenance of pregnancy in cattle and sheep has been demonstrated (Section 9–5). Protein B provides an accurate serological test for diagnosis of pregnancy in cattle and sheep (Chapter 21).

4–6 REPRODUCTIVE ROLE OF PROSTAGLANDINS

Prostaglandins are a group of biologically active lipids that have arachidonic acid, a 20-carbon, unsaturated fatty acid as their precursor. While prostaglandins have hormone-like actions, they do not fit the classic definition of a hormone. They are not produced by a specific gland or tissue. Rather, they are produced by cells throughout the body, including cells in the ovary and uterus (female) as well as the vesicular glands (male). In most cases, they act locally at the site of their production, but in some cases their site of action is in another tissue or

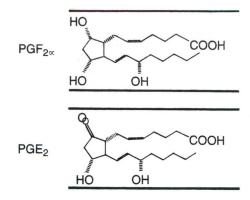

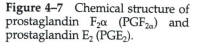

Figure 4–7　Chemical structure of prostaglandin $F_{2\alpha}$ (PGF$_{2\alpha}$) and prostaglandin E_2 (PGE$_2$).

organ. Prostaglandins are rapidly degraded in mammals, with about 90% of their activity lost in one passage through the pulmonary circulation. Based on differences in chemical structure, several parent prostaglandin compounds have been identified. Of these, prostaglandin E series (PGE) and prostaglandin F series (PGF) are of greatest biological interest. The two compounds most closely associated with reproduction are PGF$_{2\alpha}$ and PGE$_2$ (Figure 4–7).

Effects of PGF$_{2\alpha}$ are to cause luteolysis (regression of the corpus luteum) and to stimulate smooth muscle. Because of these actions, natural functions in the control of the estrous cycle, ovum transport, sperm transport, and parturition have been proposed. PGF$_{2\alpha}$ has been used in clinical situations where regression of the corpus luteum or stimulation of smooth muscle is desired.

Also, PGE$_2$ appears to have an important role in reproduction. It is a smooth muscle stimulator, but its effect on the corpus luteum is opposite to that of PGF$_{2\alpha}$. This antiluteolytic action of PGE$_2$ is a factor in the maintenance of early pregnancy by preventing PGF$_{2\alpha}$-induced luteolysis. Prostaglandins are found in the follicular fluid of Graafian follicles a few hours before ovulation and have an identified role in the ovulation process (Section 8–2). Inhibitors to prostaglandin synthesis have prevented ovulation in controlled experiments.

Little research has been reported on a role for prostaglandins in the regulation of reproductive function in males. It has been demonstrated in bulls that injection of PGF$_{2\alpha}$ will cause a surge in LH and testosterone. However, an integrative role for prostaglandins in the natural regulation of reproductive function in males has not been demonstrated.

4–7　HORMONE-LIKE FACTORS AND OTHER HORMONAL MEDIATORS

Growth factors and *cytokines* are proteins whose primary purpose is to activate cellular proliferation and/or differentiation. To identify all of the roles of the compounds classified as growth factors in reproductive processes would be far beyond the scope of this text. However, it is important to recognize the different types of growth factors that may be involved in mediating reproductive processes in a more general sense.

Growth factors that have been shown to have specific actions in male and/or female reproduction include

epidermal growth factor (EGF)	insulin-like growth factor-I (IGF-I)
platelet-derived growth factor (PDGF)	insulin-like growth factor-II (IGF-II)
transforming growth factor-α (TGF-α)	fibroblast growth factor (FGF)
transforming growth factor-β (TGF-β)	vascular endothelial growth factor (VEGF)
nerve growth factor (NGF)	platelet-activating factor (PAF)

Many of these growth factors have been shown to have synergistic effects with steroid hormones that can enhance steroidogenic effects. For example, EGF, IGF-I, TGF-α, and VEGF have all been shown to enhance the estrogenic actions of estrogen itself, as well as estrogen-like compounds such as phytoestrogens (plant estrogens) or other environmental estrogens that can be physiologically active. Many of these growth factors have steroid-responsive elements within the promoter regions of the genes that control the production (transcription of mRNA) of the various growth factors. This suggests that steroid hormones can up-regulate growth factor production, which in turn may enhance the actions of the steroid hormone itself. This relationship among growth factors, steroid hormones, steroid hormone receptors (Section 4–8), and various second messenger signaling pathways (Section 4–9) to mediate expression of steroid-responsive genes has been examined extensively in a number of reproductive tissues. In addition to this more general role of growth factors interacting with steroid hormones, each growth factor has been shown to have discrete actions within tissues of the male and female reproductive tract. Whether these actions are restricted to a given tissue or are more generalized actions throughout the reproductive system remains to be determined. Fibroblast growth factor and PDGF have been linked specifically to the differentiation and function of the CL in the bovine. *Angiogenesis,* the formation of new capillary networks and blood vessels, is an important process in tissues that reorganize during different phases of the reproductive cycle and is mediated, in part, by growth factors such as VEGF and FGF. Angiogenesis is important in the development of an ovulatory follicle and in formation of the CL, as well as during changes in the uterine endometrium throughout the estrous or menstrual cycles, and during placentation. Changes in nutrition can also influence growth factor presence and actions, as flushing (supplementing the diet to have the animal in a gaining state at the time of breeding—Section 23–3.1) can increase IGF-I in the ovary, which can reduce follicular atresia and enhance ovarian responsiveness to gonadotropins (FSH and LH). Finally, almost every growth factor identified has been added in some manner to *in vitro* cultures of sperm, oocytes, or embryos and have, in most cases, demonstrated positive effects on sperm motility, fertilization rates, and embryo development. As one can see, the actions of growth factors are diverse and are an integral component of reproductive processes mediated by their direct and/or indirect actions.

Cytokines are a unique family of growth factors that are secreted primarily by leukocytes as mediators of the humoral and cellular immune system. Cytokines that are secreted from lymphocytes are called lymphokines, many of which are further classified as *interleukins* (ILs). More than 27 ILs have been identified (IL-1 to IL-27). The potential roles of all ILs in the reproductive system or as immune factors that may influence reproductive processes have yet to be elucidated; however, some ILs have been examined extensively with respect to their roles in reproduction. Interleukin-1 (IL-1) may act at the level of the hypothalamus, modulating GnRH neuronal activity that can suppress translation of GnRH mRNA thus reducing GnRH release and gonadotropin levels. Interleukin-6 (IL-6) has been shown to inhibit gonadotropin-stimulated progesterone production in both theca and granulosa cells, suggesting that IL-6 may modulate the actions of gonadotropins on steroidogenesis. Interleukin-10 (IL-10) has been shown to be involved in placental and fetal growth and development, and it may play a role in the parturition process as well. These are only a few examples of the countless findings that have been attributed to the actions of ILs as direct or indirect (positive or negative) mediators of reproductive function.

Another classification of cytokines are the interferons. Interferons are produced by a number of different cell types, including leukocytes, fibroblasts, lymphocytes, and trophoblast cells. *Interferons (INF)* are known for their ability to alter the functions of target cells to protect against viral infections (INF-α, INF-τ, INF-γ). Most notably in reproduction, INF-τ (the τ referring to trophoblast) has been identified as an important factor in maternal recognition of pregnancy in ruminants (Section 9–4.1). Tumer necrosis factor (TNF-α and TNF-β) and colony stimulating factors (CSF) are other cytokines that also appear to play a role in reproduction, most notably in maternal immune activities supporting normal embryonic development.

In addition to growth factors and cytokines, an array of binding proteins also act as mediators of reproductive processes by shuttling hormones around the body or, in some cases, remaining bound to a hormone to prevent it from acting on a target cell. *Alphafetoprotein (α-FP, or AFP)* is an estrogen-binding protein important in the development of the GnRH neurosecretory surge center in the female hypothalamus. In females, α-FP binds estrogens, preventing them from entering the brain of the developing fetus, resulting in the full development of a GnRH surge center. In males, testosterone is able to enter the brain, where it is aromatized to estradiol, which defeminizes the brain, resulting in the absence of a surge center. Other steroid-binding proteins (SBP or sex hormone–binding globulin, SHBG) act as transport mechanisms for steroid hormones to reach their target cells. Since steroid hormones are not water-soluble, they must bind to water-soluble molecules for transport in the blood and interstitial fluids to sites of action on target cells. Androgens and estrogens can affect the amount of SHBG, with high concentrations of testosterone decreasing SHBG synthesis and high concentrations of estrogens stimulating SHBG synthesis. Thus, SHBG synthesis is regulated by the same hormones that these binding proteins will interact with and shuttle to potential sites of steroid hormone action.

4–8   REGULATION OF HORMONAL RECEPTOR SITES

Hormone action is dependent on release of the hormone in question from its gland, transport to the target cells via the circulatory system, and binding of the hormone to cellular receptor sites. After the hormone binds to the cellular receptor site, reactions are initiated within the cell to carry out the physiological response associated with the hormone.

The concentration of receptor sites for a specific hormone in a particular organ are dependent on the endocrine status of the animal. While research in this area is relatively new, and limited mostly to laboratory animals, some information is available on regulation of hormonal receptor sites. It provides a new basis for understanding how certain hormones synergize in regulating a physiological function. Patterns of regulation that can be seen are (1) hormones that regulate their own receptor sites; (2) synergism of two hormones to regulate the receptor sites of one of the hormones; and (3) hormones that regulate receptors of other hormones. *Upregulation* and *down-regulation* are terms that describe whether the number of receptors for a particular hormone is increased (induced) by the regulator or decreased by the regulator.

Up-regulation of FSH receptors is stimulated by FSH with apparent involvement of activin in the process. Up-regulation is speeded as estradiol concentrations increase. Similarly, FSH and activin up-regulate LH receptors on granulosa cells. Luteinizing hormone (LH) down-regulates its own receptors while at the same time inducing (up-regulating) receptors for prolactin. In the developing corpus luteum, prolactin increases receptors for LH and has been reported to prevent LH-induced loss of LH receptors. While this scheme of regulation was determined through research with the rat ovary, many of these principles likely apply to other species. For example, LH will down-regulate its own receptors in the ovary of the ewe.

In the male, injection of FSH will decrease (down-regulate) the number of FSH receptors in the Sertoli cells of the testes. After a transient increase, LH receptors in Leydig cells decrease in response to administration of LH. While prolactin will maintain LH receptor concentration in Leydig cells in rats, it is not clear whether this action occurs through prevention of LH-induced losses, as has been reported in the female, or by more direct up-regulation of LH receptors.

As a regulator of its own receptors in the anterior pituitary, infusion of a high concentration of GnRH will down-regulate GnRH receptors, while low-concentration infusion or intermittent doses will up-regulate GnRH receptors. The intermittent dose more closely parallels the physiological state, since intermittent surges of GnRH and LH occur in males and females. In the female, these intermittent surges are more frequent near the time of estrus, thus making the anterior pituitary more sensitive to GnRH through an increased concentration of GnRH receptors. Estradiol enhances the effect of intermittent surges of GnRH on GnRH receptors, while progesterone or a combination of estradiol and progesterone inhibits this GnRH-induced response. Estrogen receptor concentrations in the anterior pituitary vary directly with the concentration of estrogens in the blood. Estrogen and progesterone receptors are found in the hypothalamus and anterior pituitary. This lends support to the hypothesis that these steroids exert feedback control on both the hypothalamus and the anterior pituitary.

In the uterus, estrogens up-regulate both estrogen and progesterone receptors. Increased binding of estradiol in the myometrium stimulates the appearance of more oxytocin receptors. Progesterone blocks synthesis of new estrogen receptors, resulting in a reduction in their concentration. Through this mechanism, progesterone down-regulates receptors for oxytocin. Thus, estrogens enhance the effects of oxytocin on the myometrium, while progesterone inhibits the oxytocin response.

4–9 INTRACELLULAR MECHANISMS OF HORMONE ACTIONS

The mechanism by which gonadotropins stimulate a particular response from a cell involves a so-called second messenger system. The first messenger is the hormone. When the gonadotropic hormone binds to its membrane-bound receptor, it activates the membrane-bound enzyme, adenylate cyclase (Figure 4–8). The activated enzyme then stimulates the conversion of adenosine triphosphate (ATP) to *cyclic adenosine monophosphate (cAMP)* within the cytoplasm of the cell. Through a series of steps, cAMP (the second messenger) activates the enzymes needed to produce the steroid reproductive hormones. If LH binds to a membrane-bound receptor of a Leydig cell or a thecal cell, activation of the second messenger system will result in the production of testosterone. If LH binds to a membrane-bound receptor of a granulosa cell in the corpus luteum, progesterone will be produced. After stimulating the formation of cAMP within the cell, the fate of the hormone-receptor

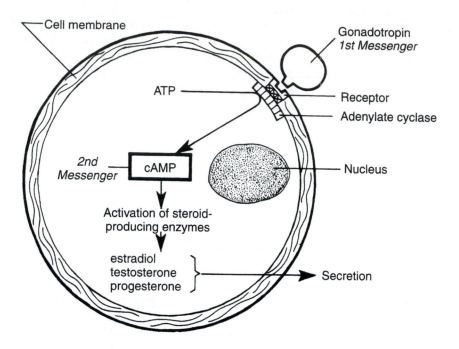

Figure 4–8 Intracellular mechanisms by which gonadotropins stimulate production of reproductive steroids.
a. The gonadotropic hormone (first messenger) binds to the membrane receptor, which
b. activates adenylate cyclase, which
c. converts ATP to cAMP.
d. cAMP (second messenger) stimulates a series of reactions, which activate steroid-producing enzymes, resulting in
e. production of estradiol, progesterone, or testosterone, which is
f. secreted into the bloodstream.

complex has not been determined. There is some evidence that it becomes internalized (taken into the cell), where it is degraded.

The intracellular mechanism of action for steroid reproductive hormones (estradiol, progesterone, and testosterone) does not involve membrane receptors or a second messenger system. Rather, the steroid hormone passes through the cell membrane and binds to a protein receptor in the nucleus of target cells (Figure 4–9). The steroid-receptor complex then initiates synthesis of specific *messenger ribonucleic acid (mRNA)* molecules from *deoxyribonucleic acid (DNA)* in chromosomes. This mRNA is then translocated to the cytoplasm, where synthesis of new proteins occurs. The newly synthesized protein is responsible for the biological activity of a steroid hormone on its target tissues.

A third intracellular mechanism of action has been proposed for GnRH. When GnRH binds to membrane receptors on anterior pituitary cells, it stimulates hydrolysis of phosphoinositides and the conversions of phosphoinositides to diacylglycerols within these cells. These diacylglycerols activate protein kinase C, which subsequently results in release of gonadotropins (LH and FSH).

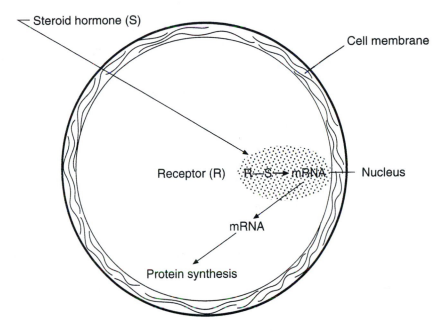

Figure 4–9 Intracellular mechanism by which steroid hormones have their action on target cells.
a. The steroid hormone (S) passes through the cellular membrane and cytoplasm and binds to a protein receptor (R) in the nucleus.
b. The protein-receptor complex stimulates synthesis of mRNA.
c. mRNA translocates to the cytoplasm, where it directs synthesis of specific proteins.
d. The new protein is responsible for the action of the steroid hormone on the target tissue.

4–10   METHODS OF HORMONE DETECTION AND MEASUREMENT

Numerous methods and procedures have been developed for the measurement of hormones (steroids and proteins) in physiological fluids—blood serum or plasma, urine, feces, and saliva. Previous methods of hormone detection primarily used radioisotope tracers to quantify hormone concentrations; however, newer methods have incorporated chemiluminescent or fluorescent means that reduce the requirement for working with radioactivity. Nevertheless, the *radioimmunoassay (RIA)* is still the mainstay for many clinical diagnostic tests and in research and have only recently begun to be replaced by nonradioisotopic *enzyme-immunoassays (EIAs)* and *enzyme-linked immunosorbent assays (ELISAs)*.

4–10.1 *Radioimmunoassays (RIAs)*

Radioimmunoassays harness the specificity of the immune system to permit the measurement of minute (nanogram, 10^{-9} to picogram, 10^{-12}) quantities of hormones. This technology was originally developed in the 1950s by Yalow and Berson for the detection of insulin, from which they collectively won the Nobel Prize for Physiology and Medicine in 1977 for the development of RIAs of peptide hormones. In a typical RIA, the unlabeled (nonradioactive) hormone will compete with the radiolabeled hormone for a limited number of antibody binding sites. Because the unlabeled and labeled hormones have an equal affinity for the antibody binding sites, they bind in direct proportion to the amount of each (labeled and unlabeled) that is present. To quantify the concentrations of a hormone in an unknown sample, the ratio of labeled versus unlabeled binding is compared with a standard curve that was created by measuring the radioactivity in a number of samples ranging from high to low concentrations in which the proportion of labeled and unlabeled bound antibody is known.

A number of radioactive tracers are used for tagging hormones to create the radiolabeled hormones. The most commonly used isotope is ^{125}I, which attaches itself easily to most antibodies and hormones, binding to tyrosine residues on protein hormones. Complexes are now also available that permit steroid hormone assays to be conducted with ^{125}I that were previously only possible for measurement with other types of radioactive isotopes. A gamma counter is used to count the gamma radiation emitted from ^{125}I. ^{125}I has a relatively short half-life of about 60 days, which makes it advantageous to use in the lab, since the quicker decay makes disposal easier, less costly, and less of an environmental or regulatory concern than other types of radioactive materials. Tritium (^3H) has also been used, but to a lesser extent in recent years than ^{125}I. Tritium requires the addition of a liquid scintillation cocktail and a beta counter to measure the beta rays emitted from this isotope. The scintillation cocktail is designed to capture the beta emission and transform it into a photon emission that can be detected via a photomultiplier tube within a beta scintillation counter. The scintillation cocktail acts as a solubilizing agent (emulsifier), keeping a uniform suspension of the sample, and contains a solvent (toluene or xylene) and a fluorescent solute which will emit light depending on the amount of beta emissions. The fact that ^3H has a long half-life of around 12.5 years adds to the costs of storage and disposal and is the primary reason many RIA procedures have been modified to incorporate the use of ^{125}I or have switched to nonisotopic means such as the EIA, which is the nonradioactive equivalent to an RIA, or the ELISA (Section 4–10.2). However, RIAs generally are more sensitive than EIAs or ELISAs for many hormones that require measurement by competitive means using hormone-antibody binding.

Another form of the RIA is the immunoradiometric assay (IRMA), which is also known as a "sandwich" assay. A sandwich assay uses at least two antibodies. The first antibody is a capture antibody in a solid phase, often covalently bonded to a test tube or plate, which binds the hormone and immobilizes it. When the second antibody that is radiolabeled is added, it binds to a different site on the immobilized hormone. The unbound reagents are then washed off and the sample measured. The benefit of this type of assay is that the signal measured is not a proportion of labeled to unlabeled hormone, as in the RIA, which is determined by subtracting the number of gamma counts emitted from the maximum number of counts for a sample that is 100% ^{125}I-labeled hormone; rather, the IRMA measures the actual hormone itself. This improves the sensitivity of detection for hormones that may be present at very low concentrations. A limitation of the IRMA is that it may not work for very small peptide hormones, since two binding sites need to be accessible for the two antibodies to bind.

4–10.2 *Enzyme-Linked Immunosorbent Assay (ELISA)*

The basic principle of an ELISA is to use an enzyme to detect the binding of the hormone to the antibody. The enzyme converts a colorless substrate (chromogen) to a colored product, which then indicates the presence of a hormone-antibody complex or that binding has occurred. Depending on the type of ELISA (competitive or sandwich), results can be read as either positive or negative, based on the presence or absence of a color change. The intensity of the color change is roughly proportional to the amount of hormone in the sample. However, because the color change is dependent on the presence of an enzyme, even small quantities of an enzyme can convert as much substrate as a large quantity of enzyme, if given enough time. Therefore, to quantify ELISA results, samples are usually read at a constant incubation time after the reactions have taken place to prevent significant drift in the color reaction, which could adversely affect the ability to accurately determine hormone concentrations. Current ELISA methods often incorporate a "stop" reaction, which will prevent further enzyme activity, allowing greater flexibility in incubation and measurement times. To quantify the hormone content of an unknown sample based on color intensity from an ELISA, a spectrophotometer is used to read light absorbance at a specific wavelength based on the substrate's color.

4–11 SUMMARY

Most of the hormonal regulation of the reproductive processes is contained in the hypothalamic-anterior pituitary-gonadal axis. Releasing hormones from the hypothalamus control the function of the anterior pituitary. Gonadotropic hormones from the anterior pituitary control the function of the gonads, in the production of both gametes and hormones. In turn, through feedback mechanisms involving the hypothalamus, the steroid hormones and proteins of the gonads regulate the release of gonadotropins. These gonadal steroids also maintain optimum conditions for fertility through their effects on mating behavior and maintenance of the female and male duct systems. While other hormones have important regulatory functions in reproduction, their function is dependent on the reciprocal balance between the gonadotropic and steroid sex hormones. A greater appreciation for and understanding of the intricate balance needed for successful reproduction should evolve as the student progresses in his or her study of reproduction.

SUGGESTED READING

ALEXANDROVA, M. and M. S. SOLOFF. 1980. Oxytocin receptors and parturition. I. Control of oxytocin receptor concentration in the rat myometrium at term. *Endocrinology,* 106:730.

ANDREWS, W. V. and P. M. CONN. 1986. Gonadotropin-releasing hormone stimulates mass changes in phosphoinositides and diacylglycerol accumulation in purified gonadotrope cell cultures. *Endocrinology,* 118:1148.

BARRACLOUGH, C. A., P. M. WISE, J. TURGEON, D. SHANDER, L. DePAULO, and N. RANCE. 1979. Recent studies on the regulation of pituitary LH and FSH secretion. *Biol. Reprod.,* 20:86.

BARTKE, A., A. A. HAFIEZ, F. J. BEX, and S. DALTERIO. 1978. Hormonal interactions in regulation of androgen secretion. *Biol. Reprod.,* 18:44.

CHANNING, C. P., L. D. ANDERSON, D. J. HOOVER, J. KOLENA, K. G. OSTEEN, S. H. POMERANTZ, and T. Y. TANABE. 1982. The role of non-steroidal regulators in control of oocyte and follicular maturation. *Rec. Prog. Hormone Res.,* 38:331.

CHARD, T. 1978. An introduction to radioimmunoassay and related techniques. Laboratory Techniques in Biochemistry and Molecular Biology. T. S. Work and E. Work, eds. North Holland Publishing Co.

CLARK, I. J., K. BURMAN, J. W. FUNDER, and J. K. FINDLAY. 1981. Estrogen receptors in neuroendocrine tissues of the ewe in relation to breed, season, and stage of the estrous cycle. *Biol. Reprod.,* 24:323.

CLAYTON, R. N. 1982. Gonadotropin-releasing hormone modulation of its own pituitary receptors: Evidence for biphasic regulation. *Endocrinology,* 111:152.

ECHTERNKAMP, S. E., H. J. HOWARD, A. J. ROBERTS, J. GRIZZLE, and T. WISE. 1994. Relationships among concentrations of steroids, insulin-like growth factor-I and insulin-like growth factor binding proteins in ovarian follicular fluid of beef cattle. *Biol. Reprod.,* 51:971.

FINDLEY, J. K. 1993. An update on the roles of inhibin, activin and follistatin as local regulators of folliculogenesis. *Biol. Reprod.,* 48:15.

KNICKERBOCKER, J. J., M. C. WILTBANK, and G. D. NISWENDER. 1988. Mechanisms of luteolysis in domestic livestock. *Dom. Anim. Endocrinol.,* 5:91.

KOLIGAN, K. B. and F. STORMSHAK. 1977. Nuclear cytoplasmic estrogen receptors in the ovine endometrium during the estrous cycle. *Endocrinology,* 101:524.

KOTITE, N. J., S. N. NAYFEH, and F. S. FRENCH. 1978. FSH and androgen regulation of Sertoli cell function in the immature rat. *Biol. Reprod.,* 18:65.

LACKEY, B. R., S. L. L. GRAY, and D. M. HENRICKS. 2000. Physiological basis for use of insulin-like growth factors in reproductive applications: A review. *Theriogenology,* 53:1147.

LIEBERMANN, J., D. SCHAMS, and A. MIYAMOTO. 1996. Effects of local growth factors on the secretory function of bovine corpus luteum during oestrous cycle and pregnancy *in vitro. Reprod. Fertil. Develop.,* 8:1003.

MATAMOROS, I. A., N. M. COX, and A. B. MOORE. 1990. Exogenous insulin and additional energy affect follicular distribution, follicular steroid concentrations and granulosa cell human chorionic gonadotropin binding in swine. *Biol. Reprod.,* 43:1.

MOSS, G. E., M. E. CROWDER, and T. M. NETT. 1981. GnRH-Receptor Interaction. VI. Effects of progesterone and estradiol on hypophyseal receptors for GnRH, and serum and hypophyseal concentrations of gonadotropins in ovariectomized ewes. *Biol. Reprod.,* 25:938.

RICHARDS, J. S. 1979. Hormonal control of ovarian follicular development: A 1978 perspective. *Rec. Prog. Hormone Res.,* 35:343.

RIEGER, D., A. M. LUCIANO, S. MODINA, P. POCAR, A. LAURIA, and F. GANDOLFI. 1998. The effects of epidermal growth factor and insulin-like growth factor I on the metabolic activity, nuclear maturation and subsequent development of cattle oocytes in vitro. *J. Reprod. Fertil.,* 112:123.

SCHALLY, A. V. 1978. Aspects of hypothalamic regulation of the pituitary gland. *Science,* 202:18.

SCHAMS, D., B. BERISHA, M. KOSMANN, R. EINSPANIER, and W. M. AMSELGRUBER. 1999. Possible role of growth hormone, IGFs, and IGF-binding protein in the regulation of ovarian function in large farm animals. *Dom. Anim. Endocrinol.,* 17:279.

SCHOMBERG, D. W. 1991. Growth factors and reproduction. Symposium on Growth Factors in Reproduction - Serono Symposia. Springer Verlag.

SCHWABE, C., B. STEINETZ, G. WEISS, A. SEGALOFF, J. K. DONALD, E. O'BYRNE, J. HOCKMAN, B. CARRIERE, and L. GOLDSMITH. 1978. Relaxin. *Rec. Prog. Hormone Res.,* 34:23.

TIJSSEN, P. 1985. *Practice and Theory of Enzyme Immunoassays. Laboratory Techniques in Biochemistry and Molecular Biology.* Vol. 15. Elsevier Science.

TINDALL, D. J., C. R. MENA, and A. R. MEANS. 1978. Hormonal regulation of androgen binding protein in hypophysectomized rats. *Endocrinology,* 103:589.

WHISNANT, C. S. and R. L. GOODMAN. 1988. Effects of an opioid antagonist on pulsatile luteinizing hormone secretion in the ewe vary with changes in steroid negative feedback. *Biol. Reprod.,* 39:1032.

YALOW, R. S. 1983. Radioimmunoassay. *Benchmark Papers in Microbiology.* Vol. 20. Hutchinson Ross Publishing Company.

ZIPF, W. B., A. H. PAYNE, and R. KELCH. 1978. Prolactin, growth hormone and luteinizing hormone in the maintenance of testicular luteinizing hormone. *Endocrinology,* 103:595.

Part 2

Reproductive Processes

The chapters in Part 2 present information that should permit students to develop a basic understanding of the physiological processes and how they are regulated. Chapters follow a logical sequence that guides students through the reproductive processes from puberty through lactation. Some instructors may wish to incorporate information from Parts 4 and 5 into these units. For example, discussion of synchronization of estrus, superovulation, treatment of cystic ovaries, and *in vitro* fertilization will serve to enhance understanding of the basic processes. Some may consider lactation to be inappropriate for a course of reproduction. However, lactation is essential for neonatal survival in all mammalian species and therefore necessary for successful reproduction.

5

The Estrous Cycle

The estrous cycle is defined as the time between periods of estrus. The average length of the estrous cycle is similar for all farm species, albeit shorter for the ewe (Table 5–1). It is about 17 days for the ewe; 21 days for the cow, water buffalo, and doe; 22 days for the mare; and 20 days for the sow. Individual variation is seen in all species. Estrous cycles ranging from 17 to 24 days are considered normal in the cow, 17 to 26 days for the water buffalo, and a range of 19 to 25 days is reported in the mare. While variation among individuals of a particular species is expected, variable cycles for one individual may indicate an abnormality.

5–1 PUBERTY

Puberty in females is defined as the age at the first expressed estrus with ovulation. It should not be considered sexual maturity. If animals are bred at puberty, a high percentage will have difficulty with parturition (Table 23–2). Most breeds of sheep will reach puberty when they are 40% to 50% of their mature weight, but breeding is not recommended until they are about 65% of their mature weight. Dairy cows reach puberty at 35% to 45% of their mature weight, with breeding not recommended until they are about 55% of their mature weight. Puberty occurs when gonadotropins (FSH and LH) are produced at high enough levels to initiate follicle growth, oocyte maturation, and ovulation. Follicle growth can be detected several months before puberty. As puberty approaches, pulsatile discharges of GnRH increase in frequency resulting in more frequent pulses of gonadotropins that provide progressively greater stimulation to the ovaries. Initially, the waves of follicle growth will be followed by atresia. When the frequency and amplitude of these pulses of gonadotropins approach the adult pattern, oocyte maturation and ovulation will occur. The more frequent pulsatile discharge of GnRH at onset of puberty appears to be at least in part due to a decreased sensitivity of the hypothalamus to the negative feedback effects of ovarian steroids which may interact with or be the result of other factors. Endogenous opioids and/or melatonin could be involved in regulation of these changing hormone patterns.

Age at puberty is affected by both genetic and environmental factors, while weight at puberty is affected more dramatically by genetic factors. Genetic factors can be seen by comparing species or breeds within a species. Average age at puberty is 5 to 7 months for sows, 5 to 7 months for does, 6 to 9 months for ewes, 8 to 11 months for European-type dairy cows, 10 to 15 months for European-type beef cows, 17 to 27 months for Zebu-type cows, 15 to 36 months for the water buffalo, and 15 to 24 months for mares. Weight at puberty for breeds within a given

Table 5–1   *Species differences in various characteristics of the estrous cycle*

	Cow	Ewe	Sow	Mare	Goat (Doe)
Estrous cycle (days)	21	17	20	22	21
Metestrus (days)	3–4	2–3	2–3	2–3	2–3
Diestrus (days)	10–14	10–12	11–13	10–12	13–15
Proestrus (days)	3–4	2–3	3–4	2–3	2–3
Estrus	12–18 hrs	24–36 hrs	48–72 hrs	4–8 days	30–40 hrs
Ovulation	10–12 hrs after estrus	late estrus	midestrus	1–2 days before estrus ends	few hrs after estrus

Table 5–2   *Species and breed differences in age and weight at puberty*

	Age (Months)	Weight (kg)
Doe	5–7	10–30
Sow	5–7	68–90
Ewe	7–10	27–34
Mare	15–24	Varies with mature size of breed
Dairy cow	8–13	160–270
Jersey	8	160
Guernsey	11	200
Holstein	11	270
Ayrshire	13	240
Beef cow (European breeds)	10–15	———
Zebu	17–27	———
Water buffalo	15–36	———

species depends on the mature size of the breed in question (Table 5–2). Jerseys reach puberty at about 8 months and 160 kg, while for Holsteins 11 months and 270 kg is the average.

A number of environmental factors have a pronounced effect on age at puberty. In general, any factor that slows growth rate, thus preventing expression of full genetic potential, will delay puberty. In an experiment, Holstein heifers on a recommended plane of nutrition reached puberty at about 11 months of age, but if raised from birth on 62% of the recommended level of energy, were over 20 months of age at puberty (Table 23–2). High environmental temperature delays puberty. For example, beef heifers, reared at 10°C, reached puberty at 10.5 months of age, while similar heifers reared at 27°C were over 13 months of age at puberty. Gilts farrowed in the late spring reached puberty at a later age than gilts farrowed in other seasons because growth before puberty was slowed by hot summer temperatures. Age at puberty in sheep and goats is affected by month of birth because it affects their age at the onset of their breeding season. For example, ewes born in January will be older at puberty than those born in March. Other environmental factors that delay puberty include poor health and poor sanitation in rearing facilities. The wide range in age at puberty that has been reported for Zebu cattle and water buffalo is probably largely due to the range in environmental factors under which they are raised, particularly nutrition and climate. While adverse environments delay puberty and reduce the mature size of animals, weight at puberty is not greatly affected. In the study with Holstein heifers, those on a low plane of nutrition were 84% older but only 7% smaller at puberty than well-fed heifers. Feeding above recommended levels resulted in earlier puberty. Holstein heifers fed at 146% of the recommended level reached puberty at an average of 9.2 months of age as compared to 11 months for controls receiving the recommended diet. Both problems associated with overconditioning and extra cost of such a diet make overfeeding undesirable. Also to be considered with the environmental factors affecting age at puberty is the effect of introduction of a reproductively active male to a group of prepubertal females. In several species, including pigs and sheep, this has induced early puberty, with more effect being seen when done a few weeks before expected onset of puberty. In one study, when mature boars were introduced to gilts at 150 days of age, puberty occurred 32 days later. In another study, mature boars introduced to gilts at 165 days of age resulted in puberty 7 days later.

5–2 PERIODS OF THE ESTROUS CYCLE

The periods of the estrous cycle are *estrus, metestrus, diestrus,* and *proestrus* (Table 5–3), which are often described in terms of the *Follicular Phase* (proestrus and estrus) and the *Luteal Phase* (metestrus and diestrus). These periods occur in a cyclic and sequential manner, except for periods of *anestrus* (absence of cycling) in seasonal breeders such as the ewe, doe, and mare, as well as anestrus during pregnancy and the early postpartum period for all species.

5–2.1 *Estrus*

Estrus is defined as the period of time when the female is receptive to the male and will stand for mating. (See Section 7–2 for expanded discussion.) The length of the period of estrus varies among species (Table 5–1). Estrus lasts for 12 to 18 hours in the cow. As in the estrous cycle, considerable variation is seen between individuals. Also, cows in hot environments have shorter periods of estrus (10 to 12 hours) than the average 18-hour period for cows in cool climates. Estrus lasts for 5 to 27 hours (average 20 hours) in the water buffalo, 24 to 36 hours in the ewe, 30 to 40 hours in the doe, 40 to 72 hours in the sow, and 4 to 8 days in the mare. The mare is the most variable of the farm species, with reported estrus ranging from 2 to 12 days. Ovulation is associated with estrus, occurring 10 to 12 hours after the end of estrus in the cow, 14 hours after the end of estrus in the water buffalo, a few hours after the end in the doe, middle to late estrus in the ewe, about midestrus in the sow, and 1 to 2 days before the end of estrus in the mare. The day of estrus in the cow (first day of estrus for other species) is usually designated either as day 0 or day 1 of the cycle, depending on individual preference.

Table 5–3 *Primary characteristics of the periods of the estrous cycle in the cow*

Period	Day(s)	Principal features
Estrus	1	Behavioral signs of estrus
Metestrus	2–4	Ovulation
		Corpus luteum formation
Diestrus	5–16	Corpus luteum function
Proestrus	17–21	Rapid follicle growth

5–2.2 *Metestrus*

The period of metestrus begins with the cessation of estrus and lasts for about 3 days. Primarily, it is a period of formation of the corpus luteum (corpora lutea with multiple ovulation). However, ovulation occurs during this period in cows, water buffalo, and does. Also, a phenomenon known as metestrous bleeding occurs in cows, appearing in about 90% of all metestrous periods in heifers and 45% in mature cows. During late proestrus and estrus, high estrogen concentrations increase the vascularity of the endometrium, this vascularity reaching its peak about 1 day after the end of estrus. With declining estrogen levels, some breakage of capillaries may occur, resulting in a small loss of blood. This will be noticed as a patch of blood on the tail approximately 35 to 45 hours after the end of estrus. It is not an indication of conception or of a failure to conceive. Also, it should not be confused with menstrual bleeding, which occurs in humans.

5–2.3 *Diestrus*

Diestrus is characterized as the period in the cycle when the corpus luteum is fully functional. In the cow, it starts about day 5 of the cycle, when an increase in blood concentration of progesterone can first be detected, and ends with regression of the corpus luteum on day 16 or 17. For the sow and ewe, it extends from about day 4 through day 13, 14, or 15. Mares are more variable because of the irregular length of estrus. For mares ovulating on day 5, diestrus will extend from approximately day 8 through day 19 or 20. It has been called the period of preparation of the uterus for pregnancy.

5–2.4 *Proestrus*

Proestrus begins with the regression of the corpus luteum and drop in progesterone and extends to the start of estrus. The principal distinguishing feature of proestrus is the occurrence of rapid follicle growth. Late during this period, the effects of estrogen on the duct system and behavioral symptoms of approaching estrus can be observed.

5–3   HORMONAL CONTROL OF THE ESTROUS CYCLE

Regulation of the estrous cycle involves a reciprocal interaction between reproductive hormones of the hypothalamus, anterior pituitary, and ovaries (Figure 4–5). An interaction between the uterus and ovaries is also important, in that $PGF_{2\alpha}$ from the uterus is the natural luteolysin that causes regression of the corpus luteum and cessation of progesterone production (Section 2–7). Removal of the uterus during diestrus will greatly prolong the life of the corpus luteum and lengthen the estrous cycle.

Concentrations of gonadotropins and ovarian steroids have been monitored for a number of species through the estrous cycle (Figures 5–1, 5–2, 5–3, 5–4). Similarities are more marked than differences when these species are compared. Progesterone concentrations are high during diestrus, with its drop signaling the start of proestrus. Small increases in FSH, LH, and estradiol during proestrus are followed by dramatic surges in these hormones near the start of estrus. Small surges of FSH and estradiol are seen again in metestrus and in mid-diestrus. A surge in prolactin occurs in late estrus. With a knowledge of the circulating concentrations of these hormones during the estrous cycle along with an understanding of the mechanisms of their release, how their receptors are regulated, and their physiological actions, a reasonably logical sequence for hormonal regulation of the estrous cycle can be set forth.

Progesterone has a dominant role in regulating the estrous cycle. During diestrus with the corpus luteum functional, high concentrations of progesterone inhibit release of FSH

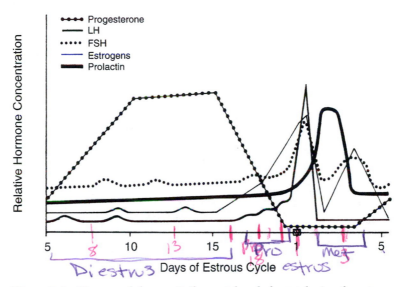

Figure 5–1 Hormonal changes in the peripheral plasma during the estrous cycle of the cow. The drop in progesterone on day 16, 17, or 18 is followed by surges in estrogens during late proestrus, FSH and LH during estrus, and prolactin during late estrus and early metestrus. (Based on literature.)

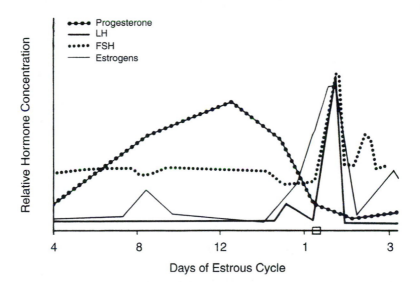

Figure 5–2 Hormonal changes in the peripheral plasma during the estrous cycle of the ewe. Patterns for the ewe are similar to those for other species. A reduction in FSH during proestrus is followed by a spike during estrus and another surge during metestrus. (Based on literature.)

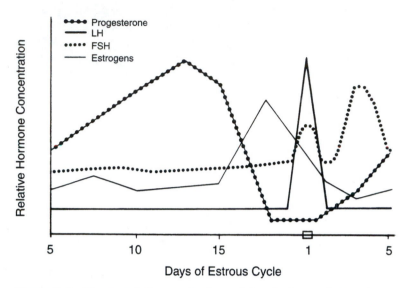

Figure 5–3 Hormonal changes in the peripheral plasma during the estrous cycle in the sow. Notable is the marked increase in FSH during metestrus. (Based on literature.)

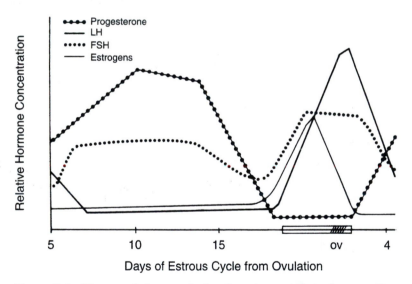

Figure 5–4 Hormonal changes during the estrous cycle in the mare. Patterns are similar to those of other species except that surges of FSH and LH during estrus last for several days. (Based on literature.)

and LH through its negative feedback control of the hypothalamus and anterior pituitary; progesterone also inhibits behavioral estrus. Likewise, during pregnancy, high concentrations of progesterone inhibit release of gonadotropic hormones as well as behavioral estrus. Small episodic increases in LH that occur during diestrus may be a factor in maintaining the function of the corpus luteum. If females do not become pregnant during the preceding estrus, $PGF_{2\alpha}$ will be released from the uterus and transported to the ovary by direct, countercurrent circulation through the utero-ovarian vein to the ovarian artery (Figure 2–12). From 10 to 14 days after formation of the corpus luteum, $PGF_{2\alpha}$ will induce regression.

The drop in progesterone removes the hypothalamus from its negative feedback inhibition. With removal of this inhibition, pulses of GnRH, FSH, and LH are released with increasing frequency and amplitude. Increased release of FSH stimulates rapid follicle growth and increased secretion of estradiol. The dominant follicle at the time of luteal regression is the follicle that is destined to ovulate. The sensitivity of the anterior pituitary to GnRH will increase through up-regulation of the GnRH receptors by the more frequent pulses of GnRH. Likewise, the increasing concentrations of FSH and estradiol will up-regulate ovarian receptors for FSH and LH. The magnitude of the increased release of FSH and LH may not be reflected in circulating blood, due to increased binding of these hormones to receptors in granulosa and thecal cells of the follicle.

Two to three days after the drop in progesterone, estradiol reaches the threshold concentration that stimulates (through a positive feedback control on the hypothalamus) the large, preovulatory surge of GnRH, FSH, and LH. The preovulatory surge of FSH stimulates more rapid growth of the follicle and greater secretion of estradiol. This high concentration of estradiol is necessary for the female to exhibit behavioral signs of estrus (Section 7–2). Release of inhibin likely modulates the release of FSH during estrus, thereby preventing overstimulation of the ovaries. Inhibin's effect on FSH may also be a factor in the atresia of follicles that are in a growing stage but do not reach the maturity necessary for ovulation. The preovulatory surge of LH stimulates final maturation of the oocyte and ovulation. The preovulatory surge of LH occurs during early estrus and lasts for 6 to 10 hours in most species. However, the mare differs in that the surge may last for several days. Ovulation follows the preovulatory LH surge by about 24 to 30 hours in cows and ewes, 30 to 36 hours in does, and 40 to 45 hours in sows.

Following ovulation a corpus luteum will form at each ovulation site. Formation occurs rapidly, and 2 to 4 days after ovulation a detectable increase in progesterone will again indicate diestrus. The dominant factor controlling formation and function of the corpus luteum is LH (a luteotropin). However, LH synergizes with other hormones in carrying out its luteotropic function. Synergism of FSH and estradiol helps up-regulated LH receptors on the granulosa cells. The surge in prolactin in late estrus helps maintain these LH receptors of granulosa cells and at ovulation initiates reactions within these cells that result in luteinization (transformation to corpus luteum cells) and production of progesterone. The likely mechanism by which LH maintains function of the corpus luteum is by increasing blood flow through this luteal structure. Conversely, $PGF_{2\alpha}$ has been reported to decrease blood flow through the corpus luteum, a possible factor in regression of the corpus luteum.

The moderate surges of FSH and estradiol that occur during metestrus and again in mid-diestrus may be factors in the selection and growth of the follicle or follicles that will ovulate during the next estrus. Also, these surges, along with the episodic surges of LH seen during diestrus, could be factors in maintenance of the function of the corpus luteum.

5–4 FOLLICULAR DYNAMICS

Ovarian follicular development in cows and ewes is a progressive and recurring process, with two to three waves of follicular growth occurring each cycle. In cows, two waves appear to be more common but three waves are frequent in long cycles and are more frequent

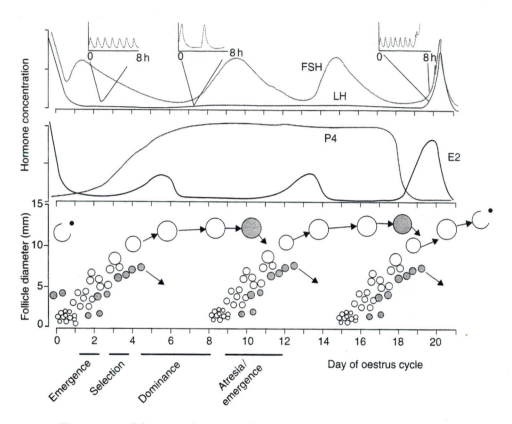

Figure 5–5 Schematic depiction of the pattern of secretion of follicle-stimulating hormone (FSH), luteinizing hormone (LH), progesterone (P4), and oestradiol (E2), and the pattern of growth of ovarian follicles during the oestrous cycle in cattle. Each wave of follicular growth is preceded by a transient rise in FSH concentrations. Healthy growing follicles are shown as open circles; atretic follicles are shaded. A surge in LH and FSH concentrations occurs at the onset of oestrus and induces ovulation. The pattern of secretion of LH pulses during an 8-hour (h) window early in the luteal phase (high frequency, low amplitude), the midluteal phase (low frequency, low amplitude), and the follicular phase (high frequency, building to the surge) is indicated in the inserts in the top panel. *Source:* Reprinted from *Encyclopedia of Dairy Sciences*, 4, Crowe, M. A., Characteristics, p. 2153, 2002, with permission from Elsevier Science.

in heifers. Patterns of follicular growth in cattle have been well characterized with the aid of transrectal ultrasonography for monitoring follicular populations during the estrous cycle. At the beginning of a follicular wave, a cohort (i.e., group) of follicles emerges and begins to develop. *Emergence* of these follicles, from which a dominant follicle of the wave will eventually develop, is also referred to as *recruitment*. The relationship between follicular emergence and the growth of follicles relative to pituitary gonadotropin and ovarian steroid hormone production is depicted in Figure 5–5 for a heifer with three fol-

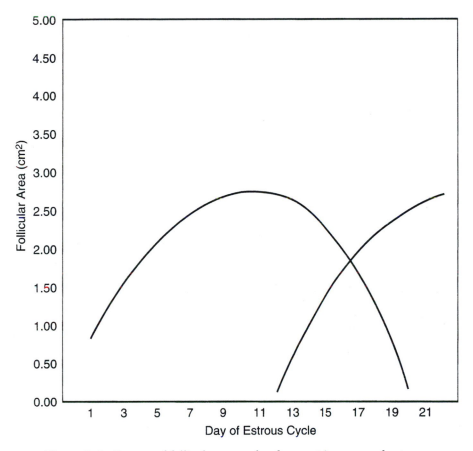

Figure 5–6 Pattern of follicular wave development in a normal estrous cycle of a cow with a two-wave cycle.

licular waves. As follicles grow to medium size (5 mm to 9 mm in diameter), a single follicle, or multiple follicles in litter-bearing species, from the pool of medium-sized follicles will be selected to become dominant. Thus, *selection* may involve one follicle or many follicles, depending on the inherent species-dependent ovulation rate. As the dominant follicle or follicles grow, they suppress the development of smaller follicles, which will eventually undergo atresia (Section 2–1). The inhibitory effects that lead to follicular atresia are due, in part, to the production of inhibin by the dominant follicle, which reduces FSH secretion. The dominant follicle has a larger, more highly developed blood supply and therefore is able to acquire gonadotropins at a sufficient level for continued growth even as FSH concentrations decline. In the last wave of the cycle, the dominant follicle is the ovulatory follicle. Two ovulatory follicles are common in ewes. For cows with a two-wave cycle (Figure 5–6), the anovulatory wave starts in early metestrus, peaks in mid-diestrus, and then regresses as atresia of the dominant follicle occurs. The ovulatory wave begins shortly after the start of regression of the first wave and will surpass the area of the regressing anovulatory wave by the end of diestrus. The area of the ovulatory wave peaks at estrus and is terminated by ovulation.

Although the first wave is anovulatory in normal cycles, the dominant follicle of this wave will become ovulatory after injection of $PGF_{2\alpha}$ in early diestrus, as in synchronization of estrus. Procedures recommended for superovulation (Section 18–2.1) result in first-wave ovulation, also. Injection of FSH in this procedure promotes growth of several follicles that would normally become subordinate and atretic. The result is a number of ovulatory follicles, rather than the one dominant follicle.

In sows, ovulatory size (8 mm to 11 mm) follicles develop only during the follicular phase after luteal regression. Prior to luteal regression, the number of small antral follicles will increase but seldom grow beyond 5 mm in diameter until after luteal regression.

5–5   SEASONAL BREEDERS

Most wild species have a breeding season that is initiated at a time when the environment will allow for the best survival of the young at their birth. These patterns have developed through natural selection over many generations. Patterns of seasonal breeding range from species that have one period of estrus each year (monoestrus) to species that have a series of estrous cycles limited to a portion of the year (seasonally polyestrus). All domesticated animals probably exhibited seasonal breeding tendencies before domestication. This has been changed by providing better environments (housing and nutrition) and by selecting for more prolific animals. Seasonal changes in fertility in cattle and swine can be related to adverse environmental conditions that are present in some years but not in others. Water buffalo are polyestrus but frequently show seasonal patterns due to limitations in feedstuffs or hot, humid climatic conditions. True seasonal breeding patterns are inherent in ewes, does, and mares.

5–5.1 *Sheep and Goats*

Most breeds of sheep and goats exhibit seasonal breeding patterns. Sheep and goats native to the tropics are an exception and cycle throughout the year. While breed differences are apparent, there is a tendency for sheep and goats native to arctic regions to have shorter, more intense seasons than those found in temperate regions.

Sheep are short-day or fall breeders (Figure 5–7). Their breeding season is initiated as the ratio of daylight to darkness decreases and ends when increasing day lengths reach a ratio of nearly equal daylight and darkness. For most breeds, the season falls between the autumnal equinox and spring equinox. However, Dorset Horn, Merino, and Rambouillet breeds have extended breeding seasons, with some individuals being polyestrus if environmental conditions (nutrition and climate) are favorable. Quiet ovulations (ovulation without behavioral estrus) occur more frequently at the beginning and at the end of the breeding season. Introduction of rams into the flock during the transition from anestrus to estrus (late summer to early fall) will result in a high degree of synchrony in first mating, with estrus peaking 15 to 20 days after introduction of the male.

As with sheep, goats are short-day breeders with cyclic activity occurring between late June and early April. Peak breeding activity usually falls between September and Jan-

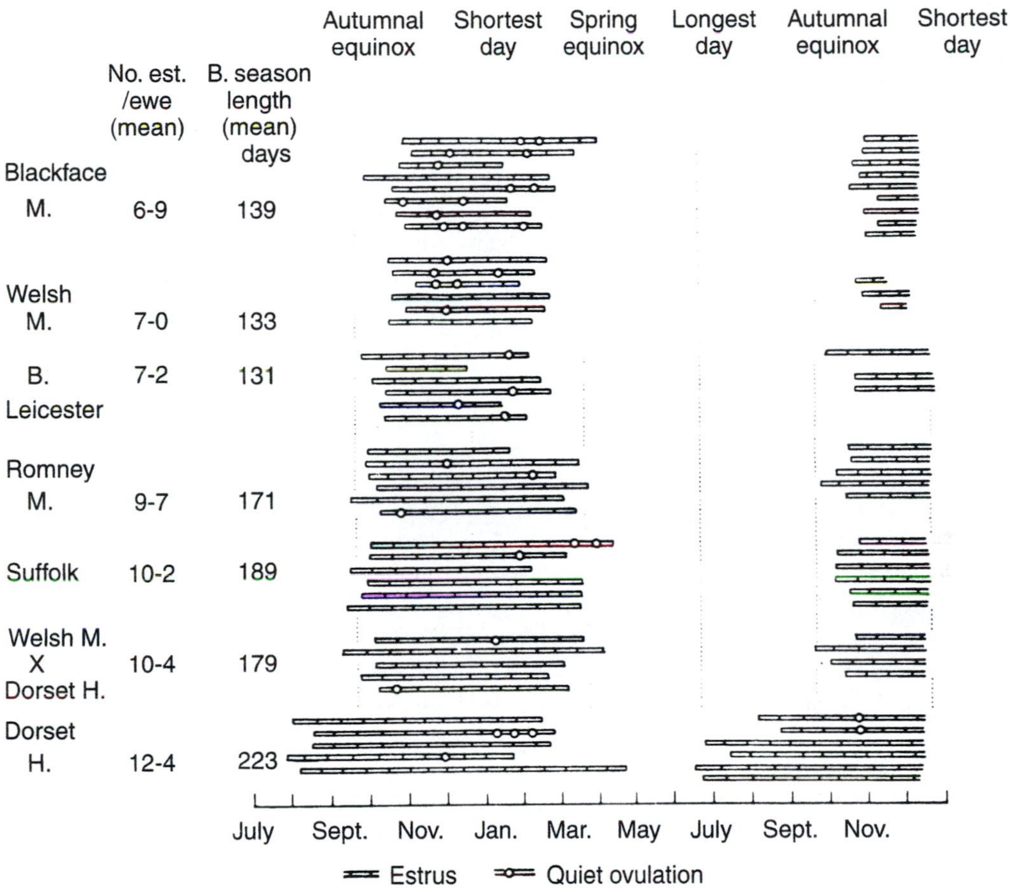

Figure 5–7 Breed differences in the duration of the breeding seasons in adult ewes in Great Britain. (Hafez. *J. Agric. Sci.,* 42:305. 1952.)

uary. Placement of bucks with does just before the start of the breeding season will stimulate estrus and result in good synchrony, with first estrus occurring as early as 5 to 10 days after introduction of males. Good response from introduction of bucks has been obtained in both lactating and nonlactating does.

Both rams and bucks are affected by photoperiod, showing highest breeding activity and fertility in the fall. Reduced sperm production, more abnormal spermatozoa, and lower fertility are characteristic of both species as photoperiod lengthens (spring and early summer). Deterioration in semen quality is more pronounced if these males are subjected to heat stress during the summer. Whereas rams will continue some sexual activity during the spring and summer, bucks become sexually inactive during this period.

The day length pattern has a dominant controlling influence on initiation and termination of breeding season. If sheep or goats are shipped from the Northern Hemisphere to the Southern Hemisphere, the breeding season will reverse. A similar reversal can be achieved by controlled artificial lighting in a room that excludes all natural light. An alternating regimen of 8 hours of light and 16 hours of darkness will induce reproductive activity during the anestrous season if it is preceded by several weeks of long photoperiod to resensitize the system. For high fertility, both sexes must be placed under the artificial light regimen. Altering the temperature in environmental control chambers does not influence estrous activity in ewes and does unless light patterns are altered also. However, high ambient temperature will lower semen quality of rams and bucks and lower fertility in ewes and does, even when they are on a short light regimen.

5–5.2 *Horses*

Mares are long-day breeders. Their season is initiated as the ratio of daylight to darkness increases and ends during decreasing day lengths. The average season for ponies is May to October but is longer in horses, extending from February to November. Peak fertility is obtained if mares are bred between May and July. Behavioral estrus occurring during short-day months (January to April) is frequently not accompanied by ovulation. Much variation in the length of the breeding season is seen in individual mares and among mares. As in the ewe, the day length pattern has the dominant controlling influence on the mare's breeding season. Following a period of short days, increased photoperiod via artificial lighting will stimulate increased reproductive capacity during the early part of the breeding season in mares. An alternating sequence of 16 hours of light and 8 hours of dark will bring mares out of anestrus.

The seasonal breeding pattern is not as well defined for the stallion. Fertile semen can be collected throughout the year. However, declines in sexual activity and semen production occur in months with short photoperiod.

5–5.3 *Photoperiod Action*

The role of photoperiod in regulation of seasonal breeding activities is well established. As breeding season approaches, there is an increase in the frequency and amplitude of episodic surges of LH. Pinealectomy has reduced the effect of changing photoperiod on LH release in rams. Also, denervation of the pineal gland has delayed onset of breeding season in mares. The retina of the eye is the photic sensor with these signals transmitted by way of the retinohypothalamic tract to the suprachiasmatic nuclei (Section 4–2.3; Figure 4–4). Diurnal signals generated by these suprachiasmatic nuclei are transmitted to the superior cervical ganglia and then to the pineal gland via sympathetic nerves.

During darkness, the sympathetic activity increases, resulting in greater activation of an enzyme needed for synthesis of melatonin. The pineal gland through the synthesis and release of melatonin serves as a mediator between the neural signals induced by changing photoperiod and the endocrine system that regulates cyclic reproductive activity. Through either direct or indirect action on the hypothalamus, melatonin modulates seasonal breeding activity in short-day and long-day breeders in concert with numerous exogenous (environmental) and endogenous (hormonal/metabolic) cues (Figure 5–8).

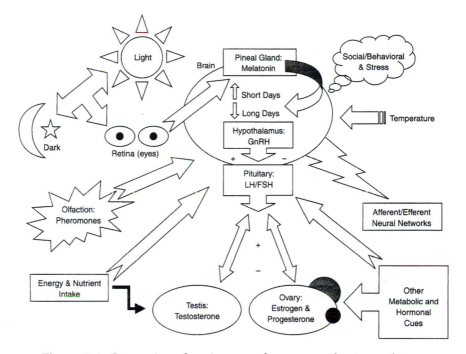

Figure 5–8 Integration of environmental cues on endocrine and neuroendocrine pathways regulating seasonal reproduction. A multitude of exogenous (environmental) factors and endogenous (hormonal and metabolic) cues coordinate the seasonal reproductive cycle in short- (e.g., sheep) and long- (e.g., horse) day breeders. Central to seasonal regulation is the role of photoperiod (light:dark cycles), which changes annually. Photic cues are relayed via the retino-hypothalamo-pituitary pathway using melatonin as a primary regulator of GnRH and LH/FSH release, either directly or indirectly, by mediating changes in the sensitivity of the hypothalamus and pituitary to the negative feedback effects of gonadal steroids. It has been said that seasonal breeders undergo an annual puberty, with spermatogenesis and estrous cycles beginning anew each breeding season as they make the transition from sexual inactivity into periods of reproductive competence and back again. While strictly seasonal breeders are driven principally by photoperiodic cues, other species may exhibit seasonal cycles directed by a variety of climatic, nutritional, metabolic, and/or behavioral indicators. GnRH = gonadotropin-releasing hormone; LH = luteinizing hormone; FSH = follicle stimulating hormone *Source:* Reprinted from *Encyclopedia of Dairy Sciences*, 4, Willard, S. T., Seasonal Breeders, p. 2166, 2002, with permission from Elsevier Science.

SUGGESTED READING

BARRELL, G. K. and K. R. LAPWOOD. 1979. Effects of pinealectomy on the secretion of LH, testosterone, and prolactin in rams exposed to various light regimes. *J. Endocrinol.*, 80:397.

CROWE, M. A. 2002. Characteristics. *Encyclopedia of Dairy Science.* eds. H. Roginski, J. W. Fuquay, and P. F. Fox. Academic Press, an Imprint of Elsevier Science.

DAELS, P. F., J. P. HUGHES, and G. H. STABENFELDT. 1991. Reproduction in horses. *Reproduction in Domestic Animals.* (4th ed.) ed. P. T. Cupps. Academic Press.

DZIUK, P. J. 1991. Reproduction in pigs. *Reproduction in Domestic Animals.* (4th ed.) ed. P.T. Cupps. Academic Press.

FORTUNE, J. E., J. SIROIS, and S. M. QUIRK. 1988. The growth and differentiation of ovarian follicles during the bovine estrous cycle. *Theriogenology,* 29:95.

GARVERICK, H. A., R. E. ERB, G. D. NISWENDER, and C. J. CALLAHAN. 1971. Reproductive steroids in the bovine. III. Changes during the estrous cycle. *J. Anim. Sci.,* 32:946.

GINTHER, O. J. 1979. Reproductive seasonality in mares. *Beltsville Symposia in Agricultural Research. 3. Animal Reproduction.* ed. H.W. Hawk. Allanheld, Osmun and Co. Publishers; Halsted Press, a division of Wiley & Sons.

GINTHER, O. J., L. KNOPF, and J. P. KASTELIC. 1989. Temporal association among ovarian events in cattle during estrous cycles with two and three follicular waves. *J. Reprod. Fertil.,* 87:223.

HANSEL, W. and E. M. CONVEY. 1983. Physiology of the estrous cycle. *J. Anim. Sci.,* 57(Suppl. 2):404.

HURNIK, J. F., G. J. KING, and H. A. ROBERTSON. 1975. Estrus and related behavior in postpartum Holstein cows. *Applied Animal Ethology,* 2:55.

L'HERMITE, M., G. D. NISWENDER, L. E. REICHERT, JR., and A. R. MIDGLEY, JR. 1972. Serum follicle-stimulating hormone as measured by radioimmunoassay. *Biol. Reprod.,* 6:325.

LINDSAY, D. R. 1991. Reproduction in sheep and goats. *Reproduction in Domestic Animals.* (4th ed.) ed. P.T. Cupps. Academic Press.

REITER, R. J. 1974. Circannual reproductive rhythms in mammals related to photoperiod and pineal function. *Chronobiologica,* 1:365.

SCHAMS, D., E. SCHALLENBERGER, B. HOFFMAN, and H. KARG. 1977. The oestrus cycle of the cow: Hormonal parameters and time relationships concerning oestrus, ovulation, and electrical resistance of the vaginal mucus. *Acta Endocrinol.,* 86:180.

SHELTON, M. 1978. Reproduction and breeding of goats. *J. Dairy Sci.,* 61:994.

WILLARD, S. T. 2002. Oestrous cycles—seasonal breeders. *Encyclopedia of Dairy Science.* eds. H. Roginski, J. W. Fuquay, and P. F. Fox. Academic Press, an imprint of Elsevier Science.

6

Spermatogenesis and Maturation of Spermatozoa

Spermatogenesis is the process by which spermatozoa are formed. This process occurs in the seminiferous tubules (Chapter 3). Output of spermatozoa per day has been reported to be 6 to 8 billion for bulls, 8 to 12 billion for rams, 5 billion for stallions, and 15 to 20 billion for boars. Actual production of spermatozoa may be 50% to 100% higher, because all that are produced cannot be collected. After formation in the seminiferous tubules, spermatozoa will be forced through the rete testis and vasa efferentia into the epididymis, where they are stored while undergoing maturation changes that make them capable of fertilization. After puberty, spermatogenesis will proceed as a continuous process throughout the life of the male. Seasonal changes in spermatozoa production may occur due to ambient temperature in all species (Section 22–1.1) and due to photoperiod in rams and bucks. Reciprocal action of FSH, LH, and testosterone is necessary for the maintenance of spermatogenesis (Section 6–2.5).

6–1 PUBERTY

In the male, puberty can be defined less succinctly than in the female. If defined as the time when fertile spermatozoa are in the ejaculate, the age will be 10 to 12 months for bulls (cattle), 3 to 5 months for bucks, 4 to 6 months for rams, 4 to 8 months for boars, 13 to 18 months for stallions, and 24 to 30 months for water buffalo bulls. However, spermatozoa are formed in the seminiferous tubules several weeks before they are seen in the ejaculate. In bulls, the time from appearance in the seminiferous tubules to appearance in the ejaculate is approximately 10 weeks.

A number of other changes can be seen in males, starting several weeks before fertile spermatozoa are in the ejaculate (Figure 6–1). These include changes in body conformation, increased aggressiveness and sexual desire, rapid growth of the penis and testes, and separation of the penis from the prepuce so that extension of the penis is possible. Timing of these events varies with species.

Development of testicular function is essential to the changes observed as puberty approaches. This development is regulated by the endocrine system. Several months before onset of puberty, pulsatile discharges of LH commence, resulting in differentiation of Leydig cells. FSH may synergize in this action by helping up-regulate receptors for LH on Leydig cells. In male rodents, prolactin helps maintain (prevents down-regulation of) receptors

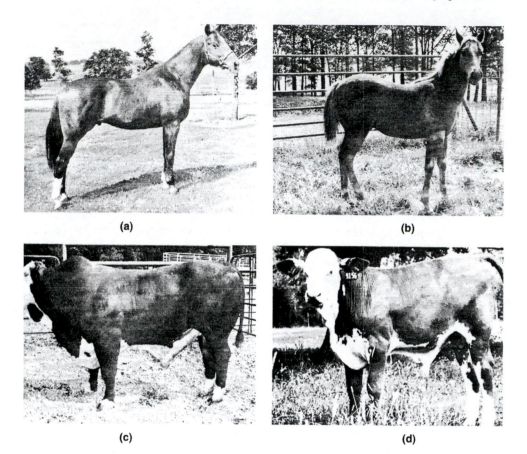

Figure 6–1   Secondary sex characteristics that develop following puberty.
(*a*) Mature stallion. Note heavy shoulders and thick neck; (*b*) 6-month-old
son of stallion; (*c*) mature beefmaster bull. Note crest, heavy front quarters,
and well-developed dewlap; (*d*) 6-month-old son of bull.

for LH. The differentiating Leydig cell initially secretes the androgen, androstenedione. As differentiation continues, LH stimulates increasing concentration of testosterone, which in turn stimulates most other changes associated with approaching puberty (see Chapter 4 for functions of testosterone). Synergistic effects from testosterone and FSH stimulate development of Sertoli cells, production of androgen-binding protein, and preparation of the seminiferous tubules for production of spermatozoa.

As with the female, puberty is not sexual maturity in the male. Some rams and boars are used for breeding and are highly fertile after about 6 months of age. However, the testes size and total production of spermatozoa increase until about 18 months of age. In bulls and stallions, total production of spermatozoa will increase at least to 3 years of age. It is recommended that stallions not be used heavily until they are 3 to 4 years old. There is a high correlation between the size of the testes and total spermatozoa production.

All factors that affect age at puberty in females will affect age at puberty in males (Chapter 5). Genetic effects on puberty are seen by comparing species or breeds within a species. Any adverse environmental factor which slows growth rate will delay puberty. For example, male lambs on a low plane of nutrition may not reach puberty until after 12 months of age.

6–2 THE PROCESS OF SPERMATOGENESIS

As stated in Chapter 3, there are two types of cells in the seminiferous tubules. These are germ cells that progress from spermatogonia to spermatozoa and Sertoli cells that are somatic cells and play a supporting role during spermatogenesis. Sertoli cells, which extend from the basement membrane to the lumen, envelop the germ cells and remain in contact until spermatozoa are released into the lumen (Figure 6–2). Sertoli cells form basal compartments (in conjunction with the basement membrane) and adluminal compartments where spermatogenesis is completed. As spermatogenesis proceeds, the developing gametes migrate toward the lumen. Between the basal and adluminal compartments, adjacent Sertoli cells form a tight junction that serves as a blood-testis barrier, therefore controlling the environment within the tubule by regulating the movement of constituents from blood into the seminferous tubules.

Spermatogenesis can be divided into three phases (Figure 6–3). The first is *spermatocytogenesis,* a series of *mitotic* divisions during which spermatogonia form primary spermatocytes. The second phase is *meiosis,* when the primary spermatocytes undergo reduction division, forming rounded spermatids with haploid nuclei. The third is *spermiogenesis,* a phase when spermatids undergo a metamorphosis, forming spermatozoa. The entire process will be completed in 46 to 49 days in rams. Time estimates are shorter for the boar (36 to 40 days) and longer for stallions (55 to 59 days) and bulls (56 to 63 days). The time needed for complete spermatogenesis is fairly equally divided among the three phases.

6–2.1 *Spermatocytogenesis*

After migrating to the embryonic testes, primordial germ cells will undergo a number of mitotic divisions before forming gonocytes. Before puberty, gonocytes will differentiate into A_0 spermatogonia, the stem cells from which all other spermatogonia arise. A_0, A_1, and A_2 spermatogonia are located in the basal compartment along the basement membrane of the seminiferous tubules. The A_2 spermatogonium will divide, forming a dormant (A_1) spermatogonium and an active (A_3) spermatogonium (Figure 6–3), which migrate through the tight junction into the adluminal compartment, starting a new generation of developing germ cells. The active spermatogonium will undergo four mitotic divisions in bulls and rams, eventually forming 16 *primary spermatocytes.* In rams, these mitotic divisions are completed in 15 to 17 days.

6–2.2 *Meiosis*

Meiosis is a two-step process. Each primary spermatocyte will undergo a meiotic division, forming two secondary spermatocytes. With this division, the chromosome complement in the nucleus is reduced by half so that nuclei in secondary spermatocytes contain unpaired

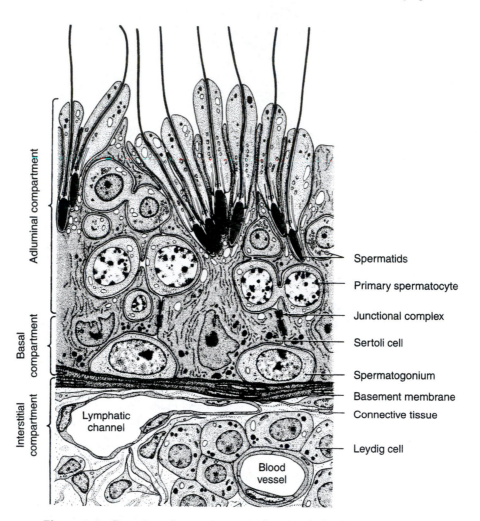

Figure 6–2   Drawing of part of a seminiferous tubule showing the relationship of the germ cells to the adjacent Sertoli cells. Formation of spermatozoa starts near the basement membrane when a spermatogonium divides to form other spermatogonia and ultimately primary spermatocytes. The primary spermatocytes are moved from the basal compartment through the junctional complexes between adjacent Sertoli cells into the adluminal compartment, where they eventually divide to form secondary spermatocytes (not shown) and spherical spermatids. The spermatogonia, primary spermatocytes, secondary spermatocytes, and spherical spermatids all develop in the space between two or more Sertoli cells and are in contact with them. During elongation of the spermatid nucleus, the spermatids are repositioned by the Sertoli cells to become inbedded within long pockets in the cytoplasm of an individual Sertoli cell. When released as a spermatozoon, a major portion of the cytoplasm of each spermatid remains as a residual body within a pocket of the Sertoli cell cytoplasm. Note the intercellular bridges between adjacent germ cells in the same cohort or generation. (Amann. 1983. *Journal of Dairy Science,* 66:2606.)

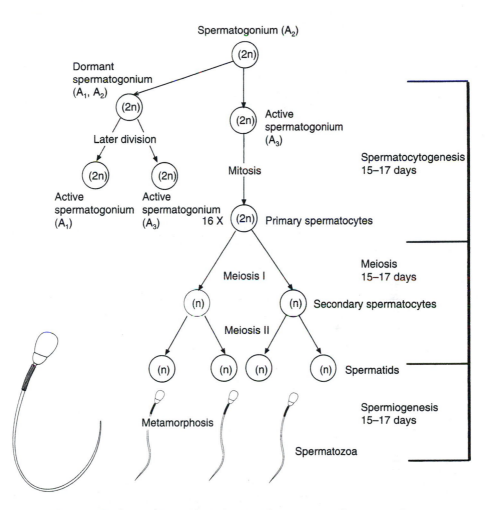

Figure 6–3 Spermatogenesis indicating the sequence of events and time involved in spermatogenesis in the ram.

a. An A_2 spermatogonium divides by mitosis, forming an active spermatogonium (A_3) and a dormant spermatogonium (A_1).

b. The active spermatogonium undergoes four mitotic divisions, forming 16 primary spermatocytes.

c. Each primary spermatocyte will undergo two meiotic divisions, forming four spermatids (a generation of 64 spermatids from the A_3 spermatogonium).

d. The dormant spermatogonium (A_1) will later divide to yield A_2 spermatogonia, which through mitosis form new active (A_3) and new dormant (A_1) spermatogonia.

e. Each spermatid undergoes metamorphosis to form a spermatozoon. (One spermatozoon is enlarged to permit more detail in morphology.)

(n) chromosomes. This step requires approximately 15 days in the ram. Within a few hours after their formation, each secondary spermatocyte will again divide, forming two *spermatids*. Thus, four spermatids form from each primary spermatocyte, or 64 from each active (A$_3$) spermatogonium, in bulls and rams. Meiosis requires 15 to 17 days in the ram. Since A$_1$ spermatogonia divide by mitosis to form A$_2$ spermatogonia, the potential yield of spermatids is higher than is actually realized. Degeneration of spermatogonia during spermatocytogenesis and meiosis accounts for most of this loss in efficiency. Sertoli cells remove degenerating germ cells by phagocytosis.

6–2.3 *Spermiogenesis*

Spermiogenesis is the process during which a haploid spermatid undergoes a metamorphosis (change in morphology) to form a mature elongated spermatid or spermatozoon (Figure 6–4; also Section 14–1.1). The process of spermiogenesis can be divided into four phases: *Golgi phase, cap phase, acrosomal phase,* and *maturation phase*. During the Golgi phase, the round spermatids are formed with initial development of the *acrosome* and acrosomic vesicles. The acrosome is a cap around the head of the spermatozoon that will form the Golgi apparatus of the spermatid. The continued development of the acrosomal cap and initiation of acrosomic vesicle spreading occurs during the cap phase. The acrosomal phases consist of nuclear and cytoplasmic elongation, which begins shaping and elongating the spermatid. The final phase, the maturation phase, is when the spermatid completely differentiates, with final formation of the flagellum (principal and end pieces), assembly

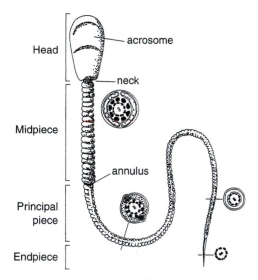

Figure 6–4   The structural features of a bovine sperm cell. Cross sections of the midpiece, principal piece, and endpiece show the fibrils surrounded by the mitochondrial sheath in the midpiece region, the fibrous sheath in the principal piece region, and the free fibrils in the endpiece (Section 14–1.1 for a description of fibril functions). (Barth and Oko. 1989. *Abnormal Morphology of Bovine Spermatozoa*. Iowa State University Press.)

of mitochondria (midpiece), neck piece, and complete condensation and shaping of the nucleus. As the cytoplasm from the spermatid is cast off during formation of the tail, a *cytoplasmic droplet* will form on the neck of the spermatozoon. The mitochondria from the spermatid will form in a spiral around the upper one-sixth of the tail, forming the *mitochondrial sheath.* Newly formed spermatozoa will then be released by a process called *spermiation* from the Sertoli cell and forced out through the lumen of the seminiferous tubules into the rete testis. Spermatozoa are unique cells in that they have no cytoplasm and after maturation possess the ability to be progressively motile. Spermiogenesis is completed in 15 to 17 days in rams.

6–2.4 *Continuation of Spermatogenesis*

Following a resting state of several weeks, the dormant (A_1) spermatogonium will divide, forming A_2 spermatogonia, which will divide, forming new active (A_3) and new dormant (A_1) spermatogonia. Even though A_0 spermatogonia (reserve stem cells) will occasionally divide, forming new A_0 and A_1 spermatogonia, formation of dormant spermatogonia from A_2 spermatogonia is the key to maintaining the continuity of spermatogenesis and thereby not diminishing the supply of potential gametes within the testes.

6–2.5 *Hormonal Control of Spermatogenesis*

The endocrinology of reproduction has not been studied in males as extensively as in females. In bulls and rams there are three to seven surges in LH per day, followed by similar surges in testosterone (Figure 6–5). The principal role of LH in regulation of spermatogenesis appears to be indirect in that it stimulates the release of testosterone from cells of Leydig. Testosterone and FSH act through cells in the seminiferous tubules to stimulate spermatogenesis. Paracrine actions of high concentrations of testosterone in fluids that bathe the seminiferous tubules (100 to 300 times higher than in peripheral plasma) are essential for normal spermatogenesis. These high concentrations are maintained through binding of testosterone to androgen-binding protein. Androgen-binding protein is secreted by Sertoli cells when stimulated by FSH. Androgen-binding protein is absorbed in the epididymis. Therefore, high concentrations of testosterone are maintained in the rete testis, vasa efferentia, and proximal portion of the epididymis as well as the seminiferous tubules. Whereas FSH release is stimulated by GnRH as is LH, episodic surges are not as apparent, possibly due to the modulating effect of inhibin on FSH secretion. Function of Sertoli cells, including secretion of inhibin, estradiol, and androgen-binding protein, is dependent on FSH. Spermatogenesis may proceed qualitatively in some species when FSH is deficient, provided testosterone concentrations in the testes are high. However, FSH is needed for normal production of spermatozoa.

Feedback controls operating among the testis, hypothalamus, and anterior pituitary in regulating the release of gonadotropins (FSH and LH) and the gonadal steroid, testosterone, are similar to those described for the female (Figures 4–5 and 4–6). Testosterone has a negative feedback effect on the hypothalamus and anterior pituitary, possibly by affecting the release of endogenous opioids. High concentrations of testosterone will inhibit the release of GnRH, FSH, and LH, whereas low concentrations permit their release.

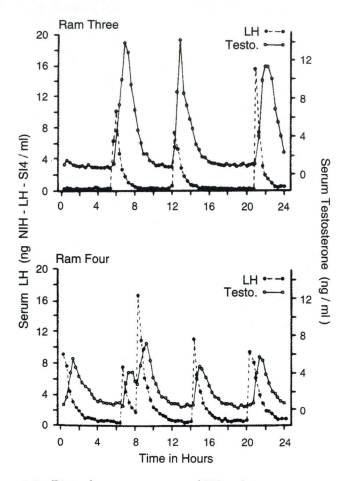

Figure 6–5   Diurnal secretory pattern of LH and testosterone in mature rams. (Sanford et al. 1974. *Endocrinology,* 95:627.) Similar patterns have been reported for the bull.

6–3   THE SEMINIFEROUS EPITHELIAL CYCLE AND SPERMATOGENIC WAVE

Spermatogenesis is not the same type of cyclic process as ovigenesis in the female. New spermatozoa are being formed and released into the duct system constantly. During the time that the generation of cells from one active spermatogonium is going through the divisions and maturation necessary to form spermatozoa, other spermatogonia in the same area will start spermatogenesis in a staggered but timed sequence. Therefore, if a transverse section is cut from a seminiferous tubule, several generations of germ cells will be found. These are arranged concentrically with layers of spermatogonia near the wall of seminiferous tubules followed by spermatocytes and spermatids in layers progressing toward the lumen (Figure 6–2).

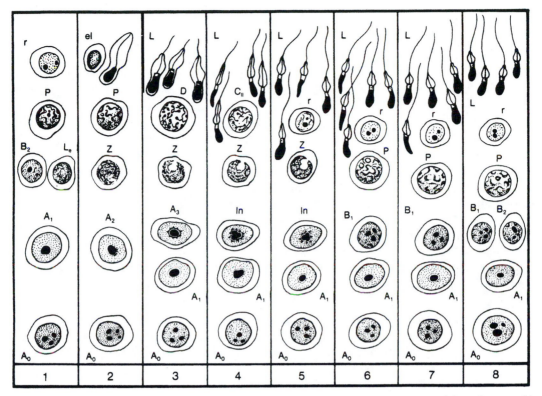

A_0, A_1, A_2, A_3, B_1, B_2, In = Spermatogonia; L_e, Z, P, D, C_{II} = Spermatocytes; r, el, L = Spermatids

Figure 6–6 Cellular composition of the seminiferous epithelial cycle in the bull. These associations or stages are identified by the morphological changes of germ cell nuclei and local arrangements of spermatids. A_0, A_1, A_2, A_3, intermediate (In), B_1, and B_2 spermatogonia are generated by mitotic divisions. Represented phases of maturation in primary spermatocytes in sequential order are leptotene (L_e), zygotene (Z), pachytene (P), and diplotene (D). C_{II} is the secondary spermatocyte. The spermatids represented are rounded (r), elongating (el), and elongated (L). (Ortavant. 1977. *Reproduction in Domestic Animals*. (3rd ed.) eds. Cole and Cupps. Academic Press.)

It has been determined that a kind of organization and synchrony exists within the seminiferous tubules of a mature male in that certain cell types are always associated together. Because these cell types are always associated together and reappear in series with cyclic regularity through a cross section of the seminiferous tubules, they can be recognized and classified. One classification system, based on developmental changes in the acrosome, has identified 12 different stages of cellular associations. Another system, based on structural changes in germ cell nuclei and local arrangement of spermatids, has identified 8 stages, which are illustrated in Figure 6–6.

The key changes in cellular association that identify a specific stage are as follows: *Stage 1* starts when spermatozoa have been released into the lumen. The rounded spermatids have spherical nuclei and are associated with two generations of primary spermatocytes, one young (L_e) and one old (P). *Stage 2* encompasses the period when spermatid nuclei are elongating. They are associated with two generations of primary spermatocytes (Z and P). *Stage 3* extends from the end of elongation of spermatids to completion of the first meiotic division. A new generation of spermatogonia (A_3) has appeared. In *Stage 4*, elongated bundles of spermatids in the cytoplasm of Sertoli cells are associated with one generation each of secondary spermatocytes (C_{II}) and primary spermatocytes (Z). In *Stage 5*, bundles of elongated spermatids in the Sertoli cell cytoplasm are associated with a new generation of spermatids (r). In *Stage 6*, dusty chromatin appears in the nuclei of young spermatids (r), and the chromatin in primary spermatocytes (P) has the networklike appearance that is characteristic of the pachytene stage. In *Stage 7*, elongated spermatids (L) are migrating to the lumen. In *Stage 8*, spermatozoa line the lumen and are released.

The time between two successive appearances of the same cellular associations (Stage 1 to Stage 1, etc.) at a given location in the seminiferous tubules is the *seminiferous epithelial cycle*. The time of the cycle is 8.6 days for the boar, 10.3 days for the ram, 12.2 days for the stallion, and 13.5 days for the bull. From the time of formation of the active spermatogonium (A_3) until it releases its generation of 64 spermatozoa into the lumen of the seminiferous tubule, between four and five seminiferous epithelial cycles will be completed.

The same eight cellular associations have been used to identify *spermatogenic waves* in the seminiferous tubules. These cellular associations occur in sequence along the seminiferous tubules, just as they do in one section of the tubules over a period of time. If the cellular association found at a specific point in a seminiferous tubule is identified as Stage 3, then Stages 2 and 4 will be found on either side of this point. A complete series of the eight cellular associations along a seminiferous tubule is called a spermatogenic wave. These stages tend to appear in a continuous manner along the seminiferous tubules, except that local reversals sometimes occur. The organization of germ cells in the seminiferous tubules through space and over time accounts for the continuous release of spermatozoa into the lumen of seminiferous tubules.

6–4   CAPACITATION OF SPERMATOZOA AND ACROSOME REACTION

After spermatozoa are produced in the seminiferous tubules, two maturation processes are necessary before they can participate in fertilization. The first of these occurs in the epididymis, as discussed in Chapter 3. This was described as (1) gaining the ability to be motile, (2) gaining the ability to be fertile, and (3) losing the cytoplasmic droplet. Spermatozoa cannot participate in fertilization until they have undergone a second maturation process in the female reproductive tract. This maturation process is known as *capacitation*.

Direct evidence for the necessity of capacitation of spermatozoa before fertilization could be completed was provided in the demonstration that capacitated sperm were essential for *in vitro* fertilization (Section 19–1.3). Estimated times for *in vivo* capacitation are 5 to 6 hours for cows and 2 to 3 hours for pigs. As illustrated in Table 6–1, best conception occurs if cows are inseminated from middle to late estrus, some 12 to 18 hours before the estimated time of fertilization. This observation relates to time needed for capacitation, time needed for transport of spermatozoa to the ampullary-isthmic junction (the site of fertilization), and to

Table 6–1 *Effect of time of insemination on ovulation and fertility in cows (cows normally ovulate 10 to 12 hours after the end of estrus)*

Time of breeding	Total cows	Cows conceiving from one service
Start of estrus	25	44.0%
Middle of estrus	40	82.5
End of estrus	40	75.0
After estrus		
6 hours	40	63.4
12 hours	25	32.0
18 hours	25	28.0
24 hours	25	12.0
36 hours	25	8.0
48 hours	25	0.0
Routine breeding	194	63.4

Source: Trimberger and Davis, *Univ. Neb. Res. Bul.* 129, 1943.

the freshness of the male and female gametes. If breeding occurs too early, the spermatozoa may capacitate and start aging before the oocyte arrives. If bred too late, the oocyte may age before spermatozoa are capacitated and transported to the ampullary-isthmic junction (Section 8–6).

Capacitation can be defined as cellular changes that spermatozoa undergo in the female reproductive tract that are necessary before the acrosome reaction and fertilization can occur. It is accompanied by hyperactive sperm motility and an influx of calcium. Based on *in vitro* studies, it appears that capacitation is accomplished through binding of glycosaminoglycans to sperm, via binding proteins on the sperm membrane.

Glycosaminoglycans (GAG) are a group of unbranched linear polysaccharides that are found in the female reproductive tract. The GAG that is most potent in capacitating sperm is heparin, but hyaluronic acid and others are found in the female tract. They are found in highest concentration in the cervix, with sequentially lower concentrations in the uterus and oviducts. Concentrations of GAG are higher around estrus than during diestrus. Bulls with high fertility have sperm-binding proteins with higher binding affinity for heparin and other GAG than bulls of low fertility. Although these GAG-binding proteins are located on the surface of spermatozoa, they are found in seminal plasma as well, but their location on the spermatozoa is necessary for high fertility. There are factors in seminal plasma that inhibit both binding of GAG to spermatozoa and capacitation. Therefore, dilution of these inhibitory factors in the female reproductive tract is necessary for spermatozoa to respond readily to GAG.

The *acrosome reaction* involves fusion of the outer acrosome membrane with the plasma membrane of the spermatozoa. This results in formation of vesicles and release of enzymes needed for sperm to penetrate the cumulus and corona radiata cells as well as the zona pellucida (Section 8–4). During the penetration process, the acrosome is lost, with only the inner acrosomal membrane remaining around the apex of the sperm head. Calcium is essential for the acrosome reaction. Although GAG do not induce the acrosome reaction, they do predispose spermatozoa to respond to calcium and subsequently bring on the membrane changes that are typical of the acrosome reaction. In *in vitro* studies with bull sperm, the time between exposure to GAG and completion of the acrosome reaction is about 9 hours.

SUGGESTED READING

AMANN, R. P. 1970. Sperm production rates. *The Testis.* Vol. 1. eds. A. D. Johnson, W. R. Gomes, and N. L. VanDemark. Academic Press.

AMANN, R. P. 1983. Endocrine changes associated with onset of spermatogenesis in bulls. *J. Dairy Sci.,* 66:2606.

AX, R. L. and R.W. LENTZ. 1987. Glycosaminoglycans as probes to monitor differences in fertility of bulls. *J. Dairy Sci.,* 70:1477.

BEDFORD, J. M. 1983. Significance of the need for sperm capacitation before fertilization in eutherian mammals. *Biol. Reprod.,* 28:108.

BELLIN, M. E., H. E. HAWKINS, and R. L. AX. 1994. Fertility of range bulls grouped according to presence or absence of heparin-binding proteins in sperm membranes and seminal fluid. *J. Anim. Sci.,* 72:2441.

DYM, M. 1977. The role of the Sertoli cell in spermatogenesis. *Reproductive Systems.* eds. R. Yates and M. Gordon. Raven Press.

DYM, M. and J. C. CAVICCHIA. 1978. Functional morphology of the testis. *Biol. Reprod.,* 18:1.

FAUCETT, D.W. 1979. The cell biology of gametogenesis in the male. *Biol. Med.,* 22:556.

GOMES, W. R. 1978. Formation, migration, maturation and ejaculation of spermatozoa. *Physiology of Reproduction and Artificial Insemination of Cattle.* (2nd ed.) eds. G. W. Salisbury, N. L. Van Demark, and J. R. Lodge. W. H. Freeman and Co.

HAFS, H. D. and M. S. McCARTHY. 1979. Endocrine control of testicular function. *Beltsville Symposia in Agricultural Research. 3. Animal Reproduction.* ed. H.W. Hawk. Allanheld, Osmun and Co. Publishers; Halsted Press, a division of Wiley & Sons.

JOHNSON, L. 1991. Spermatogenesis. *Reproduction in Domestic Animals.* (4th ed.) ed. P. T. Cupps. Academic Press.

MONESI, V. 1972. Spermatogenesis and spermatozoa. *Reproduction in Mammals. 1. Germ Cells and Fertilization.* eds. C. R. Austin and R. V. Short. Cambridge University Press.

SANFORD, L. M., J. S. D. WINTER, W. M. PALMER, and B. E. HOWLAND. 1974. The profile of LH and testosterone secretion in the ram. *Endocrinology,* 95:627.

STEINBERGER, E. 1971. Hormonal control of spermatogenesis. *Physiol. Rev.,* 51:1.

YOUNG, W. C. 1931. A study of the function of the epididymis. III. Functional changes undergone by spermatozoa during their passage through the epididymis and vas deferens. *J. Expt. Biol.,* 8:151.

7

Mating Behavior

The primary purpose of mating behavior is copulation, thus bringing male and female gametes together to ensure propagation of the species. This requires a fertile female that is sexually receptive (in estrus) near the time of ovulation and a male that is producing fertile semen and has both the desire to mate (libido) and the ability to copulate. The elements of mating behavior are sexual receptivity in females and the desire and ability to mate in males. However, fertility in both sexes and dominance in males are important factors in reproductive success. In situations of natural breeding, the male must be dominant enough to compete successfully with other males in the group for the estrous female. For males, the correlation between fertility, libido, and ability to mate is low. Therefore, when selecting breeding males for a herd or flock, these traits must be evaluated separately (Section 20–3.4). Mating behavior is first observed at the initial estrus (puberty) in females and as puberty approaches in males. Mating behavior is regulated by hormones, the senses, and other factors in an animal's environment.

7–1   REGULATION OF MATING BEHAVIOR

7–1.1 *Hormonal Influence*

High concentrations of estrogens have been associated with behavioral signs of estrus in females and are of paramount importance. As estrus approaches, the maturing follicles secrete high concentrations of estrogens, which are needed for exhibition of sexual receptivity and initiation of the hormonal changes that lead to ovulation (Section 5–3). However, sexual receptivity will not be expressed unless progesterone is low, to remove its inhibitory influence on expression of estrus. Injection of estradiol into a prepuberal female will elicit behavioral estrus, since progesterone is low in a prepuberal female. A low level of androgen is needed for normal libido in females, as well. A low concentration of testosterone is secreted by the ovaries. Although most of the testosterone produced by thecal cells is aromatized to estradiol (Section 2–1), enough is secreted into the systemic circulation to maintain libido in intact females. Clinical human studies suggest that the concentration of androgens secreted by the adrenal cortex is sufficient for this response if ovaries are not functional or have been removed surgically. Therefore, even though a high concentration of estrogens is essential for expression of estrus in females, the influences of progesterone and androgens are important as well.

Although testosterone has a dominant, controlling influence on regulation of mating behavior in males, there is evidence for interaction with estradiol. In an experiment with male red deer castrated after puberty, sexual aggressiveness was restored with injections of either testosterone or estradiol. However, only testosterone restored the social aggressiveness as seen in intact postpuberal males. In studies with rats, hamsters, and other mammals, injection of estradiol partially but not completely restored sexual activity in castrated males. It appeared that estradiol was restoring the elements of behavior regulated by the central nervous system, but androgens were needed for the peripheral elements related to tactile stimulation, penile stimulation, and erection. This suggests that aromatization of testosterone to estradiol may be necessary in the normal regulation of mating behavior that is under control of the central nervous system. In experiments with castrated male rats, a combination of estradiol and dihydrotosterone (a nonaromatizable androgen) were more effective in restoring mating behavior than estradiol alone. Overall, testosterone is the dominant hormone that regulates sexual behavior in males, but aromatization to estradiol resulting in expression through an estradiol recepter may be important for some important aspects of sexual behavior. Although testosterone and its metabolites have a major controlling influence on male sexual behavior, there is interaction with other factors (Figure 7–1).

7–1.2 *Role of the Senses*

Certain senses are important to the mating response of females and males, with the sense of smell being the most important. Both females and males secrete odorous chemicals (pheromones) that serve as sexual attractants to the opposite sex. Research evidence is stronger in sows, ewes, and does than in mares and cows, but the contribution of the senses is probably important in all species. When boars are not present, providing the smell of the

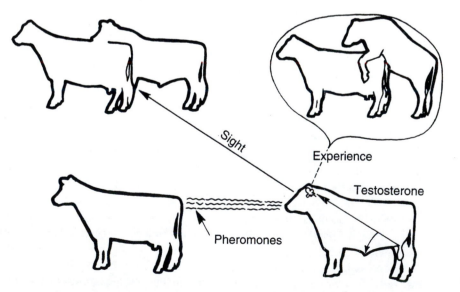

Figure 7–1   Interaction of factors that regulate sexual behavior in bulls and other species.

boar through solutions containing pheromones from glands in the sheath of the boar have elicited stronger mating responses in gilts. The "boar effect" on induction of early puberty in gilts (Section 5–1) appears to be mediated through pheromones. Similarly, ewes will not show signs of estrus when an intact ram is not present (the "ram effect"). Pheromones identified in the wax from the wool of the rams have stimulated both estrus and ovulation in ewes. Likewise, the doe seldom shows strong signs of estrus if an intact buck is not present. Scent glands located dorsally and medially from the horns are the source of these pheromones. The doe shows a clear preference for bucks with scent glands as compared with bucks whose scent glands have been removed. Rubbing a cloth over the head of a buck and then placing the scented cloth near the nose of does will make them show a stronger estrual response than when bucks are absent. Pheromones from the urine of bulls as well as the cervical mucus of cows in estrus have been reported to increase the mating response of heifers.

Pheromones found in the urine of females that are in estrus are stimulating to males. Both bulls and stallions can be trained to use a dummy mount and serve an artificial vagina when collecting semen for use in artificial insemination. When these males do not respond to the dummy mount, sprinkling urine from an estrus female on the mount will frequently elicit the desired response. On the other hand, bulls do not appear to be able to detect pheromones from distant females that are in estrus. Also, when females are restrained, bulls will mount nonestrus females as often as those in estrus. There is evidence that pheromones are detected more readily when the bull samples fluids from the genital area of the female with the tongue.

Although it is difficult to rule out an effect from the sense of sight—for example, when a boar is presented to a sow—most consider the response of the sow more related to detection of pheromones. Therefore, it has been difficult to establish that the sense of sight is of major importance to the mating response of the female. The sense of sight is of demonstrated importance in males. This sense seems related more to sexual arousal than to other aspects of mating behavior. For bulls, it is probably the most important cue in stimulating sexual interest. Sight of mounting activity, a sexually active group, an immobile castrate male, a padded dummy mount, or any object that can be mounted will usually stimulate mounting behavior. The immobility of the object, whether female in estrus, castrated male, or mounting dummy, is a strong factor in eliciting mounting. Older bulls are more discriminatory, showing a clear preference for live teaser animals. Sexually mature bulls that are wearing blindfolds will copulate normally. On the other hand, males blind from birth reach sexual maturity later than do males with normal sight.

The sense of touch is probably important to the mating response of females and males in that bunting, biting, licking, and rubbing are a part of the courtship before copulation in all species. There is good evidence in males that tactile stimulation of the penis affects copulatory behavior. When collecting semen with an artificial vagina, both bulls and rams are sensitive to the temperature of the water inside the liner of the artificial vagina. Most bulls respond best to the artificial vagina when the water temperature is approximately 45°C. If the temperature is too hot or too cold, he may not ejaculate and may become uncooperative in future attempts to collect semen. Although the temperature of the water in the artificial vagina appears to be important when collecting semen from stallions, both stallions and boars seem to be more sensitive to pressure on the penis than to temperature. For example, the boar will not ejaculate unless pressure is applied to the glans penis. This pressure can come from the hand of the attendant or the cervix of the sow as the boar's penis locks into the cervical canal during copulation.

There is some evidence that the sense of hearing is important to the mating response, especially in females. In one study, playing a recording of the grunts of a boar elicited a stronger mating response in gilts than was observed in gilts without the sound or presence of a boar. The effects of all senses seem to be interactive and additive. Usually, when one sense is eliminated, animals make use of other senses and perform normally. However, in an experiment with guinea pigs, removal of the olfactory bulbs (sense of smell) resulted in cessation of sexual activity. Therefore, interaction of pheromones with either testosterone in males or estrogens in females seems highly important to regulation of mating activity.

7–1.3 *Social and Sexual Interaction*

Most information available on the influence of social and sexual interaction during rearing on mating behavior is related to males. Although, males that are raised in isolation will sometimes show normal mating behavior when placed with a female that is in estrus, social interaction with others of the same species during development before puberty is important to attaining a high level of sexual activity in a number of species. Low libido has been reported in rams that were reared in isolation. Also, when compared with rams raised in heterosexual groups, rams raised from weaning to puberty in all-male groups have been more likely to show low sexual performance with little improvement shown over time. By contrast, rearing of bulls in all-male groups has not affected their sexual performance. Some rams show sexual preference for other rams whether reared in all-male groups or heterosexual groups. However, male mounting of other males is more frequent for rams raised in all-male groups. The social environment is a factor that must be considered when rearing males.

Lack of early sexual experience has resulted in neither serious nor permanent problems in attaining full sexual activity. In artificial insemination centers, sexually inexperienced bulls are sometimes hesitant, spend a long time exploring the genitalia of female teaser animals, and frequently have weak erections with incomplete ejaculation. However, on repeated use under the same conditions, they adjust to the surroundings and copulate vigorously.

7–2   BEHAVIORAL CHARACTERISTICS OF ESTRUS

In general, females will be more restless, irritable, and excitable during estrus. In addition, increased vocalization and interest in the male will become apparent if the male of the species is in the vicinity. Pelvic adjustments into a mating position (*lordosis*) may occur. Such indications can first be seen during late proestrus, but the female will not stand to be mounted by the male or by another female during proestrus. In recognizing the signs of estrus or approaching estrus, knowledge of the personalities of the animals in question will be beneficial. Also, it is helpful to watch for females in estrus when they are quiet. Dawn and dusk are good times to watch for estrus, especially if the animals do not know they are being watched. If the females are excited by the presence of people, noises, or anticipation of feeding, detection of estrus may be difficult. Specific behavioral and physiological patterns are characteristic of the different species.

Cows are unique in that they display rather strong homosexual tendencies, making estrus detection comparatively easy even when bulls are not present. Cows in estrus will solicit mounts and attempt to mount other cows. Cows that are not in estrus will mount cows that are in estrus. However, mounting activity is more frequent when two or more cows are in estrus than when a single cow is in estrus. Frequency of mounting is higher at night than during the day, with this being particularly true during the summer. Possibly because it is closer to the onset of estrus, more mounting activity will be seen during early morning as compared with late afternoon. Cows in estrus spend more time walking, with less time resting and feeding than when in other periods of the estrous cycle. They may smell the vulva of other cows. Frequently, they raise and switch their tail and may leave the herd in search of a bull. They will have a congested vulva and clear mucus can often be seen streaming from the vulva. Cows in other periods of the estrous cycle will not stand to be mounted. Therefore, standing for mounting is the strongest single behavioral indication of estrus.

In contrast to the cow, the ewe displays no signs of estrus if the ram is not present. The ewe will rub the neck and body of the ram. She will roam around the ram, smelling his genitalia and shaking her tail vigorously. The vulva of the ewe will not be congested, and there will be no visible mucus. If artificial insemination is being used in ewes, use of altered rams is necessary for detection of estrus. (See Chapter 20 for discussion of altered males.)

The doe in estrus will sometimes stand for mounting by another doe, but homosexual behavior is low. They will actively seek the male when in estrus. Other signs include tail wagging, bleating, and urination near the buck. Moderate swelling of the vulva and mucous discharge is seen at times. For does with weak signs of estrus, wagging of the tail and standing for mating may be the only signs. Teasing of females with bucks elicits stronger signs of estrus, especially in does that show few behavioral signs of estrus.

Homosexual activity is much less frequent in water buffalo than in cattle. In research reports, 20% to 23% have stood for herd mates. Therefore, teasing with a bull is needed for accurate detection. There is swelling of the vulva and a reddening of the mucosa of the vestibule.

Sows will assume a mating stance when pressure is applied to their loin by a boar, another sow, or the hand of an attendant. This provides some convenience in artificial insemination in that sows can be inseminated without restraint if pressure is maintained on the loin. There will be no visible mucus during estrus, but the vulva may be swollen and congested. The swollen vulva is more noticeable in gilts than sows. The vulva may become swollen after administration of certain medications, so this should be considered with other signs of estrus.

The mare will allow the stallion to smell and bite. She will extend her hind legs, lift her tail to the side, and lower her rump. The vulva will be elongated and swollen, with the labia partly everted. The erect clitoris will be exposed frequently by contractions (winking) of the labia. The mare should be teased by a stallion for accurate detection. Attempts to fight the stallion indicate she is not in estrus even though some other signs of estrus are apparent. In mares and other species, knowledge of their individual behavior during estrus will aid in detecting estrus.

Accurate detection of estrus has been listed as a major reproductive problem in farm animals. Paramount to accurate detection of estrus is an understanding of the expected behavior for the species in question and the factors that contribute to the expected response. Additional discussion on detection of estrus is found in Chapter 20.

7–3 MATING BEHAVIOR IN MALES

For males, the events in mating behavior, listed sequentially, are sexual arousal, courtship (sexual display), erection, mounting, intromission (insertion of penis), ejaculation, and dismounting. If the female is in estrus, this sequence of events takes only a few minutes in

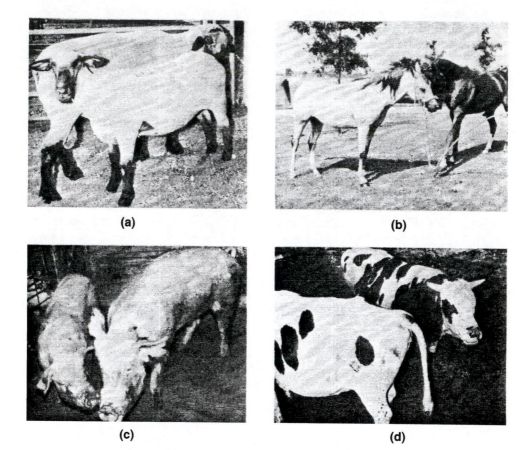

(a) **(b)**

(c) **(d)**

Figure 7–2   Courtship in farm animals: *(a)* ram sniffing vulva of the ewe; *(b)* stallion nuzzles mare's head and paws the ground; *(c)* boar and sow engage in mating grunts; *(d)* bull showing curled upper lip (flehmen).

cattle and sheep. In horses and pigs, the duration of courtship and copulation is extended, with copulation alone sometimes lasting for up to 10 minutes in pigs. After copulation, a quiescent period will follow before the male will respond again to a female that is in estrus. The length of quiescense varies with individuals and with age.

Both similarities and differences exist in the courtship patterns of different species (Figure 7–2 and Color Plate 19). Vocalization occurs in most species. This may be bellowing by the bull, neighing by the stallion, or grunts by rams and boars. Sniffing and licking of the female's genitalia and urine are seen. In cattle, sheep, and horses, the male will extend his neck and curl his upper lip (flehmen). Various tactile stimuli, including licking, bunting, and biting, are part of the courtship pattern in most males. In addition to the desired characteristics of genetic potential, strong libido, and the ability to mate, it is important that breeding males exhibit dominance. Females that are in estrus frequently seek the dominant male. In addition the dominant male will try to protect females that are in estrus, separating them from other males and females. Therefore, dominant males effactually prevent subordinate males from copulating. Two elements of male behavior that have provoked research attention because of their essentiality in successful mating are erection and ejaculation.

7–3.1 *Erection*

Erection is under control of the autonomic nervous system. With sexual excitement, blood is pumped into and temporarily trapped in the corpus cavernosum penis and corpus spongiosum penis (Section 3–6). The penis of the stallion has large, cavernous areas which account for the increase in size of the penis during erection. In the bull, ram, and boar, erection results in extension of the penis with little increase in size. They have fibroelastic penises with small areas of cavernous tissue. The corpus cavernosum penis is larger and more important in attaining an erection than the corpus spongiosum penis. Pressure in the corpus cavernosum penis just before ejaculation may exceed 15,000 mm mercury in bulls and 6,500 mm mercury in stallions. The energy for this pressure comes from the ischiocavernosus muscle, which contracts to pump blood into and traps blood in the corpus cavernosum penis. The corpus cavernosum penis is a closed system with no venous outlet to bleed off the pressure. However, cartilage damage from injury sometimes results in development of venous outlets that impair erection.

7–3.2 *Ejaculation*

Ejaculation is defined as the ejection of semen from the body. The ejaculate includes spermatozoa from the vasa deferentia and epididymides and fluids from the accessory glands. Ejaculation is initiated by stimulation of sensory nerves in the glans penis, which triggers a series of peristaltic contractions involving smooth muscles in the epididymides, vasa deferentia, and urethra. In addition, fluids from the accessory glands are pumped into the urethra. Peristaltic contractions move spermatozoa concentrate and accessory gland fluids through the ducts leading to the external urethral orifice. The final discharge of semen is brought about by a wave of contractions involving the smooth muscles lining the urethra and in bulls by pressure from the corpus spongiosum penis, which collapses the urethra in a wave. The pressure from the corpus spongiosum penis is generated by the bulbospongiosum muscle and proceeds from the penile bulb toward the glans penis.

Ejaculation varies among species in a number of aspects (Table 7–1). Ejaculation occurs almost instantaneously with the thrust of the penis in bulls, bucks, and rams. Ejaculation time is about 10 to 15 seconds in stallions and 3 to 10 minutes in boars. Volumes of ejaculates vary considerably, being smaller in bucks and rams (1.5 ml) and bulls (6 ml) and much larger in stallions (75 ml) and boars (200 ml). Concentration of spermatozoa ranges from a low of approximately 150 million per ml in stallions to a high of 2 billion per ml in bucks and rams. Boars (200 million per ml) and bulls (1.2 billion per ml) are intermediate in spermatozoa concentration. The consistency of the ejaculate varies among species. In bulls, bucks, and rams, there is a complete mixing of spermatozoa concentrate with fluids

Table 7–1 *Characteristics of average ejaculate of semen for different species*

Species	Ejaculation time	Volume (ml)	Concentration
Bull	Less than 1 second	6	1.2 billion/ml
Ram and buck	Less than 1 second	1.5	2.0 billion/ml
Boar	3–10 minutes	200	200 million/ml
Stallion	10–15 seconds	75	150 million/ml

from the accessory glands in the urethra before expulsion of the semen. Dribblings from the prepuce of the bull before copulation, thought to be from the bulbourethral glands, are quite low in volume. Both boars and stallions have a segmented ejaculate. A spermatozoa-free segment will be followed by a spermatozoa-rich segment and a spermatozoa-poor segment. When collecting boar semen for artificial insemination, the initial spermatozoa-free segment can be discarded without influencing fertility (Chapter 13).

7–3.3 *Maintaining Libido*

Maintaining *libido* (sex drive) in males is of concern in both range (or farm) conditions and with artificial insemination organizations. The problem has been studied more extensively in bulls than in other farm species.

Providing a balanced diet is very important. This means to neither underfeed nor overfeed. As mentioned in Chapter 6, underfeeding will delay puberty. It has also been demonstrated that underfeeding young bulls between the age of puberty (10 to 12 months) and the end of their growth period (30 to 36 months) will reduce libido and total semen production. In mature bulls, overfeeding is more likely to be a problem. If mature bulls are overweight, the increased likelihood of foot, leg, and joint problems may shorten their reproductive life. Adequate but restricted diets do not reduce libido or semen production in mature bulls.

Diseases and injuries will reduce libido. Neither of these conditions has to be serious to reduce sexual activity. A seemingly minor problem, such as a swollen joint or mild respiratory infection, may reduce the overall vigor of the male as well as his libido. When males are confined to small areas, special attention must be given to hoof care (trimming, etc.) and moderate exercise to help maintain a state of good health and prevent conditions that make copulation unpleasant. If copulation is unpleasant or causes pain, voluntary retirement from sexual activity is not uncommon.

7–3.3a Sexual Exhaustion

Sexual exhaustion can be a problem when males run with females for a prescribed breeding season. A primary effect of sexual exhaustion is loss of libido. This is more likely to happen with a dominant male during the heavy part of the breeding season under range conditions. Subsequent gestations have been delayed because dominant but sexually exhausted males have prevented subordinate males from copulating. If a number of females are in estrus, or if at least two other males are running with the herd or flock, the dominant but sexually exhausted male will be less able to prevent breeding of estrous females. After adequate rest, males that have been sexually exhausted will regain their libido. One mature bull or one mature ram for 40 to 50 breeding-age females is usually considered adequate for a normal breeding season under range conditions. In pigs, one mature boar is needed for 10 sows during an intensive breeding program. During the first breeding season after puberty, it is recommended that matings be limited (e.g., 3 to 4 mares or 10 to 15 cows).

It has been reported that excessive copulation by a stallion will reduce fertility and in some cases cause sterility. However, mature stallions in good health have been used daily and sometimes more frequently for extended periods without loss of fertility. Reduced libido occurs before reduced fertility in other species and this may be true in stallions. One report indicates that a seminal plasma protein associated with fertility in bulls is reduced with successive ejaculates over a short period of time (Section 14–2.1). Although this makes predicted fertility lower, enough sperm seem to be deposited into the female tract to compensate for the change in this protein during natural service.

7–3.3b Sexual Satiety Whereas sexual exhaustion is a physical problem that can be cured with rest, sexual satiety is a mental problem. It is a term used to describe a sexual indifference that results when a bull has copulated with the same cow under the same conditions for an extended period. It is a problem which has been encountered by organizations where bulls are maintained exclusively for the purpose of providing semen for artificial insemination. In most cases, sexual satiety can be cured by providing variety in the collection procedure. This might be done by changing the teaser animal, bringing out a second teaser, or moving to another collection area (Section 13–2.1). Using a female that is in estrus or sprinkling the collection area with urine from a female in estrus will help frequently.

SUGGESTED READING

ALLRICH, R. D., 1994. Endocrine and neural control of estrus in dairy cows. *J. Dairy Sci.,* 77:2738.

BECKETT, S. D., R. S. HUDSON, D. F. WALKER, R. I. VACHON, and T. M. REYNOLDS. 1972. Corpus cavernosum penis pressure and external penile muscle activity during erection in the goat. *Biol. Reprod.,* 7:359.

CHENOWETH, P. J. 1981. Libido and mating behavior in bulls, boars and rams: A review. *Theriogenology,* 16:155.

HAFS, H. D. and M. S. McCARTHY. 1979. Hormonal control of testis function. *Beltsville Symposia in Agricultural Research. 3. Animal Reproduction.* ed. H.W. Hawk. Allanheld, Osmun and Co., Halsted Press, Wiley & Sons.

HALE, E. B. and J. O. ALMQUIST. 1960. Relation of sexual behavior to germ cell output in farm animals. 4th Biennial Symp. on Animal Reproduction. *J. Dairy Sci.,* 43 (suppl.):145.

HULET, C. V., S. K. ERCANBRACK, R. L. BLACKWELL, D. A. PRICE, and L. O. WILSON. 1962. Mating behavior of the ram in the multi-sire pen. *J. Anim. Sci.,* 21:865.

HURNIK, J. F., G. J. KING, and H. A. ROBERTSON. 1975. Estrus and related behavior in postpartum Holstein cows. *Appl. Anim. Ethology,* 2:55.

KATONGOLE, C. B., F. NAFTOLIN, and R. V. SHORT. 1971. Relationship between blood levels of luteinizing hormone and testosterone in bulls and the effects of sexual stimulation. *J. Endocrin.,* 50:458.

KATZ, L. S., E. O. PRICE, S. R. J. WALLACH, and J. J. ZENCHAK. 1988. Sexual performance of rams reared with or without females after weaning. *J. Anim. Sci.,* 66:1166.

LINDSEY, D. R. 1965. The importance of olfactory stimuli in the mating behavior of the ram. *Animal Behavior,* 13:75.

MELROSE, D. R., H. C. B. REED, and R. L. S. PATTERSON. 1971. Androgen steroids associated with boar odour as an aid to the detection of oestrus in pig artificial insemination. *Brit. Vet. J.,* 137:497.

SCORDALAKES, E. M., D. B. INWALLE, and E. F. RISSMAN. 2002. Oestrogen's masculine side: Mediation of mating in male mice. *Reproduction,* 124:331.

SEIDEL, G. E., JR. and R. H. FOOTE. 1969. Motion picture analysis of ejaculation in the bull. *J. Reprod. Fert.,* 20:317.

WIERZBOWSKI, S. 1966. The scheme of sexual behavior in bulls, rams and stallions. *World Rev. Animal Prod.,* 2:66.

Ovigenesis and Fertilization

8–1 OVIGENESIS

Formation and maturation of the gametes must be completed for both the male and female before the reproductive processes can be initiated. *Ovigenesis* (or *oogenesis*) is the formation and maturation of the female gamete.

Ovigenesis (Figure 8–1) begins in the prenatal period. Formation of primary follicles has been described in Chapter 2. The potential gamete associated with the primary follicle when first formed is the oogonium. Oogonia originate from an extension of the yolk sac, which forms from the hindgut of the embryo. Following initial formation, proliferation of oogonia by mitotic division occurs within the parenchyma of the ovary. As previously stated in Chapter 2, this proliferation ceases before birth so that the ovaries, at birth, contain a fixed number of potential ova, or *oocytes*. Oocytes enter prophase of the first meiotic division during the fetal period with meiosis I being arrested in late prophase shortly after birth. These oocytes in this dormant (arrested) state are referred to as *dictyate oocytes*.

During the prenatal period and continuing postnatally, a cyclic pattern in oocyte growth and maturation has been reported. However, until the female reaches puberty, no oocytes will reach full maturity. Those oocytes that start development before puberty and most that start development after puberty become atretic and are lost as potential ova. It has been estimated that fewer than 1% of all oocytes reach maturity and are released during ovulation.

Growth and maturation of oocytes will continue in a cyclic manner after puberty. During the waves of follicular growth that occur during each estrous cycle (Section 5–3), groups of oocytes associated with these follicles start growth and maturation (most become atretic) while the others remain dormant. However, at the time of luteal regression, the oocyte associated with the dominant follicle reaches maturity and is released through ovulation to the duct system for possible fertilization in the cow, ewe, doe, and mare. In sows, 10 to 25 oocytes may reach maturity and be released through ovulation.

Following arrested meiotic development, maturation resumes with growth of the oocyte and formation of the *zona pellucida,* a gel-like outer membrane, around the oocyte (Figures 8–1 and 8–2). Growth of the oocyte is followed closely by growth of the associated follicle. FSH stimulates proliferation of the granulosa cells that surround the oocyte, with the follicle progressing from a primary to a secondary follicle. Continued stimulation from FSH results in continued proliferation of granulosa cells and formation of an antrum.

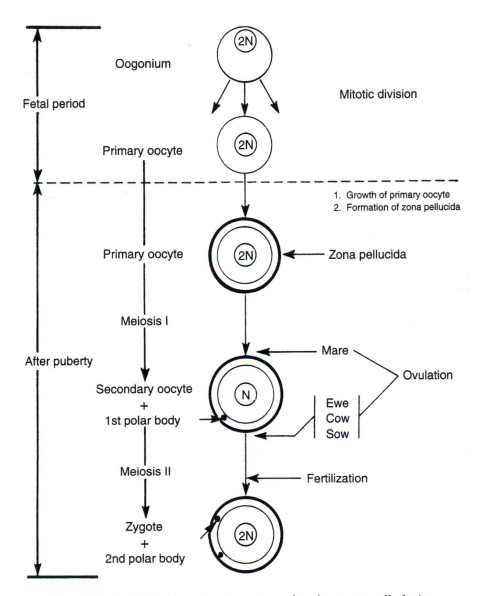

Figure 8–1 Principal maturation stages for the germ cell during ovigenesis.

a. During the fetal period, mitosis of oogonia is completed and meiosis I starts.

b. Meiosis I is arrested shortly after birth at prophase I.

c. Growth of the oocyte and formation of the zona pellucida are followed closely by growth of the follicle.

d. The preovulatory surge of LH initiates a resumption of meiosis.

e. Meiosis I is completed but meiosis II is arrested at metaphase II.

f. During fertilization, meiosis II resumes and is completed with formation of the zygote.

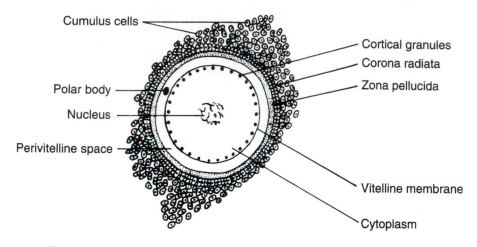

Figure 8–2   Oocyte and its associated cells soon after ovulation. Cumulus and corona radiata cells are shed before fertilization in some species.

Less pronounced proliferation of thecal cells outside the basement membrane occurs under the influence of LH. During this development, the follicle or follicles destined to ovulate become dominant. When the dominant follicle and other antral follicles secrete enough estrogen, the preovulatory surge of LH is triggered. High LH concentrations release the associated oocyte into the follicular fluid and from its arrested state. Thereafter, meiosis I continues to completion. The products of the first meiotic division are the *secondary oocyte* and the *first polar body,* which is trapped between the *vitelline membrane* (plasma membrane) and the zona pellucida in the perivitelline space. With this division, the chromosome numbers in the oocyte are changed from the *diploid* (2n) to the *haploid* (n) state. The secondary oocyte retains all of the cytoplasm and half of the nuclear material (chromosomes) of the primary oocyte. The other half of the nuclear material is extruded as the first polar body. This first meiotic division is completed just before ovulation in the cow, sow, and ewe and shortly after ovulation in the mare.

The second meiotic division (meiosis II) begins immediately after completion of the first division. This division is arrested at metaphase II. The second meiotic arrest will be released and meiosis II initiated again during the fertilization process. It will not be completed without interaction of the oocyte with the fertilizing sperm. With fertilization, the products of the second meiotic division are the *zygote* (fertilized egg) and the *second polar body.* It should be noted that the *true ovum* never exists in the cow, sow, ewe, or mare or, if so, only in a transient state. The true ovum would be the product of the second maturation division if the division were completed before fertilization.

8–2   OVULATION

Farm animals are spontaneous ovulators rather than having ovulation induced by copulation, as in the cat, rabbit, camel, llama, and a number of other species. For induced ovulators, copulation stimulates sensory neurons in the vagina and/or cervix with direct neural links to the neurons of the hypothalamus. This neural stimulation results in the increased release of GnRH, which produces the LH surge requisite for ovulation to occur. With maturation of the oocyte and follicle in either spontaneous or induced ovulators, the preovulatory surge of LH will initiate a sequence of events that leads to ovulation some 24 to 45 hours later. Following the surge of LH, the concentration of progesterone in follicular fluid increases immediately, to be followed some hours later by increases of estradiol and prostaglandins ($PGF_{2\alpha}$ and PGE_2). Inhibition of either ovarian steroid or prostaglandin secretion will block ovulation. The role of the prostaglandins in ovulation appears to be that of rupturing lysosome-like vesicles, containing proteolytic enzymes, which are located just outside the follicle between the surface epithelium and tunica albuginea, as well as that of activating plasmin, a proteolytic enzyme found in follicular fluid. Proteolytic enzymes from the lysosomes cause a localized degeneration of the tunica albuginea, theca externa, and theca interna, whereas plasmin acts on the basement membrane. The walls of the follicle become thin and weakened. A bulge (the *stigma*) which appears at the apex of the follicle is the point where the follicle will rupture. The general weakening of the walls of the follicle permits plasma to escape into the spaces between the thecal cells, causing edema, and eventually capillaries penetrate beyond the basement membrane into the granulosa layer.

When the follicle ruptures, follicular fluid, the secondary oocyte, and loosened granulosa cells will be extruded into the peritoneal cavity near the infundibulum. Contractions of the ovary to include the walls of the follicle, which are stimulated by prostaglandins, likely contribute to both rupture of the follicle and expulsion of the oocyte. Spontaneous contractions of the ovary increase as time of ovulation approaches. Ovulation can occur anywhere on the ovarian surface for most species but occurs at one site, the *ovarian fossa,* in mares. The ovarian fossa causes a depression in the mare ovary that gives it the kidney-shaped appearance. The oocyte will be embedded in the cumulus mass, a sticky, loose matrix of cumulus cells around the more tightly packed corona radiata cells that surround the oocyte (Figure 8–2). These granulosa cells (cumulus and corona radiata) are shed quickly in some species and are not believed to be present at time of fertilization. They appear to be a factor in capture of the oocyte by the infundibulum and in its movement into the ampulla.

8–3 GAMETE TRANSPORT

Movement of viable gametes to the site of fertilization is an essential part of successful reproduction. It is notable that these gametes are transported in opposite directions. From the ovary, the oocyte moves through the infundibulum and ampulla while spermatozoa move from the vagina or cervix through the uterine horn and isthmus to the ampullary-isthmic junction, where fertilization occurs. An understanding of the mechanisms involved in gamete transport along with its associated timing is important because of the essential role of transport in successful reproduction.

8–3.1 *Oocyte*

Following ovulation, the oocyte with its associated cumulus mass is picked up by ciliated epithelial cells of the infundibulum. Most of the epithelial cells in the infundibulum and ampulla are ciliated. These cilia beat in the direction of the uterus. In addition to a role in actively moving the oocyte toward the ampullary-isthmic junction, cilia in beating toward the

Table 8–1   *Transport time of oocytes in the oviduct of farm animals*

Species	Time (hours)
Cattle	90
Sheep	72
Horse	98
Swine	50

Adapted from Hafez. *Reproduction in Farm Animals.* (3rd ed.) Lea and Febiger, 1974.

uterus create a directional flow in oviductal fluids which may aid transport. Currents caused by the beating of the cilia may facilitate movement of the oocyte from the ovary to the surface of the infundibulum. Although it has been demonstrated that cilia can move the oocyte to the ampullary-isthmic junction independently, cilia may not be the major means of oocyte transport through the ampulla. Segmented, peristaltic contractions of the ampulla proceed in the direction of the uterus, milking the oocyte through. These segmented, peristaltic contractions are likely the most important mechanism for normal transport of the oocyte through the ampulla to the site of fertilization. The oocyte passes through the ampulla to the ampullary-isthmic junction rapidly, then remains at that point for 2 to 3 days before moving through the isthmus to the uterus (Table 8–1). Thus, fertilization occurs at the ampullary-isthmic junction. Estrogens have been reported to cause retention of the oocyte in the oviduct, whereas progesterone hastens transport. Epinephrine has been reported to hasten transport, also.

8–3.2 *Spermatozoa*

Mechanisms for transport of spermatozoa to the site of fertilization are more speculative than oocyte transport. Some spermatozoa reach the ampullary-isthmic junction within a few minutes after deposition of semen in the female tract. This rapid phase transport of sperm has been attributed to a series of copulation-induced peristaltic contractions involving smooth muscle in the cervix, uterus, and oviduct. Both oxytocin, which is released after stimulation of sensory nerves near the cervix during copulation, and prostaglandins from the semen could be involved in stimulating these contractions. Both dead and motile sperm reach the oviduct during this rapid transit phase. These uncapacitated sperm are probably not involved in fertilization and likely pass on through the oviduct into the peritoneal cavity. The rapid transport phase is followed by a slower, sustained transport of sperm to the oviduct. Both barriers to transport and mechanism of transport must be considered for the sustained transport phase.

For those species (cows, ewes, does) with deposit of semen in the vagina during natural service, the cervix is the greatest barrier to transport. The billions of spermatozoa deposited in the vagina are probably reduced to thousands actually reaching the uterus. The cervical mucus has a biophysical configuration during estrus that helps channel spermatozoa along the cervical folds through the cervix into the uterus. In the bovine, two types of cervical mucus have been identified as important to sperm transport: *sialomucins,* low-viscosity mucus produced by cells in the basal portions of the cervical folds, and *sulfomucins,* high-viscosity mucus produced in the apical portions of the cervical folds. The highly viscous sulfomucins cause sperm to be washed out of the reproductive tract (i.e., away from the cervix toward the vestibule), whereas sperm in the low-viscosity sialomucins, while also flowing in a vaginal direction, facilitate sperm passage through the cervix (i.e., sperm swim into the low-viscosity current). This orientation of sperm in the basal passages of the cervix has also been referred to as the "privileged pathway," as many sperm gain entry to the uterus through the cervix via this route. The movement of spermatozoa through the cervical mucus requires an interaction between spermatozoa and cervical mucus, with sperm motility an apparent necessity. In addition to helping channel spermatozoa through the cervix, cervical mucus also helps filter out dead and abnormal sperm. The concept of a filtering process is supported by the high concentration of dead and abnormal sperm found in the cervix a few hours after copulation, even though cervical mucus during estrus has been identified as providing a favorable environment for sperm. It is likely that some spermatozoa are also temporarily trapped in the folds of the cervix with these spermatozoa being fed into the uterus slowly, thus feeding fertile spermatozoa into the uterus for some hours after copulation. This barrier is bypassed by artificial insemination in cattle.

However, even with artificial insemination retrograde transport of spermatozoa can occur. If semen is deposited in the uterine body or in the uterine horns following artificial insemination, retrograde loss of spermatozoa within the first 12 hours has been reported to be around 18% to 30% of that deposited. In contrast for semen deposited in the cervix by artificial insemination, retrograde loss within the first 12 hours may be as high as 60% of that deposited. The potential for such great losses in spermatozoa as a result of retrograde transport demonstrate the importance of using experienced personnel as part of artificial insemination programs (Chapter 17).

When spermatozoa reach the body of the uterus via either natural transport or direct deposition during artificial insemination, they likely move along the liquid interface of the endometrial lining toward the oviducts. An interaction of spermatozoa with the uterus seems necessary, with both sperm motility and tonic contractions of the uterus aiding transport. It is not known if sperm are preferentially routed toward the oviduct containing the oocyte. Therefore, approximately equal numbers may move up each uterine horn and oviduct. However, more spontaneous contractility has been observed in the oviduct adjacent to the ovulating ovary in cows. Therefore, preferential routing is possible. Random movement of sperm may result in some movement back into the cervix as well as toward the oviduct.

The uterotubal junction is another major barrier for spermatozoa in their transit to the site of fertilization. Either the uterotubal junction or the lower isthmus also appears to serve as a filter, since a higher concentration of nonviable sperm is found in this region than in the uterus or near the ampullary-isthmic junction. The isthmus has been identified as a second reservoir for pooling of spermatozoa (the cervix being the first reservoir). This isthmic reservior may be created by the binding of viable sperm to the epithelium. Sperm retain their viability longer when in contact with the oviductal epithelium. There is evidence in sheep and cattle that viable sperm from the isthmic pool are transported more rapidly to the site of fertilization near the time of ovulation. The isthmic epithelium appears to regulate the release of sperm, allowing only a few to move the site of fertilization at one time. Both $PGF_{2\alpha}$ and estradiol have speeded sperm transport in inseminated rabbits. Therefore, the high concentration of estradiol during estrus likely contributes to this transit from the isthmic pool. Interaction of motile sperm in oviductal fluid with a spontaneously contracting oviduct appears to facilitate movement of sperm through the uterotubal junction and finally

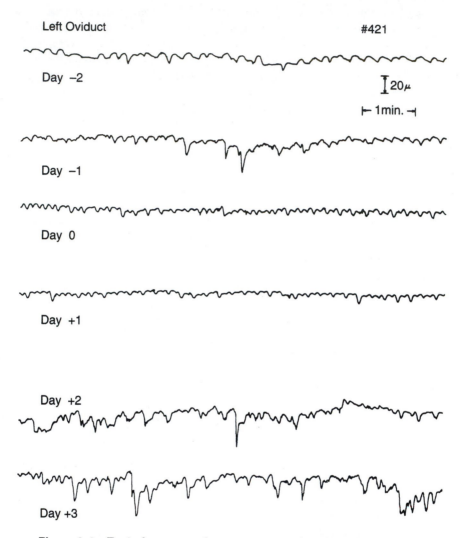

Figure 8–3   Typical patterns of spontaneous oviductal motility in a cow during proestrus, estrus (day 0), and metestrus. High-amplitude contractions of longitudinal muscles (indicated by downward deflections) are seen more frequently during proestrus and metestrus. During estrus, low-amplitude contractions of high frequency in circular muscles (indicated by upward deflections) are predominant. (Bennett, W.A. Master of Science Thesis. Mississippi State University. 1974.)

from the isthmic reservoir to the ampullary-isthmic junction, the site of fertilization. Patterns of oviductal motility change around the time of estrus (Figure 8–3). During proestrus and metestrus, high-amplitude pulses associated with contraction of longitudinal muscles are prominent in the isthmus. At estrus, low-amplitude but high-frequency activity associated with contraction of circular muscle is dominant. The precise relationship of these contractions to movement of gametes or the zygote has not been established. The slower, sustained phase of transport provides viable sperm at the site of fertilization about 8 hours after natural mating in cows and ewes. This timing seems compatible with providing viable and recently capacitated sperm at the site of fertilization at the approximate time of arrival of the oocyte, if animals are bred at the recommended time during estrus.

In the sow and to a large extent in the mare, semen is deposited directly into the uterus. Therefore, the cervix is neither a barrier to transport nor a filter to remove dead sperm as occurs in ruminant species. The larger volume in their ejaculates (Table 14–3) likely ensures rather rapid and uniform distribution of semen throughout the uterus. This appears particularly likely in pigs, where the volume (150 ml to 300 ml) is sufficient to cause distention of the uterus. Therefore, the uterotubal junction is the primary barrier to sperm transport to the ampullary-isthmic junction where fertilization occurs. In pigs, whole semen does not enter the oviduct and sperm motility appears to be essential for passage through the mucosal folds of the isthmus to the ampullary-isthmic junction. Thus, dead sperm are filtered out at the uterotubal junction or lower isthmus. Sperm transport is more rapid than in cattle or sheep. In pigs, a sufficient sperm population to ensure fertilization will be established near the fertilization site in 1 to 2 hours after semen is deposited into the uterus. Injection of oxytocin, a smooth muscle stimulator, has improved farrowing rate and increased litter size in pigs. Nevertheless, irrespective of how fast sperm traverse the female reproductive tract to the oocyte, sperm fertilization ability is still dependent on sperm maturation and capacitation, which requires several hours to complete (Section 6–4).

8–4 FERTILIZATION

The process of fertilization starts with a collision between the oocyte and a spermatozoon and ends when their pronuclei have merged. The resulting diploid cell containing the genetic code for a new individual is the zygote. Even though the corona radiata and other granulosa cells may be shed before this process begins, fertilization will be described as though they remain around the oocyte. Features of the oocyte which are important to the process of fertilization are illustrated in Figure 8–2. These include the cumulus; the zona pellucida, the gel-like outer membrane of the oocyte; the vitelline membrane, which is the true plasma membrane of the oocyte; cortical granules—small, rounded bodies which lie just beneath the vitelline membrane; and the haploid nucleus of the oocyte. Major steps in fertilization are illustrated in Figure 8–4.

The first step in fertilization involves penetration of the spermatozoon through the cumulus and corona radiata cells, with its head sticking to the zona pellucida. Two enzymes, hyaluronidase and corona-penetrating enzyme, aid this passage. Both are associated with the head of the sperm. Release of these enzymes is made possible by capacitation and the acrosome reaction (Section 6–4).

During the second step, the spermatozoon must bind to the zona pellucida, penetrate the zona extracellular matrix, and gain entry into the perivitelline space, where it will fuse with the vitelline membrane. More than 20 years ago, it was identified that a "sperm receptor" was present on the zona pellucida, referred to as zona pellucida protein-3 (ZP3). There are, of course, other zona proteins (ZP1, ZP2, etc.), however these proteins function more to maintain the integrity of the zona pellucida matrix and structure than for initial sperm binding. It is generally accepted that ZP3 is an initiator of sustained acrosome reaction processes once binding of sperm to the zona pellucida has occurred. Sperm may also

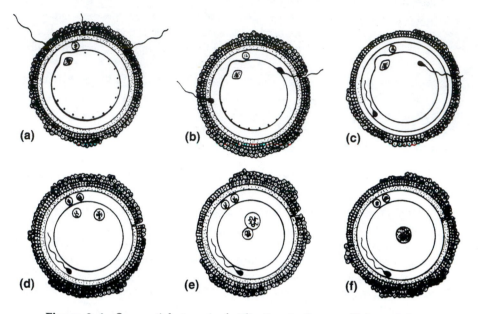

Figure 8–4 Sequential steps in fertilization in the rat. (Adapted from Austin and Bishop, 1957. *Biol. Rev.,* 32:296.):

a. A spermatozoon penetrates the cumulus and corona radiata cells, sticking to the zona pellucida.
b. A spermatozoon penetrates the zona pellucida and fuses with the vitelline membrane. The zona reaction is initiated as the cortical granules disappear.
c. The spermatozoon is engulfed by cytoplasm in the oocyte. The vitelline block is evoked.
d. The cytoplasm shrinks; a second polar body is pushed into the perivitelline space; the male and female pronuclei form.
e. Syngamy occurs.
f. The zygote is formed, completing fertilization.

possess so-called egg-binding proteins (EBPs), which further assist in the fusion of sperm to the zona membrane. It is has been suggested that the presence of specific "sperm receptors" on the zona pellucida and corresponding EBPs on spermatozoa may aid in conferring species specificity, much the same way as a hormone binds to its own receptor. Penetration of the zona pellucida is assisted by the secretion of acrosin, a trypsinlike enzyme associated with the head of the sperm, and a slit is left in the zona pellucida at the point of entry. Following passage of the spermatozoon, the *zona reaction* occurs. When the plasma membrane of the head of a spermatozoon fuses with the vitelline membrane, the cortical granules also fuse with the vitelline membrane and empty their contents into the perivitelline space. The spilling of the contents of the cortical granules into this space seems responsible for the zona reaction. The zona reaction guards against penetration of the zona pellucida by other spermatozoa and is the most important protection in cattle, sheep, and swine against *polyspermy* (Section 8–5). In cattle, a number of accessory sperm may be trapped in the zona pellucida after fertilization and this has been positively associated with fertility and embryo quality. The zona reaction is not an absolute safeguard, since other spermatozoa can

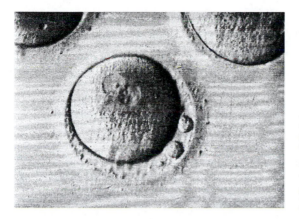

Figure 8–5 The fusion of the male and female pronuclei (syngamy). The first and second polar bodies are clearly visible within the perivitelline space. (Courtesy of S. Jindal, Hackensack Medical Center, Hackensack, NJ.)

sometimes be seen in the space between the zona pellucida and vitelline membrane. This does not happen frequently in farm species but does occur frequently in rabbits.

The spermatozoon then penetrates the vitelline membrane by phagocytosis and enters the cytoplasm. After this entry, the *vitelline block,* which is a second reaction to guard against fertilization by other spermatozoa, occurs and is most important in rabbits. Cortical granules may participate in the vitelline block, also. Upon entering the cytoplasm, the tail of the spermatozoon separates from the head. Mitochondria associated with the tail degenerate and other parts appear to dissolve in the cytoplasm. The cytoplasm shrinks and the second polar body is extruded. Both the male and the female pronuclei form. This involves an unfolding of the chromosomes in preparation for pairing. *Syngamy,* a merging of the pronuclei then occurs (Figure 8–5). When syngamy is complete, the zygote has been formed, thus completing fertilization.

8–5 POLYSPERMY

Polyspermy is a term used to describe fertilization by more than one spermatozoon. The result is a zygote with a polyploid nucleus. Embryos with cells containing polyploid nuclei will develop normally for a period of time and then will die and degenerate. Therefore, a major disadvantage of polyspermy is that it results in embryo loss. With the zona reaction and vitelline block guarding against polyspermy, it seldom occurs (1% to 2% in mammals). It is more likely to occur if the secondary oocyte is either aged or heated. Delayed mating in pigs has resulted in rates of up to 15%. Therefore, polyspermy is more likely if the animal is bred too late or if her body temperature is elevated by fever or high ambient temperature. Polyspermy could account for some of the reduction in conception rate and increase in early embryonic mortality under such conditions.

8–6 AGING OF GAMETES

To achieve optimum conception during controlled natural breeding or AI, it is essential that fertilization take place before either gamete has aged (Section 6–4). For species other than the horse, some loss in fertility of spermatozoa can be expected after about 24 hours following

Table 8–2   *Estimated fertile life of sperm and ova in farm animals*

Species	Fertile life in hours	
	Spermatozoa	Ova
Cattle	24–48	8–12
Swine	24–48	8–10
Sheep	30–48	16–24
Horse	72–120	6–8

Adapted from McLaren. *Reproduction in Farm Animals.* (3rd ed.) ed. Hafez. Lea and Febiger. 1974.

Table 8–3   *Effect of age of the ovum on fertility in cattle*

Hours from ovulation to insemination	Fertility observed at 2–4 days		Fertility observed at 21–35 days	
	Total animals	Animals with fertile ova	Total animals	Animals with normal embryos
2–4	4	75%	4	75%
6–8	4	75	10	30
9–12	5	60	13	31
14–16	4	25	8	0
18–20	5	40	6	17
22–28	1	0	11	0

From Nalbandov. *Reproductive Physiology of Mammals and Birds.* (3rd ed.) W.H. Freeman and Co., copyright © 1976.

Table 8–4   *The effect of the length of time of storage of extended semen on its fertility level and the difference between 1-month and 5-month nonreturns*

	Age of extended semen when inseminated in relation to day of collection				
	Same day	2nd day	3rd day	4th day	5th day[a]
No. of inseminations	12.0	726.0	756.0	970.0	56.0
1-month nonreturns (%)	58.3	67.0	62.8	54.3	57.2
5-month nonreturns (%)	50.0	57.0	50.7	41.5	39.3
Difference (%)	8.3	10.0	12.1	12.8	17.9

From Salisbury, Bratton, and Foote. *J. Dairy Sci.,* 35:256. 1952.

[a]5th day or more.

mating (Table 8–2). The fertile life of the ovum is usually less than 12 hours, except possibly for the ewe. In Tables 8–3 and 8–4, the two-fold problem of aged gametes is illustrated. (1) Fertilization rates are lower when the gametes have aged. (2) Subsequently, both embryo and fetal death losses are higher whether the aged gamete is of male or female origin. It should be noted that the semen used in the research reported in Table 8–4 was diluted in egg yolk–citrate diluter and presumably stored at 5°C. Therefore, aging was slower than would occur in the reproductive tract of the cow. When one considers the inability to estimate the time of ovulation due to lack of knowledge of the exact hour that estrus begins and the variability of the female, the critical nature of diligent management during the breeding season becomes apparent.

While not a physiological function of traditional livestock, with the exception of poultry, the concept of *delayed fertilization* is important to note with respect to gamete aging. In the hen and various species of bats, snakes, and fish, among other species in the wild, spermatozoa deposited in the female reproductive tract following mating can remain viable for extended periods of time. In the hen, fertile eggs may be laid for more than 20 days following mating; in bats, mating occurs before hibernation but the female does not ovulate until after the hibernation period some 2 to 6 months later, depending on the species; and some snakes maintained in isolation in captivity have been known to lay fertile eggs up to 4 to 6 years later. Some species have specialized utero-vaginal glands for storing sperm, yet the mechanisms that permit sperm to be stored and remain viable for such extended periods of time remains unclear. It is tempting to speculate that what might be learned from species that demonstrate delayed fertilization, in the form of protective proteins or other mechanisms, might have relevance for use in livestock to extend the fertile life of gametes in the female reproductive tract postmating to improve chances for conception.

SUGGESTED READING

BAKER, T. G. 1982. Oogenesis and ovulation. *Reproduction in Mammals. 1. Germ Cells and Fertilization.* (2nd ed.) eds. C. R. Austin and R. V. Short. Cambridge University Press.

BEDFORD, J. M. 1982. *Fertilization. 1. Germ Cells and Fertilization.* (2nd ed.) eds. C. R. Austin and R. V. Short. Cambridge University Press.

BENNETT, W. A., T. L. WATTS, W. D. BLAIRS, S. J. WALDHALM, and J. W. FUQUAY. 1988. Patterns of oviductal motility in the cow during the estrous cycle. *J. Reprod. Fert.,* 83:537.

BYSKOV, A. G. 1982. Primordial germ cells and regulation of meiosis. *Reproduction in Mammals. 1. Germ Cells and Fertilization.* (2nd ed.) eds. C. R. Austin and R. V. Short. Cambridge University Press.

COONS, L. W. and A. JOHNS. 1982. Effects of ovulation on the conduction and contraction velocities in rabbit oviduct: Contrast between longitudinal and circular muscles. *Biol. Reprod.,* 27:440.

DEJARNETT, J. M., R. G. SAACKE, J. BAME, and C. J. VOGLER. 1992. Accessory sperm: Their importance to fertility and embryo quality, and attempts to alter their number in artificially inseminated cattle. *J. Anim. Sci.,* 70:484.

ERICKSON, G. F. 1978. Normal ovarian function. *Clin. Obst. Gynecol.,* 21:31.

GALLAGHER, G. R. and P. L. SENGER. 1989. Concentrations of spermatozoa in the vagina of heifers after deposition of semen in the uterine horns, uterine body or cervix. *J. Reprod. Fertil.,* 86:19.

HAFEZ, E. S. E. 1987. Folliculogenesis, egg maturation and ovulation. *Reproduction in Farm Animals.* (5th ed.) ed. E. S. E. Hafez. Lea and Febiger.

HAFS, H.D. 1978. Ovigenesis, ovulation and fertilization. *Physiology of Reproduction and Artificial Insemination of Cattle.* (2nd ed.) eds. G. W. Salisbury, N. L. VanDemark, and J. R. Lodge. W. H. Freeman and Co.

HAWK, H. W., B. S. COOPER, and H. H. CONLEY. 1982. Effect of acetylcholine, prostaglandin F_2, and estradiol on number of sperm in the reproductive tract of mated rabbits. *J. Anim. Sci.,* 55:891.

HUNTER, R. H. F. and L. WILMUT. 1983. The rate of functional sperm transport into the oviducts of mated cows. *Anim. Reprod. Sci.,* 5:167.

HUNTER, R. H. F., L. BARWISE, and R. KING. 1982. Sperm transport, storage and release in the sheep oviduct in relation to time of ovulation. *Brit. Vet. J.,* 138:225.

HUNTER, R. H. F., B. COOKS, and N. L. POYSER. 1983. Regulation of oviduct function in pigs by local transfer of ovarian steroids and prostaglandins: A mechanism to influence sperm transport. *Europ. J. Obstet., Gynec. Reprod. Biol.,* 14:225.

SAUREZ, S. S., K. BROCKMAN, and R. LEFEBVRE. 1997. Distribution of mucus and sperm in bovine oviducts after artificial insemination. *Biol. Reprod.,* 56:447.

SAUREZ, S. S., K. REDFERN, P. RAYNOR, F. MARTIN, and D. M. PHILLIPS. 1991. Attachment of boar sperm to mucosal explants of oviduct *in vitro:* Possible role in formation of reservoir. *Biol. Reprod.,* 51:222.

WASSERMAN, P. M., L. JOVINE, and E. S. LITSCHER. 2001. A profile of fertilization in mammals (review). *Nature Cell Biol.,* 3:E59.

9

Gestation

Gestation is the period of pregnancy. It starts with fertilization, which has been described, and ends with *parturition* (the birth process). The average length of the gestation period is 114 days for the sow, 148 days for the ewe, 149 days for the doe, 281 days for the cow, 320 days for the water buffalo, and 337 days for the mare. Both individual and breed differences exist, except that gestation length seems to vary little for different breeds of goats and domestic pigs (Table 9–1). Gestation is a little longer when a cow is carrying a male than when carrying a female. With twins, gestations are shorter in cows.

During the early part of gestation, the embryo remains free, first in the oviduct and then the uterus. Its nutrients are those which are stored in its own cytoplasm and those that can be absorbed from uterine milk. Only after placentation, the process by which chorionic villi extend into the endometrium forming a union (Section 2–3), can the embryo derive nutrients and transfer waste products through maternal blood. In sows, this process starts about day 12 and will be completed by 18 to 24 days. In ewes, a transitory attachment will occur about day 15, with chorionic villi extending into caruncles by day 30. Early during the course of placentation, the placental attachments are quite fragile. In the cow between 30 and 35 days after fertilization, there will be 3 or 4 fragile cotyledonary attachments in the pregnant horn. Before 40 days, fragile attachments will be present in both horns. There will be 40 to 50 cotyledonary attachments in both horns by 70 days, and this figure increases to approximately 120 by the middle of the pregnancy. A transitory attachment occurs in mares after day 24, with chorionic villi extending into the endometrium by days 37 to 45. Endometrial cups, which secrete PMSG, form about day 37 or 38. The timing of these placentation events is more difficult in the sow and mare with diffuse placental attachments than in cows and ewes with cotyledonary attachments. Before the embryo can derive benefit from placentation, organ development will have to occur to the point that the embryo's circulatory system is functional.

Migration and spacing of embryos, which occurs before placentation in sows, is completed by 12 days. After entry into the uterus, embryos migrate freely from one side to the other. Even though about 55% of the ova come from the left ovary, embryos will be distributed equally between the two uterine horns of the sow after spacing is completed. Embryos migrate freely in mares between days 10 to 16 and sometimes to day 25, with the fetus frequently found on the side opposite to the corpus luteum of pregnancy. By day 25, the embryo will have become stabilized at one location. In cows and ewes, transuterine migration of embryos is less frequent than in mares. In ewes with a single ovulation, less than 10% of

Table 9–1   *Species and breed differences in gestation length*

Breed	Average length (days)
Cattle	
Ayrshire	278
Guernsey	283
Jersey	279
Holstein	279
Brown Swiss	290
Angus	279
Hereford	284
Shorthorn	283
Brahman	293
Sheep	
Hampshire	145
Southdown	145
Merino	151
Horse	
Belgium	335
Morgan	342
Arabian	337
Goat	149
Swine	114

the fetuses are found in the opposite uterine horn and no migration has been reported for cows with a single ovulation. With two ovulations on one ovary, migration of one fetus to the opposite horn occurs frequently in ewes and occasionally in cows. After fertilization, the conceptus develops through periods of cleavage, differentiation, and growth. Until differentiation is completed, the conceptus is called an embryo. After differentiation, it is called a fetus.

9–1   CLEAVAGE

After fertilization the zygote will divide and redivide many times without any increase in cytoplasm (Figure 9–1). The overall size may increase due to absorption of water, but the total cellular material will decrease. This process of cell division without growth is *cleavage*. The first cleavage will result in a 2-cell embryo. This is followed by additional cleavages, resulting in 4-cell, 8-cell, 16-cell, 32-cell embryos, and so on. (Figure 9–2). With each cleavage, cells become smaller. In sows, a 4-cell embryo will enter the uterus at 46 to 48 hours after ovulation. In ewes and cows, an 8- to 16-cell embryo will enter the uterus 3 to 4 days after ovulation. The 8- to 16-cell stage embryo is called a morula. By the 32- to 64-cell stage, the morula will compact with gap junctions forming between interior cells and tight junctions forming between cells on the outside of the embryo, a necessary step in blastocyst formation. During the next few days, fluid collecting in the intercellular spaces will push to the center, forming a *blastocyst,* a structure with a fluid-filled cavity (the blastocoele) surrounded

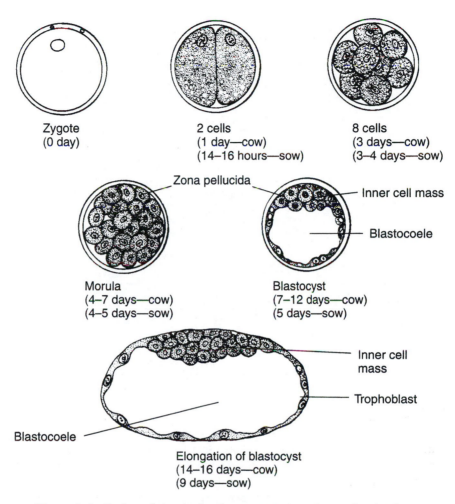

Figure 9–1 Early embryonic development at given times after fertilization in the cow (281-day gestation) and the sow (114-day gestation).

by a layer of trophoblast cells. The blastocyst stage will be reached by day 5 in pigs, day 6 in horses and sheep, and day 7 in cattle (Table 9–2). The embryo enters the uterus at this stage in horses. The development that occurs in the oviduct is critical to survival of the embryo.

While not seen in most domesticated species, embryos having undergone initial stages of cleavage to the blastocyst stage can remain free-floating in the uterus without further development for a period of time, referred to as *delayed implantation* or *embryonic diapause*. Delayed implantation has been reported to occur in bears, otters, mink, weasels, badgers, seals, and roe deer, among other species. The advantages of delayed implantation are similar to those of delayed fertilization (Section 8–6), which assures that mating and birthing seasons correspond to periods when external conditions are favorable for conception and/or offspring survival following birth. In delayed implantation, fertilization occurs

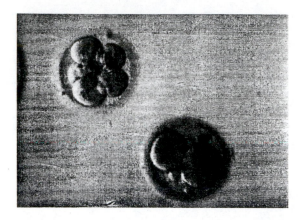

Figure 9–2 Embryos at the 2-cell (bottom) and 8-cell (top) stages of development. (Courtesy of S. Jindal, Hackensack Medical Center, Hackensack, NJ.)

Table 9–2   *Time comparisons during early embryonic development for different farm species*

Species	1-cell (hours)	8-cell (days)	Blastocyst (days)	Enter uterus (days)
Cattle	24	3.0	8	3.5
Horse	24	3.0	6	5.0
Sheep	24	2.5	7	3.0
Swine	14–16	2.0	6	2.0

Adapted from McLaren. *Reproduction in Farm Animals.* (3rd ed.) ed. Hafez. Lea and Febiger. 1974.

normally with early cell cleavage and then the embryonic development is arrested at the blastocyst stage until a more suitable time for development to continue. Blastocyst dormancy in bears may last 5 to 6 months, whereas the longest period of blastocyst dormancy is seen in otters, lasting 10 to 11 months. Again, while such phenomena have not been observed in domesticated livestock, much could be gained from a greater understanding of the physiological mechanisms mediating these processes if they could be practically applied to the long-term storage of gametes or embryos.

9–2   DIFFERENTIATION

Differentiation might be called the true period of the embryo. It is a period when the cells are in the process of forming specific organs in the body of the embryo. Notable events during differentiation include the formation of the *germ layers, extraembryonic membrane,* and *organs.* In addition, rapid changes in relative size occur during differentiation.

9–2.1 *The Blastocyst*

The blastocyst stage is a transitory stage that prepares the embryo for formation of germ layers. There is some differentiation as a group of cells will congregate at the polar end of the blastocyst, forming the *inner cell mass* (Figure 9–1). The inner cell mass will, with time, form the body of the embryo. However, cells in this mound are still indeterminate and cannot be associated with formation of any specific organs. The remaining cells in the blastocyst form a wall, the trophoblast, around the blastocoele. When formed, the blastocyst is contained within the zona pellucida. As the blastocyst expands, it will press against the zona pellucida, causing it to thin. Cracks will appear in the zona pellucida and the blastocyst will escape (hatch) from the zona. This will occur by day 6 in sows, day 8 in ewes and mares, and day 12 in cows. Loss of the zona pellucida will permit the blastocyst to elongate. An exception is in mares, where the zona pellucida is replaced by an embryonic capsule that helps maintain the embryo in a spherical form until days 17 to 19, after which its membranes conform to the shape of the lumen of the uterus. Elongation of the blastocyst in cows and pigs is quite rapid.

9–2.2 *Germ Layers*

True differentiation begins with the appearance of the germ layers (Figure 9–3). These germ layers are the start of formation of organs and extraembryonic membranes. As these germ layers are differentiating in the inner cell mass, the germ cell layers that will form extraembryonic membranes push out from either end of the inner cell mass. The *endoderm*, the innermost germ layer, first appears when a single layer of cells pushes out from the inner cell mass and grows around the blastocoele. The endoderm is the origin of the digestive system, liver, lungs, and most other internal organs (Table 9–3). The *mesoderm*, the middle germ layer, arises from the inner cell mass, pushing between the endoderm and *ectoderm*. The mesoderm is the origin of the skeletal system, muscles, circulatory system, and reproductive system. The ectoderm, the outer germ layer, is the origin of the nervous system, sense organs, hair, skin, mammary glands, and hooves.

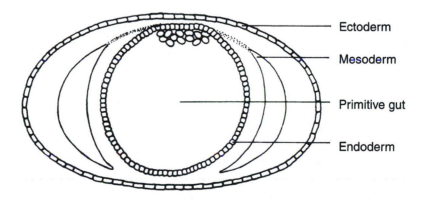

Figure 9–3 Germ layers as they appear in a section of an embryo 2 to 3 days after the start of differentiation. Not detailed in this illustration is the differentiation of these germ layers within the inner cell mass.

Table 9–3   *Certain organs that have been identified as forming from
specific germ layers*

Germ layer	Organs
Ectoderm	1. Central nervous system 2. Sense organs 3. Mammary glands 4. Sweat glands 5. Skin 6. Hair 7. Hooves
Mesoderm	1. Circulatory system 2. Skeletal system 3. Muscle 4. Reproductive systems (male and female) 5. Kidneys 6. Urinary ducts
Endoderm	1. Digestive system 2. Liver 3. Lungs 4. Pancreas 5. Thyroid gland 6. Most other glands

9–2.3 *Extraembryonic Membranes*

Soon after the appearance of the germ layers, formation of the extraembryonic membranes
will begin (Figure 9–4). Two extraembryonic membranes, the *amnion* and *allanto-chorion,*
will form during this period and function throughout the remainder of gestation. A third extraembryonic membrane, the *yolk sac,* is seen early during differentiation but will have dis-
appeared by the end of this stage of development. Endodermal and mesodermal layers form
the yolk sac and allantois while mesodermal and ectodermal layers form the amnion and
chorion (Figure 9–4). The yolk sac contains an early source of nutrients for the developing
embryo. As the yolk is depleted, the yolk sac regresses. A portion of the yolk sac is folded
into the embryo, forming its primitive gut.

The amnion, the inner extraembryonic membrane, forms as the *trophoderm* (outer
layer formed by fusion of ectoderm and mesoderm) folds around the embryo (Figure 9–4),
leaving an ectodermal layer on the inside of the amnion. The amnion contains fluids which
suspend the embryo, protecting it and permitting its free growth. During the period of differentiation, the fluid in the amnion will make it turgid. The amnion can be palpated by way
of the rectum in cows between 30 and 45 days, but its turgidity will not permit palpation of
the embryo. Since the embryo is quite fragile during this early period, the turgidity helps
maintain its shape and prevents injury during rectal palpation for pregnancy. As the amnion
enlarges, it becomes less turgid. By 60 days postfertilization, it will have softened enough
for the fetus to be palpated by rectal palpation. The amnionic fluid will continue to bathe
and suspend the fetus throughout gestation.

With formation of the amnion, the outer layer of extraembryonic membranes is called
the *chorion* rather than the trophoderm. The allanto-chorion, the outer extraembryonic mem-

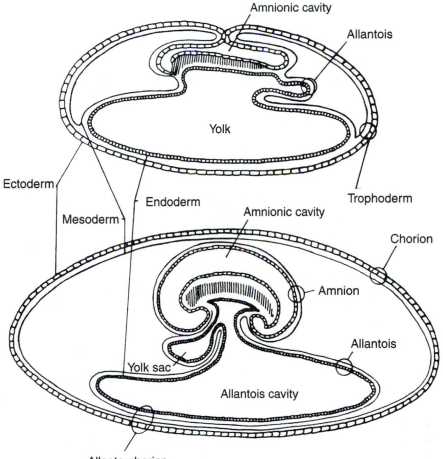

Figure 9–4 Progressive development of the extraembryonic membranes, including fusion of the chorioamnionic folds and the allantois with the chorion. (Redrawn from Patten. 1964. *Foundations of Embryology.* McGraw-Hill.)

brane, forms by a fusion of the chorion with the *allantois.* The beginning development of the allanto-chorion is illustrated in Figure 9–4. The allantois is a vascular membrane that is first seen as an outpouching of the hindgut. It connects to the embryonic bladder and contains fluids high in waste products. As the allantois enlarges, it fuses with the chorion until the allanto-chorion has completely formed around the amnion. The allanto-chorion becomes attached to the endometrium during placentation, forming the *placenta* (Color Plate 6). After placentation, oxygen and nutrients from maternal blood pass through the placental attachments into the embryonic circulation, which transports them to the developing embryo. Waste products, including ammonia and carbon dioxide from the embryo, are transported from embryonic blood through the placental attachments to maternal blood for elimination through the maternal system. Should the allanto-chorion not develop properly, the embryo would soon die from deprivation of oxygen and nutrients and/or buildup of toxic waste products.

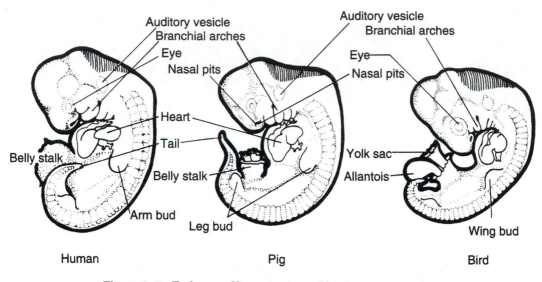

Figure 9–5 Embryos of human, pig, and bird at corresponding stages of development. (Redrawn from Patten. 1964. *Foundations of Embryology.* McGraw-Hill.)

9–2.4 *Organ Formation*

As formation of the extraembryonic membranes progresses, cells within the inner cell mass are differentiating. A neural plate forms from ectodermal cells as the beginning of the central nervous system. The primitive brain and spinal cord are quickly discernible. The circulatory system develops rapidly from mesodermal cells and by day 16 in the sow and by day 22 in the cow an embryonic heartbeat can be detected. The liver, pancreas, lungs, and digestive system can be identified as they differentiate from endodermal cells. Within a few days, limb buds, which will form legs, a tail bud, and the lens of the eye can be identified. At this stage of development, embryos from most species (including human embryos) are so similar in appearance that they cannot be distinguished as to species (Figure 9–5).

During the period when other organs are developing, the reproductive system will form. A dual duct system, the *Müllerian ducts* and the *Wolffian (mesonephric) ducts,* will appear in all embryos. Sexual differentiation will not have occurred. If the embryo is a genetic female, the pair of Müllerian ducts will develop into the female duct system. This includes the oviducts, uterus, cervix, and vagina. The Wolffian ducts will regress and disappear. If the embryo is a genetic male, the pair of Wolffian ducts will develop into the male duct system. The male duct system includes the vasa efferentia, epididymis, vas deferens, and urethra (Chapter 3). The Müllerian ducts regress and disappear in the male.

The embryonic gonads arise on either side of the dorsal wall of the abdomen. These first appear as *genital ridges,* slight thickenings near the kidneys. The indifferent gonad soon differentiates into an inner medulla and outer cortex. In the genetic male, *primary sex cords* arise and extend into the medulla, which develops into the testes as the cortex regresses. Primordial germ cells migrate from the hindgut of the embryo into the primary sex cords, which will later differentiate into seminiferous tubules and the rete testis. Primordial germ cells undergo mitotic divisions in the fetal testes. They form gonocytes, which differentiate into spermatogonia just before puberty.

In the genetic female, appearance of primary sex cords will be followed by *secondary sex cords,* which arise from the surface epithelium and remain in the cortex, which develops into the ovaries. Primordial germ cells from the hindgut are incorporated into the secondary sex cords. These cords later break up into isolated clusters of cells called primary follicles. As described in Chapter 2, they consist of an oogonium surrounded by a single layer of granulosa cells. A period of mitosis follows in the fetal period, during which thousands of primary follicles are formed. The ovaries form later and develop more slowly than the testes. In the female, the primary sex cords and medulla regress. Appearance of the secondary sex cords is an early distinguishing feature of the female.

The undifferentiated embryo is programmed to develop sexually as a female if no Y chromosome is present. The Y chromosome has an SRY gene (sex determining region Y), which stimulates the medulla of the embryonic gonad to differentiate into a testis with both Sertoli and Leydig cells as ovarian development is inhibited (Figure 9–6). This sets into motion the machinery for differentiation of the male reproductive system while inhibiting differentiation of female organs.

Sertoli cells in the embryonic testis secrete Müllerian inhibiting factor, which inhibits differentiation of Müllerian ducts while simultaneously Leydig cells are secreting testosterone, which initiates differentiation of Wolffian ducts into the male duct system.

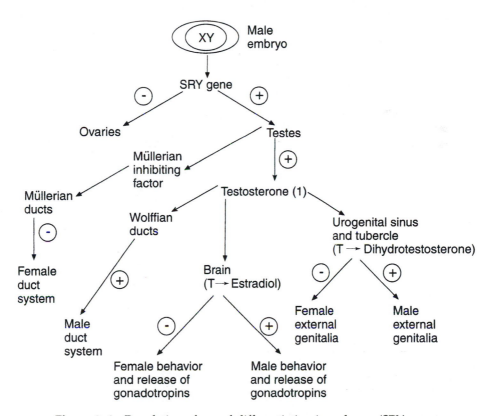

Figure 9–6 Regulation of sexual differentiation in embryos (SRY = sex determining region Y). (⊖ = inhibition; ⊕ = activation)

Cells in the urogenital sinus and genital tubercle have the enzyme 5α-reductase, which converts testosterone to dihydrotestosterone. Dihydrotestosterone stimulates differentiation of the urogenital sinus and genital tubercle into the external genitalia of the male. This entails migration of the genital tubercle from below the anus to the inguinal region. If either testosterone or 5α-reductase is deficient, the external genitalia will be female in appearance. With a 5α-reductase deficiency and normal testosterone, an individual otherwise differentiated as a male would have the external genitalia of the female. Cells in the brain associated with sexual behavior and the pattern of the release of GnRH have the enzyme aromatase, which converts testosterone to estradiol. This masculinizes the brain, resulting in development of male sexual behavior and a male pattern of release of gonadotropins. If testosterone or presumably aromatase is deficient, female behavior will be present, as will a cyclic release of gonadotropins as in the female. While the majority of this research has been done in the rat, it serves as a useful model for other mammalian species. Sexual differentiation of the brain occurs later in gestation than differentiation of reproductive organs.

Both relative rate of growth and formation of organs proceed rapidly during differentiation (Table 9–4). The period of differentiation starts about day 7 in the sow, 11 in the ewe, and 13 in the cow. It will be completed by day 28 in the sow, by day 45 in the ewe and the cow, and by day 50 in the mare. Primitive organs that appear early in the period of differentiation will be completely formed at the end of the period. The embryos at the end of this period will appear as miniature pigs, cows, sheep, or horses (Figure 9–7). The head will have filled out and facial features will be distinct. Legs, hooves, and tail will have formed. In the male, a scrotum can be identified. In the female, mammary buds and the vulva can be seen. The function of organs is limited at the end of differentiation, but everything necessary for the development into functional organs will be present. The period of differentiation is a critical period. Anything that interferes with normal differentiation will not be corrected later in the gestation after differentiation is completed. Drugs that interfere with normal differentiation of legs or eyes will appear as defects in the offspring after parturition. Likewise, therapy with reproductive hormones may interfere with normal sexual differentiation.

Table 9–4   *Developmental features in cattle and swine during differentiation*

Identifiable characteristics	First appearance	
	Cattle (days)	Swine (days)
Germ layer	14	8
Open neural tube	20	13
Fusion of chorioamnionic folds	18	16
Heartbeat	22	16
Allantois prominent	23	17
Fore limb bud	25	18
Hind limb bud	28	19
Lens of eye	30	21
Placentation	33	12
Facial features distinct	45	28

Adapted from Hafez. *Reproduction in Farm Animals.* (3rd ed.) Lea and Febiger. 1974.

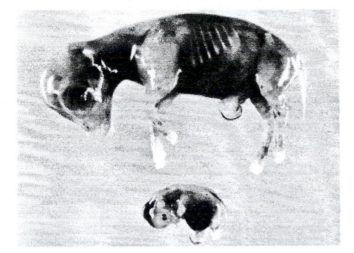

Figure 9–7 Fetal calf at 75 days of the gestation, compared with a 42-day embryo.

9–3 FETAL GROWTH

After differentiation is completed, the product of conception is called a *fetus* rather than an embryo. This portion of gestation, between the completion of differentiation and parturition, has been termed "the period of the fetus." The principal developmental feature of this period is growth.

Several landmarks in the development of the fetal calf have been identified. Calcification of bone matrix will start at about 70 days, with extensive bone formation having occurred by 180 days. Tooth formation will begin at about 110 days. Hair can be seen around the eyes and muzzle at 150 days (Color Plate 5), with hair covering the entire body by 230 days. In males, the testes will descend from the body cavity, through the inguinal canals into the scrotum. Descent of the testes will be completed by midgestation in bulls, but not until near the time of parturition in stallions.

The pattern of growth is interesting. If growth is expressed as relative change in size over a specified period, growth rate in the fetal calf increases for 2 to 3 months and then declines gradually for the rest of the gestation (Table 9–5). In one study, fetuses between 61 and 90 days into the gestation period averaged 72.6 g, as compared with 5.9 g for those between 31 and 60 days, a greater than 1,100% increase in size. When comparing fetuses between 241 and 270 days (28.6 kg) with those between 211 and 240 days (17.7 kg), the relative increase was about 62%. Male fetal calves are heavier than females before 100 days and maintain a higher rate of gain thereafter. Even though the relative rate of growth is slower during late gestation, over half of the total weight of the fetal calf at term is gained during the last 2 months. It is only during the last 2 months that the mother must be given an added increment of nutrients to account for the growing fetus.

Similar patterns of growth have been reported in sheep, with slower relative growth rates in late gestation than early gestation. Relative growth rate declines to a greater degree during late gestation when ewes are carrying twin fetuses (Table 9–6). If rate of growth is expressed as grams of gain per day, growth rate continues to increase to the end of gestation for single fetuses. If ewes are carrying twin fetuses, growth rate declines during the last month of the gestation period for ewes fed at 1.5 times maintenance, but continues to increase when

Table 9–5   *Weight changes of the bovine uterus and its contents during pregnancy*

Stage of gestation (days) (kg)	Total uterus and contents (gm)	Embryo or fetus (gm)	Amnionic fluids (gm)	Fetal membranes (kg)	Empty uterus
0–30	.9	.5	——	4.5	.9
31–60	1.6	5.9	181.6	49.5	1.4
61–90	2.3	72.6	590.2	149.8	1.5
91–120	4.0	531.4	1,600.0	258.8	1.7
	(kg)	(kg)	(kg)		
121–150	10.1	1.6	5.0	.7	2.8
151–180	14.6	3.8	5.5	1.3	4.1
181–210	23.8	9.5	6.4	2.5	5.5
211–240	37.4	17.7	10.0	2.4	7.3
241–270	53.8	28.6	11.8	3.4	10.0
271–300	67.8	39.9	15.4	3.8	8.6

From *Physiology of Reproduction and Artificial Insemination of Cattle.* G. W. Salisbury, N. L. VanDemark, and J. R. Lodge. W. H. Freeman Co., copyright © 1978.

Table 9–6   *Average daily growth rates and relative growth rates for single and twin fetal sheep at different stages of gestation*

Stage of gestation (days)	Avg daily growth rate (g/day)		Relative growth rate (%)	
	Singles	Twins	Singles	Twins
80–85	31	47	50.2	54.7
100–105	71	153	29.5	35.6
120–125	129	236	21.0	19.9
140–145	199	167[a]	16.4	8.2[a]
140–145		271[b]		12.0[b]

From Rattray et al. *J. Animal Sci.,* 38:613, 1974.

[a]Level of nutrition 1.5 × maintenance.

[b]Level of nutrition 2.0 × maintenance.

ewes are fed 2.0 times maintenance. This emphasizes the need for feeding pregnant females at a level well above maintenance during late gestation. If an adequate level of nutrition is maintained, rate of gain will be greater during late gestation than in earlier stages of gestation.

The weights of the fetal fluids, fetal membranes, and maternal uterus increase as gestation progresses. There is evidence that increases in fetal weight lag behind expansion of the allanto-chorion and accumulation of allantoic fluids within this membrane. This is logical in that the allanto-chorion is the medium of nutrient transfer from maternal blood. The expanded allanto-chorion provides more surface area for this exchange, thereby ensuring an adequate supply of nutrients to support growth of the fetus. Just before parturition in the cow, the fetal fluids weigh about 15.5 kg and the fetal membranes weigh about 3.8 kg. The uterus will increase from about 1.0 kg to 10 kg during the course of pregnancy. Even with the tenfold increase in the size of the uterus, the fetus and its associated fluids and membranes will account for about 85% of the total weight of the uterus and its contents.

9–4 MAINTENANCE OF PREGNANCY

Maintenance of pregnancy is largely dependent on a proper balance of hormones. This is evidenced by the fact that disturbance of the normal balance frequently results in abortion. Maintenance of the proper balance of hormones throughout the gestation period is dependent on an interplay among the mother, the placenta, and the conceptus (embryo or fetus).

9–4.1 *Maternal Recognition of Pregnancy*

Progesterone has a dominant role in maintenance of pregnancy, particularly during the early stages. If the uterus is not presented with an embryo by day 11 to 13 in pigs and sheep or 15 to 17 in cattle, $PGF_{2\alpha}$ will be released from the endometrium and be transported by a countercurrent circulation pattern to the ovary, where it causes regression of the corpus luteum (Section 2–7). If $PGF_{2\alpha}$ is injected during early pregnancy, the pregnancy will be terminated in all species. Therefore, the embryo must communicate its presence to the maternal system in some manner that prevents $PGF_{2\alpha}$-induced luteolysis. The biochemical process by which the embryo signals its presence is termed "maternal recognition of pregnancy."

In cattle and sheep, the embryonic unit produces a protein, called bovine interferon-τ and ovine interferon-τ, respectively (Section 4–5). In both species, these proteins have antiluteolytic properties through alteration of prostaglandin biosynthesis and regulation of uterine oxytocin receptors (Figure 9–8). Both bovine interferon-τ in cows and ovine interferon-τ in ewes have been reported to at least partially inhibit endometrial synthesis of $PGF_{2\alpha}$, possibly to levels below the luteolytic concentration. In ewes, ovine interferon-τ has been reported to increase the concentration of PGE_2 (an antiluteolytic hormone) in the venous plasma of pregnant sheep by day 13. Therefore, either through increased synthesis of PGE_2 or inhibited synthesis of $PGF_{2\alpha}$, the higher ratio of PGE_2 to $PGF_{2\alpha}$ would likely favor the corpus luteum-protecting properties of PGE_2. The current model of interferon-τ signaling in the cow, doe, and ewe is depicted in Figure 9–8 and includes those mechanisms described here as well as additional pathways through which interferon-τ may exert its conceptus-protective effects.

For mares, the critical period for the maternal recognition of pregnancy is 14 to 16 days after ovulation. The embryonic signal to the maternal unit appears to involve inhibition of synthesis and/or release of $PGF_{2\alpha}$ by the endometrium. The nature of this embryonic signal has not been identified. Both proteins and estrogens are secreted by the embryo during the critical period.

In the sow as in other species, $PGF_{2\alpha}$ is the luteolytic substance produced by the uterus that causes regression of the corpus luteum in nonpregnant animals. However, estradiol is the antiluteolytic signal from the embryo to the maternal unit that is needed for maternal recognition and maintenance of pregnancy. Pig blastocysts produce estrogen on days 11 and 12 and pseudopregnancy can be induced in sows by administering estrogens during days 11 to 15. A minimum of four blastocysts is needed to maintain pregnancy.

Estrogens do not alter the synthesis of $PGF_{2\alpha}$ by the endometrium. Rather, estrogens cause it to be excreted into and sequestered in the lumen of the uterus, as opposed to being secreted into the utero-ovarian vein as an endocrine product. Therefore, $PGF_{2\alpha}$ does not reach the ovary by the countercurrent route that functions during a normal estrous cycle (Section 2–7), and the corpus luteum is maintained.

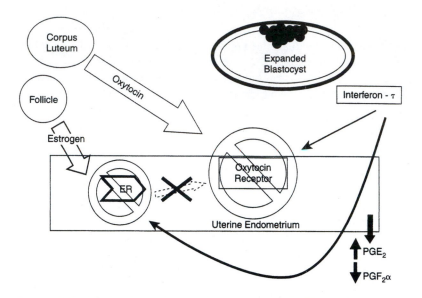

Figure 9–8   Mechanisms of action for interferon-τ (INF-τ) on the uterine endometrium of the cow, doe, and ewe. The expanded blastocyst (conceptus) secretes INF-τ, which prevents luteolysis and establishes maternal recognition of pregnancy. The primary mechanism for doing this appears to be mediated through INF-τ inhibition of oxytocin receptors on uterine endometrial cells. This may come about directly or indirectly via the inhibition of estrogen receptor (ER) synthesis. Estrogens, acting though the ER, can up-regulate oxytocin receptors. By inhibiting the synthesis of estrogen receptors, this pathway is effectively blocked. The reduction or absence of oxytocin receptors results in an inability of oxytocin to be received by the endometrial cells, thus decreasing oxytocin-induced prostaglandin $F_{2\alpha}$ ($PGF_{2\alpha}$) production. Inhibitory actions of INF-τ on enzymatic pathways (cyclooxygenases) important for $PGF_{2\alpha}$ conversion from arachidonic acid have also been confirmed (not depicted). In the ewe, prostaglandin synthesis appears to be redirected to also increase the production of PGE_2, an antiluteolytic hormone.

9–4.2 *Functions of Hormones*

High concentrations of progesterone decrease the tone of the myometrium and inhibit uterine contractions. The role of progesterone in down-regulating receptor sites for estradiol and oxytocin in the myometrium is largely responsible for these effects. In addition to its effect on the myometrium, high progesterone will stop cyclic estrus by preventing the cyclic release of gonadotropins. Progesterone is produced by both the corpus luteum and the placenta.

The sow and doe are completely dependent on the corpus luteum as the primary source of progesterone throughout most of gestation. In the cow, lutectomy (removal of the corpus luteum or an injection with $PGF_{2\alpha}$) late in gestation, after 6 to 8 months of pregnancy, may not always cause abortion as a result of sufficient placental steroidogenesis. In the ewe, placental take-over can occur as early as 50 days of gestation; in the mare, by 70 days of gestation. While the placenta may take over as a primary source of progesterone early in gestation for some species, the corpus luteum continues to secrete progesterone throughout gestation

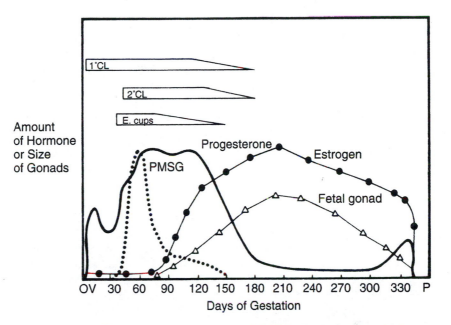

Figure 9–9 Progesterone, estrogen, and PMSG concentrations during pregnancy in the mare. (Stabenfelt and Hughes. 1977. *Reproduction in Domestic Animals.* (3rd ed.) eds. Cole and Cupps. Academic Press.)

and contributes to the maintenance of pregnancy regardless. Pregnancy-specific protein, protein B (Section 4–5) may help maintain the corpus luteum of pregnancy in cows and ewes. This reproductive function is more complex in mares (Figure 9–9). The corpus luteum which forms at the ovulation site is active for 150 to 180 days. Secretion of PMSG by the endometrial cups results in formation of accessory corpora lutea by luteinization of small tertiary follicles. These form by 40 days postfertilization and actively secrete progesterone until 150 to 180 days. After 150 to 180 days postfertilization, progesterone necessary for maintenance of pregnancy in the mare must come from the placenta. All corpora lutea regress at this time. A drop in progesterone at this time corresponds to an increase in estrogen.

Relaxin and relaxin-like factors, polypeptides produced by the corpus luteum (sow and cow) and the placenta (mare), are important during gestation. Their primary role appears to be the softening of connective tissue, which permits the uterine muscles to stretch to accommodate the growing fetus. Relaxin will cause the pelvic canal to expand, particularly during late gestation. There is greater increase in pelvic width, but pelvic height is increased, also. In the pig, relaxin secretion increases above basal concentration but remains relatively low during most of the gestation period. At about 100 days, it surges, reaching a peak about 14 hours prepartum. Thereafter, it drops but is still fairly high at time of parturition. Concentrations, while lower in cows than sows, increase during late gestation.

Concentrations of estrogens are low during early gestation but increase during middle and late gestation. In mares, estrogen levels are quite high during the latter half of gestation. The primary source of these estrogens is the placenta. Estrogens are a regulator of the progressive increases in uterine blood flow that occur as gestation progresses. Also, estrogens synergize with progesterone in development and preparation of the mammary gland for synthesis of milk after parturition. Placental lactogen likely has a role in development of the mammary gland as well as being a regulator of fetal growth.

Other primary hormones of reproduction do not appear to have a dominant role during gestation. Low concentrations with little variation are usually found in the blood. Normal function of the thyroid, parathyroid, adrenal cortex, and other endocrine glands which produce secondary hormones of reproduction are important to maintenance of a metabolic state in the mother which permits proper embryonic and fetal development.

A number of endocrine changes occur near the end of the gestation period. These will be discussed in the next chapter as they relate to parturition.

9–4.3 *Immunological Considerations*

A major concern when foreign tissues (e.g., organs) are transplanted into an animal is that an immune response will occur which results in rejection of that tissue. This occurs because the foreign tissue has proteins that are antigenic (initiate an immune reaction) and stimulate production of host lymphocytes that cause the rejection. This is a potential problem with maintenance of pregnancy because the embryo/fetus inherits antigens from the father that could potentially lead to activation of tissue rejection responses by the mother, resulting in loss of the pregnancy.

Several factors guard against the tissue rejection response when the embryo/fetus joins with the uterus during placentation. The most important factor may be that the parts of the placenta that contact the endometrium have low antigenicity because the major histocompatibility antigens are absent. This is a result of fetal gene expression in the placenta. Progesterone, also, is a regulator of immune function and plays a role. Although progesterone can directly inhibit lymphocyte function, placental progesterone is probably not high enough during placentation to have this effect. There is evidence that progesterone from the corpus luteum does stimulate secretion of molecules from the endometrium that block lymphocyte proliferation. Interferon-τ, which is secreted by the trophoblast and plays a key role in preventing regression of the corpus luteum in cattle and sheep (Section 9–4.1), has been shown to block lymphocyte proliferation. Therefore, the low antigenicity of the placenta and the inhibitory properties of progesterone and interferon-τ on lymphocytes appear sufficient to prevent the immunological reactions that would result in rejection and loss of the pregnancy.

9–5   TWINNING

Twinning sometimes occurs in monotocous species. It occurs more frequently in sheep and goats than in cattle. The percentage of lambs per lambing may exceed 150% for some flocks, and lambing rates of 120% to 140% are not uncommon. Twinning rate is higher for October and November matings than for those made earlier in the breeding season or in the spring (late in the breeding season). Some breeds have higher twinning rates than others. For example, the Finn breed has a twinning rate greater than 150%.

Twinning is not considered undesirable in sheep, in that it increases the number of lambs that are weaned in a given year. Double ovulations occur in about 25% of all estrous cycles in the mare, but twinning in mares is very undesirable. Only 9% of the conceived twins are carried to term. Of those, both foals are born dead 64.5% of the time, one foal is born alive 21% of the time, and live twins are born 14.5% of the time. Both of the live twins are small and weak and one usually dies in 3 or 4 days. Approximately 60% of mares with twin embryos give birth to a single, live foal, while 31% lose both fetuses, usually by abortion. Current recommendations are to breed mares that have two large follicles, which increases initial pregnancy rate from 50% to 75%. The embryonic vesicle becomes fixed in the uterus between 15 and 17 days, so ultrasound can be used at that time to determine whether twins are present. If so, and if they are fixed separately, one can be manually destroyed by pinching. Those that are fixed together should be left and 75% to 90% will be naturally reduced to a single by 40 days. This group of mares should be reexamined by ultrasound at 40 days and the few mares still carrying twins should be aborted with $PGF_{2\alpha}$. Twinning rates in cattle are relatively low, ranging from 0.5% to 4% for different breeds (Color Plate 6). In some herds, rates of 8% to 10% have been reported. Twinning rates for Brown Swiss and Holsteins are higher than for Jerseys and Guernseys, and dairy cows have higher twinning rates than beef cows. The twinning rate in most beef breeds is less than 1%. Twinning has not been considered desirable in cattle because of increased incidence of retained placentae, reduction in future reproductive efficiency, weaker calves that are more difficult to raise, and reduced milk production by cows after twinning.

The heritability of twinning is low. A higher incidence of twinning has been reported for certain cow families, but long-term selection studies to increase twinning have not greatly increased the twinning rate. Twinning seldom occurs in *primiparous* (first gestation) females. The incidence of twinning increases with age for the next several years and then declines. These age effects are reported for both cattle and sheep. Increasing the level of nutrition will increase the incidence of twinning in sheep. While not clearly demonstrated, level of nutrition may be a factor in cattle and could account for some of the difference between dairy and beef breeds. Seasonal effects on twinning have been reported but may be related to seasonal changes in available feed. Increased twinning can be expected after hormone therapy for cystic ovaries or for other reproductive disorders.

Most twins are of the *dizygous* type. That is, they result from ovulation of two oocytes during the same estrous cycle. These oocytes are fertilized and eventually implanted in the uterus, where they are carried until parturition. They may be the same sex or opposite in sex. They are no more alike than siblings with the same parents born from different gestations.

Some twins are *monozygous*, resulting from fertilization of a single oocyte. Monozygous twins are always the same sex and are genetically and phenotypically identical, except that one is frequently larger than the other. The means by which a single zygote can result in twins is not known. Theories that have been advanced include both (1) separation of the zygotic cells after the first cleavage with each cell developing independently and (2) formation of two inner cell masses within the same blastocyst (Figure 9–10). Other theories involving aberrations in differentiation have been advanced. About 8% to 10% of all twin births in cattle are monozygous. About 30% of all human twins are monozygous with a higher loss during the gestation than with dizygous twins. Embryo loss and abortion may account for the lower percentage of monozygous twins in cattle.

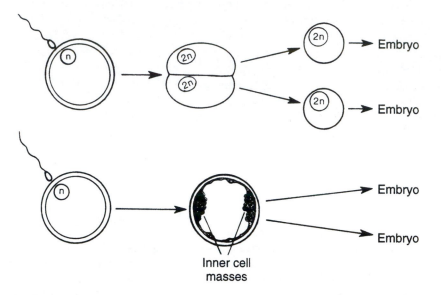

Inner cell
masses

Figure 9–10   Two theories on development of monozygous twins.

SUGGESTED READING

ANDERSON, G. B. 1991. Fertilization, early embryo development and embryo transfer. *Reproduction in Domestic Animals* (4th ed.) ed. P. T. Cupps. Academic Press.

AREY, L. B. 1974. *Developmental Anatomy.* (7th ed.) W. B. Saunders Co.

BETTERIDGE, K. J. 1995. Phylogeny, ontogeny and embryo transfer. *Theriogenology,* 44:1061.

ELEY, R. M., W. W. THATCHER, F. W. BAZER, C. J. WILCOX, R. B. BECKER, H. H. HEAD, and R. W. ADKINSON. 1978. Development of the conceptus in the bovine. *J. Dairy Sci.,* 61:467.

ELLINWOOD, W. E., T. M. NETT, and G. D. NISWENDER. 1979. Maintenance of the corpus luteum of early pregnancy in the ewe. II. Prostaglandin secretion by the endometrium *in vitro* and *in vivo. Biol. Reprod.,* 21:845.

GOMES, W. R., 1978. Gestation. *Physiology of Reproduction and Artificial Insemination of Cattle.* (2nd ed.) eds. G. W. Salisbury, N. L. VanDemark, and J. R. Lodge. W. H. Freeman and Co.

GROSS, T. S., M. C. LACROIX, F. W. BAZER, W. W. THATCHER, and J. P. HARVEY. 1988. Prostaglandin secretion by perfused porcine endometrium: Further evidence for an endocrine versus exocrine secretion of prostaglandins. *Prostaglandins,* 35:327.

HANSEN, P. J., 2002. Pregnancy—Physiology. *Encyclopedia of Dairy Sciences.* eds. H. Roginski, J. W. Fuquay, and P. F. Fox, Academic Press, an imprint of Elsevier Science.

KING, G. 2002, Pregnancy—Characteristics. *Encyclopedia of Dairy Sciences.* eds. H. Roginski, J. W. Fuquay, and P. F. Fox. Academic Press, An Imprint of Elsevier Science.

LUKASZEWSKA, J. and W. HANSEL. 1980. Corpus luteum maintenance during early pregnancy in the cow. *J. Reprod. Fertil.,* 59:485.

McLAREN, A. 1982. The embryo. *Reproduction in Mammals. 2. Embryonic and Fetal Development.* eds. C. R. Austin and R.V. Short. Cambridge University Press.

RATTRAY, P. V., W. N. GARRETT, N. E. EAST, and N. HINMAN. 1974. Growth, development and composition of the ovine conceptus and mammary gland during pregnancy. *J. Anim. Sci.,* 38:613.

ROBERTS, R. M., P. V. MALATKY, T. R. HANSEN, C. E. FARIN, and K. IMAKAWA. 1990. Bovine conceptus products involved in pregnancy recognition. XIX Biennial Symposium on Animal Reproduction. *J. Anim. Sci.* (Suppl. 2). 68:28.

SHARP, D. C., M. T. ZAVY, M. W. VERNON, F. W. BAZER, W. W. THATCHER, and L. A. BERGLUND. 1984. The role of prostaglandins in maternal recognition of pregnancy in mares. *Anim. Reprod. Sci.,* 7:269.

SHORT, R. V. 1982. Sex determination and differentiation. *Reproduction in Mammals. 2. Embryonic and Fetal Development.* eds. C. R. Austin and R. V. Short. Cambridge University Press.

SWETT, W. W., C. A. MATHEWS, and M. H. FOHRMAN. 1948. Development of the fetus in the dairy cow. *U.S. Dept. Agr. Tech. Bull.* 964.

VALLET, J. L., F. W. BAZER, M. F. V. FLISS, and W. W. THATCHER. 1988. Effect of ovine conceptus proteins and purified bovine trophoblast protein-1 on interoestrus internal and plasma concentrations of prostaglandin $F_2\alpha$ and E and of 13, 14-dihydro-15-keto prostaglandin $F_2\alpha$ in cyclic ewes. *J. Reprod. Fert.,* 84:493.

WILSON, J. D. 1978. Sexual differentiation. *Ann. Rev. Physiol.,* 40:279.

10

Parturition and Postpartum Recovery

10–1 OVERVIEW OF THE PARTURITION PROCESS

Parturition is the birth process. It begins with softening and initial dilation of the cervix along with the start of uterine contractions. It ends when the fetus and its associated placental membranes are expelled. The time required for parturition varies among individuals and among species (Table 10–1).

Parturition can be divided into three stages. Stage 1 starts with softening and initial dilation of the cervix and ends with complete dilation of the cervix and entry of the fetus into the cervix. Uterine contractions start during this stage. The time required for this stage is 1 to 4 hours in mares, 2 to 6 hours in cows and ewes, and 2 to 12 hours in sows.

Stage 2 extends from complete dilation of the cervix until the fetus is expelled. During this period, uterine contractions are regular and strong. In all species, less time is required for this stage than for the first stage, usually taking no more than 2 hours in cows and ewes. A similar time is required in sows, but the time varies with the size of the litter. The second stage is completed in 15 to 20 minutes in mares. In the mare, fetal expulsion must be rapid (Color Plate 10). The placental membranes become separated from the uterus, and the foal will suffocate if a longer time is required. The first two stages take longer in first-gestation females of all species than in *multiparous* (second or later gestation) females.

Expulsion of the placenta occurs during Stage 3. Uterine contractions continue during this phase, although less intensely than during Stage 2. Expulsion is rapid in mares, frequently being completed in less than 30 minutes. In sows, this phase is completed in 1 to 4 hours after expulsion of the last piglet. In cattle and sheep, expulsion may occur in as little as 30 minutes after expulsion of the fetus but is more likely to occur 3 to 5 hours later.

10–2 APPROACHING PARTURITION

Signs of approaching parturition can be seen during the last month of the gestation. Careful evaluation of these signs will indicate when the female will need to be observed closely.

10–2.1 *Rotation to Birth Position*

For monotocous species such as the ewe, doe, mare, and cow, the first event signaling parturition may be the rotation of the fetus into the birth position. During most of the gestation

Table 10–1   *Average time required for the three stages of parturition for different species of farm animals*

Animal	Stage		
	1 (hours)	2 (hours)	3 (hours)
Cow	2–6	0.5–2	4–5
Ewe	2–6	0.5–2	0.5–8
Sow	2–12	1–4	1–4
Mare	1–4	0.15–0.5	0.5–3

Compiled from Roberts. *Veterinary Obstetrics and Genital Diseases.* Pub. by author. Ithaca, N.Y. 1971.

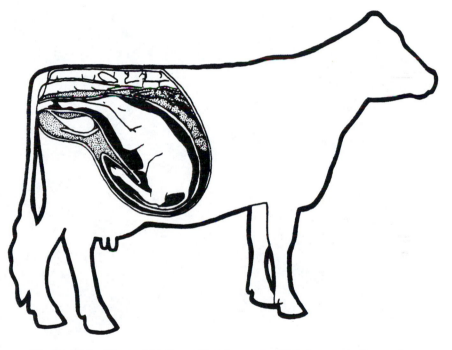

Figure 10–1   Normal birth position in cows which is assumed near the end of the gestation period. (G.W. Salisbury, N.L. VanDemark, and J.R. Lodge. *Physiology of Reproduction and Artificial Insemination of Cattle.* (2nd ed.) W.H. Freeman and Co., copyright © 1978.)

in these species, the fetus will be on its back, with its feet pointing up. After rotation into the birth position, it will be resting on its thorax or abdomen, with its forefeet positioned at the uterine end of the cervix and its nose resting between the forefeet (Figure 10–1). Parturition proceeds more easily when the fetus is in this position, except in pigs, where both front and back delivery proceed with equal ease.

Abnormal positions are sometimes seen and occur more frequently with twins. The incidence of abnormal presentations is about 5% in cattle, with a variety of abnormalities

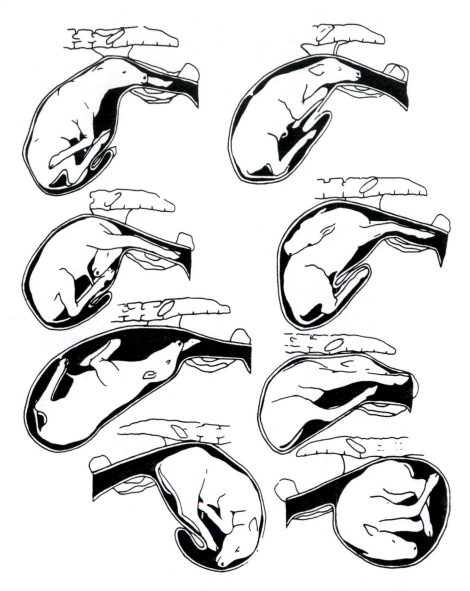

Figure 10–2   Abnormal birth positions that may be seen in cows. (*Diseases of Cattle.* 1942. USDA Special Report.)

possible (Figure 10–2). This ranges from one leg to both legs or the head turned back to several breech positions with the tail pointed toward the cervix. In those cases where the normal birth position is not assumed, assistance in delivery of the fetus is usually required. This involves repositioning the fetus to the normal position. The process of repositioning the fetus may break the umbilical cord. Should this happen, the fetus will suffocate if it is not quickly removed from the uterus. Assistance from a veterinarian is advised in cases of abnormal presentations. The cause (or causes) of rotation of the fetus into normal or abnormal positions is not known. The action of relaxin in expanding the pelvis may facilitate this movement, in addition to providing a larger birth canal.

10–2.2 *Mammary Gland Changes*

Growth of the mammary glands can be seen during the last part of the gestation. This is likely caused by the synergistic actions of estrogens and progestins, which stimulate development of both ducts and secretory tissue in the mammary glands. As parturition approaches, the mammary glands will enlarge as they fill with milk. Synthesis of milk is a function of prolactin in synergism with other hormones (Chapter 11). As oxytocin is released during labor, milk letdown will occur, frequently causing milk to leak from the teats.

10–2.3 *Other Changes*

With parturition imminent, relaxin synergizing with estrogen will cause further expansion of the pelvis, enlarging the birth canal to facilitate passage of the fetus. A sinking around the tailhead due to relaxation of pelvic ligaments will make the tailhead appear more prominent. The vulva will soften and become swollen. Mucus may be seen stringing from the vulva as estrogen causes the epithelial cells of the cervix to secrete new mucus, loosening the mucous plug. A "nesting instinct" thought to be stimulated by prolactin will be seen. The sow will actually build a nest. While cows do not build nests, they will try to leave the herd, seeking a place of seclusion during parturition.

10–3 PARTURITION

Approximately 2 days before the start of parturition a rapid sequence of changes in hormone levels involving both the fetus and mother can be seen (Figure 10–3).

10–3.1 *Hormonal Initiation*

The hormone pattern established during the latter part of the gestation period sets the stage for parturition. High levels of progesterone, relaxin, and estrogen are present during late gestation. About 48 hours before parturition, there is a rapid changes in the patterns of these maternal hormones. The concentration of progesterone drops precipitously, while estrogens and relaxin increase in concentration, as do $PGF_{2\alpha}$ and oxytocin. The signal that triggers these changes is a surge in fetal cortisol; therefore, the fetus initiates the start of parturition. This was first discovered in sheep in the 1960s, when it was observed that removal of the fetal pituitary gland, and therefore ACTH, prevented the surge of cortisol from the fetal adrenal and resulted in abolition of the initiation of parturition. Subsequently, the concept of fetal initiation of parturition through secretion of cortisol was demonstrated in a number of other mammalian species. In cows, does, and sows, the rise in fetal cortisol causes production and greater release of estrogens by the placenta, which initiates release of $PGF_{2\alpha}$ from

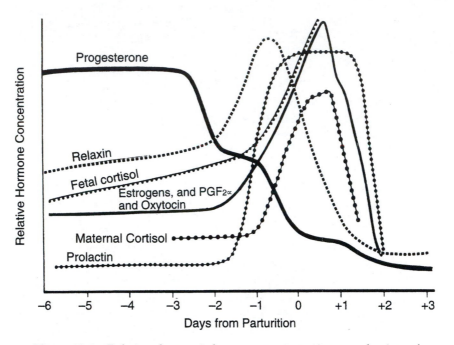

Figure 10–3   Relative changes in hormone concentration near the time of parturition. (From literature.)

a. Fetal cortisol is released, resulting in a higher concentration of estrogens (all species) and a lower concentration of progesterone (ewes).

b. Estrogens stimulate greater synthesis and release of $PGF_{2\alpha}$ from the endometrium, which reduces progesterone secretions in sows, does, and cows.

c. Relaxin in sows increases sharply, reaching a peak about 14 hours prepartum, and then declines rapidly.

d. Oxytocin release increases tend to parallel that of $PGF_{2\alpha}$ and reach a peak during expulsion of the fetus.

e. Surges in maternal cortisol and prolactin do not have direct roles in the parturition process.

the uterus, causing regression of corpora lutea and a marked drop in progesterone concentration. In ewes, a similar sequence is seen, but the order differs. The placenta is the major source of progesterone in the ewe during late pregnancy. It appears that the rise in fetal cortisol causes changes in placental enzymes, which result in conversion of placental progesterone to estrogens. Placental estrogens cause release of $PGF_{2\alpha}$ from the uterus of the ewe, but the decrease in progesterone is seen before the rise in $PGF_{2\alpha}$. Thus, for all species studied, fetal cortisol will initiate a sequence of changes that includes a sharply reduced level of progesterone with increased concentrations of estrogen and $PGF_{2\alpha}$ in the blood serum of the mother prior to the start of parturition.

In one research report, relaxin in sows increased prior to parturition and then decreased rapidly. The concentration 3 days prepartum was 12 ng/ml but increased to 145 ng/ml by 14 hours prepartum. Just preceding parturition, it decreased to 42 ng/ml and at 1 hour postpartum the level was 1 ng/ml.

Less is known about relaxin concentrations in other species, but higher concentrations have been reported during late pregnancy than during early or midpregnancy in cows. Oxytocin is released as movement of the fetus stimulates sensory nerves in the cervix and vagina. The highest concentration is seen during expulsion of the fetus, with a small surge seen during expulsion of the placenta. The greater release of $PGF_{2\alpha}$ at this time may be caused by oxytocin. An increase in maternal cortisol near the start of parturition is probably due to the stress of parturition on the mother and is not involved in the regulation of parturition. Surges in maternal cortisol and prolactin near the start of parturition are stress responses that have positive regulatory influences on milk synthesis.

Less is known about endocrine patterns near time of parturition in mares, but some differences are apparent. Progesterone concentrations remain low in late gestation, whereas an increase in total progestins occurs during the last 20 prepartum days. A marked drop in progestins and estrogens occurs a few hours before parturition. Dexamethasone (a synthetic glucocorticoid), progesterone, and $PGF_{2\alpha}$ will induce parturition. Based on this, it appears that fetal cortisol and $PGF_{2\alpha}$ play roles similar to that for the ewe during the parturition process. The role of progesterone is in contrast to most other species, where infusion of progesterone will delay parturition.

10–3.2 *Regulation of the Physiological Events*

The main physiological events in parturition are (a) dilation of the cervix, which permits the fetus to pass, and (b) uterine contractions, which forcefully expel the fetus and placental membranes.

As parturition approaches, the cervix changes from a firm and inelastic organ to one that is soft and distensible. This change, called "cervical ripening," is a result of remodeling of connective tissue from tight bands to dispersed fibers, which with the increased uptake of water softens the cervix and allows for cervical expansion. The initial dilation of the cervix is caused by relaxin as it synergizes with rising levels of estrogen. Working together, these hormones soften the cervix and cause the epithelial cells to secrete mucus. Further dilation occurs as uterine contractions force the allanto-chorion and later the amnion against the cervix. Complete dilation occurs as the fetus is forced into the cervix. The allanto-chorion may break during this process, but the amnion usually does not break until after the fetus enters the cervix.

A number of factors contribute to the initiation and continuation of uterine contractions which occur concurrently with dilation of the cervix and then continue for several hours after expulsion of the fetus. The reduced level of progesterone removes the inhibition to contractions. With progesterone low, rising levels of estrogens up-regulate uterine receptors for both estradiol and oxytocin in the myometrium, thus increasing the responsiveness of the myometrium to oxytocin.

The initial uterine contractions are probably caused by $PGF_{2\alpha}$ as it is released from the endometrium by rising estrogen levels. These early contractions are weak and irregular, occurring at about 15-minute intervals. They become progressively stronger and more frequent as parturition proceeds. As the fetus is pushed into the cervix, stimulation of sensory nerves causes release of oxytocin from the posterior pituitary. The increased release of oxytocin is accompanied by greater release of $PGF_{2\alpha}$. Oxytocin, by direct action on the myometrium and/or indirectly through stimulation of greater release of $PGF_{2\alpha}$, causes uterine contractions to be stronger, more rhythmic, and more frequent. Concentrations of both oxytocin and $PGF_{2\alpha}$ peak during expulsion of the fetus. Since both have similar release patterns and similar effects on the myometrium, the question of whether their actions are dependent or independent has not been resolved.

Fetal motility due to anoxia (low oxygen) may be another factor contributing to stronger contractions near the completion of the stage when the fetus is expelled. As uterine muscles contract, reducing the blood flow to the fetus, its oxygen supply will be reduced, causing the increased activity associated with anoxia. The mechanical movement of the fetus pushing against uterine muscles that are in a sensitized and contracting state evokes a stronger contractile response from these muscles. Just before expulsion of the fetus, uterine contractions will be regular, strong, and frequent, occurring at about 2-minute intervals and lasting for approximately 1 minute. Contraction of abdominal muscles will aid final expulsion. Following expulsion of the fetus, the strong uterine contractions subside. However, diminished contractions will continue for another 1 or 2 days. The continued contractions are responsible for expulsion of the placental membranes as well as fluids and fragments of placental tissues that may remain in the uterus. A secondary surge in oxytocin is associated with expulsion of the placenta.

10–3.3 *Induced Parturition*

Livestock managers have indicated a need for a safe and effective means of inducing parturition. While marginal, some possible advantages are

1. To group parturitions for cows that would normally be spread over 1 or 2 weeks and for sows that would normally be spread over 3 or 4 days into 24 hours to facilitate closer observation. $PGF_{2\alpha}$ can be safely used to induce parturition in sows, if given no more than 3 days before expected parturition. It is important to know the average gestation length for the herd involved?
2. To have more offspring of a uniform age and size at time of marketing
3. To shorten gestation and generation interval
4. For medical reasons such as pregnancy toxemia or large fetuses

10–3.3a Advantages and Disadvantages   At the present time, the disadvantages far outweigh the advantages. In sheep, the treatments for inducing parturition are effective only when administered very near to term. This requires that the exact breeding dates be known and even then only very small groupings can be accomplished. In cattle, the incidence of retained placentae is very high following induced parturition. In some studies, more than 50% of treated cows retained their placentae. One study utilizing a small number of cows indicated that an injection of 6 mg of estradiol benzoate IM at the time of induction treatment reduced the incidence of retained placentae. Another, more complete study showed that estradiol-17β, estradiol-17α, and estrone were not effective in reducing the incidence of retained placentae.

10–3.3b Techniques   It has been established that the fetus initiates parturition in sheep and that an intact hypothalamic-pituitary-adrenal axis in the fetus is required. This and other data have led scientists to accept fetal cortisol as the compound that triggers parturition (Section 10–3.1).

Induction of parturition has been accomplished in both cattle and sheep by IM injections of dexamethasone and other corticoids into the dam. $PGF_{2\alpha}$ and its more potent analog will also induce parturition in these species, but these materials are less reliable and predictable. A thorough understanding of the endocrinology of parturition will help one visualize means by which parturition may be induced.

10–4 DYSTOCIA

Dystocia is defined as prolonged and difficult parturition, with assistance frequently being required. It is common with oversized fetuses in cattle (46% of all dystocias in beef cattle) and in sheep and cattle with twin pregnancies, which often result in abnormal birth positions. For beef cattle, abnormal birth positions represent 26% of all dystocias, but only about 5% of all parturitions with abnormal presentations of the fetus require assistance. Dystocias due to an oversized fetus or abnormal birth position can be the result of cattle with a small pelvic diameter, especially in primiparous females (heifers). It is common in 2-year-old heifers that were bred below their recommended weight for breeding to experience dystocia at calving, as compared with heifers bred above their recommended breeding weight. Dystocias are also more frequent with male fetuses than with female fetuses.

Dystocia is a major cause of calf losses around the time of birth in beef cows. Further, retained placentae and postpartum reproductive problems are more frequent after dystocia. Postpartum estrus is delayed, fertility is reduced, calving interval is extended, and fewer calves are born the next year after dystocia. Calf size at birth is a heritable trait and artificial insemination businesses have identified calving ease bulls that are recommended for use on heifers. Another safeguard is to not breed young females when below their recommended breeding weight (55% of mature size in cattle and 65% of mature size in sheep).

10–5 CARE OF THE NEWBORN

Reproduction is not successfully completed unless the neonate (newborn) survives. The first few hours after expulsion from the uterus are critical to its survival. It has been transferred from a germ-free environment in which its temperature regulation, nutrient, and oxygen requirements have been dependent on the maternal system to an environment where it must survive independently.

Immediate changes must occur in the circulatory and respiratory systems. The umbilical artery has been taking blood saturated with carbon dioxide to the placenta, where the carbon dioxide is exchanged for oxygen and then returned to the fetal heart through the umbilical vein to be pumped throughout the fetus. Fetal lungs have been present but have not been functioning as a respiratory organ. Most of the blood reaching the fetal heart bypasses the lungs by diversion into a parallel system that functions in the fetus. As the fetus passes through the vulva, its umbilical cord breaks, severing the neonate from the maternal system. Immediate survival depends on the cessation of circulation in the umbilical vessels along with the routing of blood through the lungs rather than through the parallel system that functioned in the fetus. In addition, respiration must start to oxygenate the blood as it circulates through the lungs. Increasing levels of carbon dioxide stimulate the respiratory center in the brain, thus initiating respiration.

The neonate is more susceptible to extremes in environmental temperature than is an older animal whose thermoregulatory mechanisms have had time to adjust to fluctuating environmental temperatures. In cold environments, the rectal temperature of some species has been reported to drop several degrees within a few hours after birth. In both extremely hot and extremely cold environments, neonatal survival is reduced.

A time for adjustment to absorption of nutrients from the digestive system, along with their metabolism and utilization, is needed, also. A neonate has a relatively large amount of glycogen stored in its liver and muscles to be utilized during this adjustment period. Climatic stress speeds the depletion of these reserves.

The neonate's immune system has not been challenged. Therefore, it does not have circulating antibodies to ward off diseases. Maternal antibodies do not pass through the placental barrier to fetal blood in cattle, goats, sheep, swine, or horses. Maternal antibodies can be absorbed through the intestines if the newborn receives a meal of *colostrum* (the first milk) from its mother soon after parturition. There is evidence that the newborn loses the ability to absorb maternal antibodies through the intestines as early as 6 hours after birth. Stress from high temperature reduces absorption of maternal antibodies. Other stresses may also reduce antibody absorption.

An animal caretaker who is aware of the challenges to the survival of the neonate will likely take steps to increase the chances of survival. When the umbilical veins and arteries break, they will be retracted into the stump of the umbilical cord. Very little loss of blood will occur. The umbilical stump should be painted with an antiseptic solution such as iodine to lessen the chance of infection. The respiratory passages should be checked for pieces of placental membrane or mucus that could prevent respiration. If breathing has not started, it might be stimulated by slapping the neonate or by giving artificial respiration. One should not expect a high success rate in cases where respiration has not started spontaneously.

In cold weather, the newborn should be dried and if possible placed in a clean, dry shelter. In the summer, a shade will be beneficial to survival. If the newborn has not nursed within the first hour, it should be assisted in obtaining a meal of colostrum, to provide both nutrients and antibodies. If the mother dies during parturition, colostrum from another female of the same species should be provided in a pail or bottle with a nipple. Normal milk will provide most needed nutrients but will not contain the needed antibodies (Chapter 11).

10–6   RETAINED PLACENTAE

During normal parturition in the sow and mare, the placental membranes become separated from the endometrium during fetal expulsion. The continued contractions of the uterus expel these membranes, with retention seldom occurring. Although rare in mares, it is considered serious if it occurs because of the resulting toxemia. In ewes, does, and cows, removal of blood from the cotyledons and continued contractions of the uterus loosen the chorionic villi from the caruncles, with expulsion occurring shortly thereafter. Retention is rare in ewes but sometimes occurs in cows.

Retained placentae (also called retained afterbirths) will occur in from 5% to 15% of the parturitions in healthy herds of cows. They occur when separation of the chorionic villi from the caruncles is delayed. Many of these can be associated with short gestations (270 to 275 days) and twin births, which result in shorter gestation periods. They are more likely to occur in high milk producers than low producers, which may account for the higher incidence in dairy cows than is seen in beef cows. Also, retained placentae are more common after difficult births (dystocia) than after uncomplicated births.

In herds where the incidence is over 15% to 20%, a problem is indicated. Nutritional deficiencies of either selenium or vitamin A have caused a much higher rate of placental retention. In selenium-deficient regions, a prepartum injection of selenium and vitamin E will frequently reduce the incidence. Vitamin E is needed for utilization of selenium. If ruminant animals have not had access to green forage for several months, feeding a vitamin A supplement is a good prophylaxis for preventing retained placentae and other problems associated with deficiency of vitamin A. If placental retention is associated with a higher than expected abortion rate, reproductive diseases may be involved (Chapter 26). Assistance from a veterinarian will be needed in identifying and treating disease problems.

If the placenta of a cow has not been expelled 24 hours after expulsion of the fetus, it will likely be retained another 5 to 6 days. The decaying placental tissues make excellent media for microbial growth. Uterine infections occur in conjunction with many retained placentae. Lower fertility after retention is a frequent problem. The stress associated with this problem sometimes will reduce milk production below anticipated levels.

Several alternatives are available in the management of the retained placenta problem. None are as satisfactory as measures that would prevent the problem. Manual removal 48 to 72 hours after parturition, followed by intrauterine treatment with antibiotics was used by veterinary practitioners for many years. Because of complications which reduced reproductive efficiency, it is no longer recommended. Manual separation of the chorionic villi from the caruncles frequently causes tears in the uterus, which create reproductive problems.

A current recommendation on treatment of retained placentae is to use a lukewarm water lavage (flushing out) of the uterus, with the last part of this lavage having iodine added to bring its concentration up to about 1%. This is then followed with an intramuscular injection of estradiol cypionate (ECP), which increases the tone of the myometrium, resulting in expulsion of the water and loose placental tissue. Some animal managers use an alternate procedure of infusing the uterus with a 2% lysol solution. Because of concerns about contamination of milk and meat, antibiotic treatment is not recommended unless metritis develops. Some have suggested that antibiotic infusions may even slow the recovery process in uncomplicated cases. There are proponents of no treatment in uncomplicated cases. If no treatment is given, cows should be observed closely for signs of metritis with or without toxemia and treated appropriately with antibiotics if symptoms develop.

10–7 POSTPARTUM RECOVERY

Following parturition, the next successful gestation depends on both return to normal estrus and return of the uterine environment to a state that will support another pregnancy. Sows frequently have a "farrowing estrus" a few days after parturition. This estrus is infertile because of failure to ovulate. Mares have a "foaling estrus" 8 to 15 days after parturition. They should be bred at this time only if a careful examination indicates a complete recovery from gestation. A bruised or torn cervix, vaginal discharge, or lack of uterine tone are good reasons not to breed at foaling estrus. Normally, mares will return to estrus again by 30 days postpartum and will have higher fertility than when bred at the foaling estrus.

10–7.1 *Postpartum Ovulation and Estrus*

After parturition, many dairy cows will ovulate in 15 to 30 days. However, a high percentage of these ovulations will occur without evidence of estrus. These are called "quiet ovulations." When these cows ovulate again at 40 to 50 days postpartum, the majority will show signs of estrus. Such cows are less likely to become reproductive problems than those that have an extended period of *anestrus* (absence of cycling). Several factors can extend postpartum anestrus.

Suckling the young will delay return to estrus. Beef cows that are suckling a calf may have a postpartum anestrus that is two to three times longer than cows that are not suckling a calf. Removal of the calf for 48 hours beyond 45 days postpartum as well as limiting calves to one period of suckling per day after 21 to 30 days postpartum has shortened the postpartum anestrus period in beef cows. In one experiment involving Hereford-Brahman cross first calf heifers on common Bermuda grass pastures, limiting calves to one 30-minute period of suckling per day after 30 days postpartum, as compared with conventional suckling, shortened postpartum anestrus by an average of 99 days. Neither weaning weights nor milk production was affected by limited suckling. The cause of the delay is not understood fully, but stress of *lactation* (milk production) does not appear to be a major factor. Dairy cows being milked twice daily are apparently not delayed. On the other hand, milking a dairy cow four times per day has delayed return to estrus. A similar effect is seen in sows. After the farrowing heat, most sows stay in anestrus until their pigs have been weaned. If their pigs are removed after 1 week, sows will return to estrus in 3 weeks. Therefore, factors associated with frequent stimulation of the mammary gland appear to cause extended postpartum anestrus. By either neural or chemical (hormonal) means, pulsatile increases in GnRH are inhibited by suckling. In ewes, it has been demonstrated that β-endorphin, an opioid (Section 4–2.2), is released in the hypothalamus in response to suckling. It seems likely that this release prevents the episodic surges of GnRH and consequently gonadotropins, thus inhibiting growth and maturation of ovarian follicles. In sows, the prolactin released by the suckling stimulus has an inhibitory effect on release of LH. If the suckling stimulus is removed or limited, more frequent pulses of GnRH, FSH, and LH will result in return to estrus.

A low level of nutrition, either during the gestation or after parturition, will delay return to estrus. Quiet ovulations are also more frequent for cows on a low plane of nutrition. Cows most affected seem to be those in thin condition at time of calving. A combination of low nutrition and suckling will compound the problem, as can be noted in Table 10–2. Hereford-Brahman cross heifers fed to gain weight during late gestation and at above maintenance after parturition had an average postpartum anestrus period of 124 days with normal suckling, as compared with 32 days with one 30-minute period of suckling per day after 21 days postpartum. Similar heifers fed below maintenance during late gestation and postpartum and suckled once daily had a postpartum anestrus period of 71 days.

Table 10–2 *Interaction of energy level and suckling on postpartum anestrus in beef cows*

	High energy		Low energy
	1/day suckling	Normal suckling	1/day suckling
Number of heifers	17	17	16
Days to 1st estrus	32.1	124.2	71.4

Compiled from Randel and Webber. *Beef Cattle Research in Texas.* Progress Report No. 3599, p.19, 1980.

Many beef cows that calve in thin condition and suckle their calves will stay in anestrus well beyond 150 days. Some will not have a calf the next year because of failure to show estrus and ovulate while running with bulls during the next breeding season. The pattern for postpartum return to estrus in water buffalo is similar to beef cows nursing a calf. Conception may not occur until 4 to 6 months postpartum.

Other factors that may extend postpartum anestrus include infectious diseases, metabolic disorders, uterine infections, and other health problems.

10–7.2 *Involution of the Uterus*

Involution of the uterus implies the return to the normal, nonpregnant state. This includes return to the nonpregnant size as well as recovery and repair of the endometrium. Return to nonpregnant size is quite rapid in mares, being completed in less than 2 weeks.

A similar period of involution has been reported for sows. However, if pigs are weaned at less than 3 weeks and sows are bred at the next estrus, they will have smaller litter sizes than when weaning occurs between 5 and 8 weeks. Embryo loss attributed to disturbances in the implantation process has been implicated as a cause. Therefore, complete involution may not be as rapid as has been reported. In ewes, the uterus returns to the nonpregnant size in approximately 2 weeks, but another 2 weeks is needed for complete recovery of the endometrium.

Uterine involution has been studied more extensively in cows than in other species. This is partly because it is easy to follow the course of involution by rectal palpation. Criteria for involution include (a) return of the uterus to the pelvic area; (b) return to the nonpregnant size; and (c) recovery of normal uterine tone. Using these criteria, uterine involution in cows following uncomplicated parturitions requires an average time of 45 days (Figure 10–4). Histological studies have shown that another 15 days may be required before the endometrium is histologically normal. The reader is referred to Color Plates 11 through 16, which accompany Figure 10–4, and characterize the changes that occur within the uterus from day 20 to day 60 after calving.

The authors have found that uteri of cows return to the nonpregnant size in about 30 days. The tone of the nonpregnant horn may be normal at that time. However, another 2 weeks may be needed for normal tone to return to the pregnant horn. Periods of estrus seem to speed the return of normal tone. It should be noted that one uterine horn may be larger than the other after complete involution. Also, in older cows, uteri may not return to the pelvic area. Therefore, as determined by rectal palpation, tone is a more precise indicator

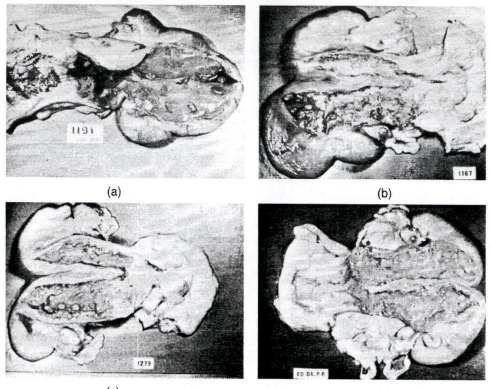

Figure 10–4 Uteri from cows slaughtered at intervals postpartum: (*a*) No. 1191, 10 days; (*b*) No. 1167, 20 days; (*c*) No. 1279, 46 days; and (*d*) 60 days. (Courtesy of N.L. VanDemark and Univ. of Ill., Urbana, Ill.)

of involution. Following placental retention and/or uterine infection, involution of the uterus may be delayed by several weeks.

Induction of early cycling has been shown to speed uterine involution in cattle. This has been accomplished by injecting GnRH at about 15 days postpartum followed by $PGF_{2\alpha}$ 10 days later. In one study, cows that were induced to cycle early had excellent uterine tone as determined by palpation by day 45 postcalving. Tone was good but not excellent in a similar group that was not induced to cycle early. Average days to first estrus for the two groups was 27 and 36 days.

SUGGESTED READING

BUTLER, W. R., R. W. EVERETT, and C. E. COPPOCK. 1981. The relationship between energy balance and milk production in postpartum Holstein cows. *J. Anim. Sci.,* 53:742.

CASIDA, L. E. 1971. The postpartum interval and its relation to fertility in cow, sow and ewe. *J. Anim. Sci.,* 32(Supp. I):66.

CHAMLEY, W. A., J. M. BUCKMASTER, M. E. CERINI, I. A. CUMMINGS, J. R. GODING, J. M. OBST, A. WILLIAMS, and C. WINFIELD. 1975. Changes in the level of progesterone, corticosteroids, estrone, estradiol-17β, luteinizing hormone and prolactin in the peripheral plasma of the ewe during late pregnancy and at parturition. *Biol. Reprod.,* 9:30.

COX, N. M. and J. H. BRITT. 1982. Relationship between endogenous gonadotropin-releasing hormone, gonadotropins and follicular development after weaning in sows. *Biol. Reprod.,* 27:70.

GIER, H. T. and G. B. MARION. 1968. Uterus of the cow after parturition: Involution changes. *Amer. J. Vet. Res.,* 29:38.

INSKEEP, E. K. 1979. Factors affecting postpartum anestrus in beef cattle. *Beltsville Symposia in Agricultural Research. 3. Animal Reproduction.* ed. H. W. Hawk. Allanheld, Osmun and Co. Publishers; Halsted Press, a division of Wiley & Sons.

LASTER, D. B., H. A. GLIMP, L. V. CUNDIFF, and K. E. GREGORY. 1973. Factors affecting dystocia and the effects of dystocia on subsequent reproduction in beef cattle. *J. Anim. Sci.,* 36:695.

LIGGINS, G. C. 1982. The fetus and birth. *Reproduction in Mammals. 2. Embryology and Fetal Development.* eds. C. R. Austin and R. V. Short. Cambridge University Press.

MORROW, D. A., S. J. ROBERTS, K. McENTEE, and H. G. GRAY. 1966. Postpartum ovarian activity and uterine involution in dairy cattle. *J. Amer. Vet. Med. Assoc.,* 149:1596.

PEREZGROVAS, R. and L. L. ANDERSON. 1982. Effect of porcine relaxin on cervical dilation, pelvic area and parturition in beef heifers. *Biol. Reprod.,* 26:765.

RYAN, P. L. 2002. Parturition. *Encyclopedia of Dairy Science.* eds. H. Roginski, J. W. Fuquay, and P. F. Fox. Academic Press, an Imprint of Elsevier Science.

THOMPSON, J. R., E. J. POLLACK, and C. L. PELLISIER. 1983. Interrelationships of parturition problems, production of subsequent lactation, reproduction, and age at first calving. *J. Dairy Sci.,* 66:1119.

THORNBURN, G. D. and J. R. G. CHALLIS. 1979. Endocrine control of parturition. *Physiological Reviews,* 59:863.

WALTERS, D. L., R. E. SHORT, E. M. CONVEY, R. B. STAIGMILLER, T. G. DUNN, and C. C. KALTENBACK. 1982. Pituitary and ovarian function in postpartum beef cows. III. Induction of estrus, ovulation and luteal function with intermittent small dose injections of GnRH. *Biol. Reprod.,* 26:655.

WILTBANK, J. N., W. W. ROWDEN, J. E. INGALLS, K. E. GREGORY, and R. M. KOCH. 1962. Effect of energy level on reproductive phenomena of mature Hereford cows. *J. Anim. Sci.,* 21:219.

Lactation

Lactation is the production of milk by *mammary glands,* which develop for the purpose of nourishing the young. Therefore, mammary glands can be considered accessory reproductive organs. Their development and function coincides precisely with parturition. The initial secretions of the mammary gland, colostrum, provides the neonate with an array of nutrients as well as immunoglobulins (antibodies), which can be absorbed during the first few hours of life. This provides the neonate with the nutrients and the passive immunity (through antibody absorption) that are necessary for both early development and good health. The "normal" milk that is secreted after a few days continues to meet the nutritional needs of the offspring during the first few weeks of life. In most species, when the offspring no longer nurse their mothers, lactation ceases and the secretory tissue in the mammary gland involutes but will again develop during the next pregnancy. In certain breeds of cattle, goats, and sheep, selection and breeding for higher milk production has provided an excess of milk over that needed by the young and with extended periods of lactation. This has permitted milk from these species to become an important part of the diet of both young and adult humans throughout the world.

11–1 STRUCTURE OF MAMMARY GLANDS

When comparing the mammary glands various species, certain anatomical and morphological differences can be noted (Table 11–1).

11–1.1 *Anatomy*

The cow has four mammary glands (quarters) fused together into a single structure, the *udder* (Figure 11–1). They are located in the inguinal region, with two glands lined up on either side of the midline. Each gland has a single teat. A *streak canal* through the teat permits removal of milk which has been produced and stored in that gland. Even though fused together, each gland is a separate unit. For example, dye injected into a single teat will be found only in the gland drained by that teat.

    The mammary system of the mare appears as two glands with two teats. However, as in the cow, the mare has four separate areas of secretory tissue located in the inguinal region. On either side of the midline, two secretory areas are fused into a single gland com-

Table 11–1 *Comparison of the mammary glands of various species*

Species	Number of glands	Number of teats	Streak canals in teats	Position of glands
Cow	4	4	1	Inguinal
Mare	2 gland complexes	2	2	Inguinal
Ewe	2	2	1	Inguinal
Doe	2	2	1	Inguinal
Sow	4–9 pairs	4–9 pairs	2	Abdominal

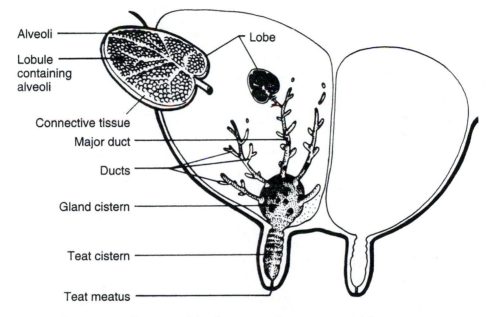

Alveoli

Lobule containing alveoli

Lobe

Connective tissue

Major duct

Ducts

Gland cistern

Teat cistern

Teat meatus

Figure 11–1 Diagram of the duct system in one quarter of the mammary gland of the cow, with a single lobe illustrated. Four quarters are fused into a single gland complex.

plex, which is drained by a single teat (Figure 11–2). Each teat has two streak canals, one draining each secretory area.

Both the ewe and doe have two mammary glands, with one teat for each gland. These glands are fused together, with one on either side of the midline in the inguinal region. Each teat has a single streak canal.

The sow has from four to nine pairs of mammary glands, which are located on either side of the midline along the entire abdominal wall. Each gland has a teat, with two streak canals, which drain separate secretory areas in the individual glands.

11–1.2 *Morphology*

Lactation has been studied more extensively in cows than in other species. Therefore, the cow will be used as a model in discussing both morphology and function of the mammary gland.

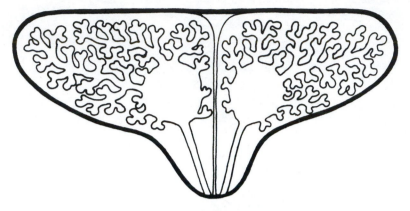

Figure 11–2   Diagram of the gland complex found in the mare.

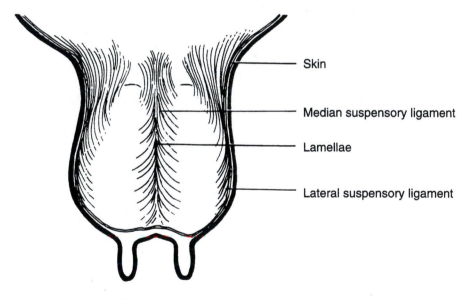

Skin

Median suspensory ligament

Lamellae

Lateral suspensory ligament

Figure 11–3   Diagram of a cross section of the supporting structures of
the mammary glands of the cow as viewed from the rear.

The mammary gland can be divided into supporting tissues and those tissues involved in synthesis and transport of milk. The supporting structures are skin, ligaments,
and connective tissue. The major support comes from *lateral suspensory ligaments,* which
are not elastic, and the *median suspensory ligament,* which is elastic (Figure 11–3). The
lateral suspensory ligaments are over the outside of the udder just under the skin. In addition to enveloping the udder, the lateral suspensory ligament sends *lamellae* (thin, con-
vex layers of connective tissue) into the udder. These lamellae become continuous with
the interstitial framework of the udder, adding to its support. The median suspensory ligament forms longitudinally between the two halves of the udder and is fused on the ab-

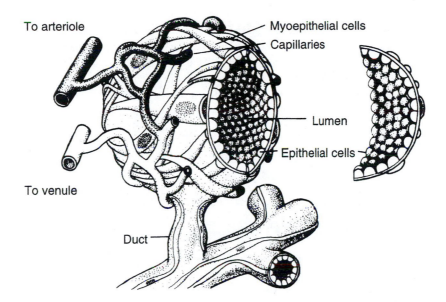

To arteriole

Myoepithelial cells

Capillaries

Lumen

Epithelial cells

To venule

Duct

Figure 11–4 Diagram of alveolus, showing lumen, epithelial cells, myoepithelial cells, and capillaries.

domen. Since it is elastic, it will stretch as the udder fills with milk. Lamellae are given off by the median suspensory ligament, also. The role of skin in support of mammary glands is small when compared with lateral suspensory ligaments and the median suspensory ligament.

Connective tissue divides the milk synthesis and transport system into many subdivisions. The larger of these subdivisions is the *lobe*. The lobe is further divided into small subdivisions called *lobules*. Lobules are not further divided by connective tissue and each has one drainage duct. Each lobule contains from 150 to 225 *alveoli*. Alveoli are tiny, saclike structures, which are spherical in shape (Figure 11–4). They have a lumen and are lined with epithelial cells. These epithelial cells are the basic milk secretion units in the mammary gland. Over half of all of the milk stored in a mammary gland will be stored in the lumen of alveoli. The rest will be stored in the ducts leading from the lobules and lobes (Figure 11–1).

An adequate blood supply to the mammary gland is necessary for the production of milk. Nutrients which are utilized in the synthesis of milk come from blood. Approximately 400 volumes of blood must pass through the mammary gland for the synthesis of 1 volume of milk. The primary blood supply for mammary glands in cows, mares, sheep, and goats is from the *external pudic* artery. In sows, mammary glands are supplied by both external pudic and *external thoracic arteries*. Arteries that penetrate mammary glands branch and follow the connective tissue septa which forms lobes and lobules. Alveoli will be surrounded by a fine network of arterial capillaries where the transfer of nutrients used in milk synthesis takes place. The venous return from the mammary gland is through both the external pudic and *subcutaneous abdominal* veins in those species with mammary glands in the inguinal region. In sows, return is through external pudic and external thoracic veins.

A network of *myoepithelial cells* covers the surfaces of alveoli and small ducts down as far as ducts draining the lobules. They have a smooth, musclelike function but are of ectodermal rather than mesodermal origin. They originate from epithelial cells. Myoepithelial cells are the contractile tissues which play a major role in milk ejection ("letdown" of milk).

Smooth muscle fibers are found in mammary glands. They regulate the size of small arteries and veins, thus controlling the blood supply to the secretory cells. They appear to be too sparse and too irregular to play a major role in the letdown of milk.

11–2   HORMONAL REGULATION OF THE DEVELOPMENT AND FUNCTION OF THE MAMMARY GLAND

11–2.1   *Mammary Development*

Development of the mammary gland (*mammogenesis*) can be divided into four phases. These are embryonic development, fetal development, postnatal growth period development, and development during pregnancy. Differences occur in the regulation of each phase. The first evidence of mammary development in the embryo is the *mammary band,* a small, thickened area of epithelial cells that is seen at about 30 days in cattle. The mammary gland is of ectodermal origin. The developmental stages that follow are the *mammary line, mammary crest, mammary hillock,* and *mammary bud.* Mammary buds can be seen by the early part of the "period of the fetus." In cattle, mammary buds will be found on either side of the ventral midline of the embryo and will later give rise to the fore and rear quarters. There is little evidence that the embryonic development of the mammary gland is under endocrine control. Mammary buds are seen in both males and females but also mark the beginning of the differential patterns of devlepment for female and male glands.

In the female, the mammary bud stage is followed by teat development. In addition, invaginations of ectodermal cells form cores which develops into primary sprouts. A *primary sprout* will form in the mammary tissue of the fetus by the third month of gestation. The primary sprout is the beginning of the milk secretion tissue that will form. Before the end of gestation, *secondary sprouts* and possibly *tertiary sprouts* will have formed. The mammary fat pad, important to postnatal development, starts forming at this time as well and by the end of gestation will make up a majority of the udder's mass. While regulation of this phase in development is not completely understood, there is evidence for endocrine influence. Prolactin in synergism with insulin, steroid hormones of the adrenal cortex, and possibly progesterone stimulates this development.

After birth, mammary growth will continue at a growth rate similar to that of general body growth until about 3 months of age. From about 3 months until just before puberty, mammary growth rate will be faster than body growth. Most of the mammary enlargement during this period is from continued enlargement of the fat pad. Growth hormone has been implicated as a regulator of this growth.

After puberty, the mammary gland will be exposed to cyclic increases in estrogens and progesterone. In response to these increases, surges of development are seen in mammary ducts and lobular structures which will eventually contain alveoli. The principal effect of estrogens is on duct development, while progesterone stimulates lobular development.

Following pregnancy, mammary development will continue, with the most rapid growth occurring during late pregnancy, paralleling the most rapid period of absolute fetal growth. The most extensive development during pregnancy is growth of the lobules and alveoli, including development of the epithelial cells that line the alveoli. Growth of these epithelial cells requires the presence of the fat pad, which to a large extent regulates the number of epithelial cells in the mammary gland. Synergy between estrogens and progesterone establishes the conditions required for the mammary development that occurs during pregnancy. Progesterone is elevated throughout the pregnancy, although higher during early pregnancy, whereas estrogens are much higher during late pregnancy, the period of greatest mammary growth. Together, these hormones are important regulators for development of functional mammary tissue with potential for secreting milk. It has been demonstrated that nonpregnant cows and heifers can be induced into lactation with a 7-day treatment of high concentrations of a specific estrogen (estradiol-17β) and progesterone injected subcutaneously. The hormone concentrations given mimic levels seen in the plasma of cows during the last month of pregnancy. Other hormones that synergize with estrogens and progesterone in preparing mammary tissue for secretion of milk include growth hormone (through stimulation of the secretion of insulin-like growth factor I), prolactin, glucocorticoids, and insulin. Prolactin and glucocorticoids have been identified as major positive regulators of structural differentiation of secretory cells. Placental lactogen, which has been identified in some mammals, has effects similar to those of growth hormone and prolactin. It should be noted that, while mammary tissue is prepared for milk synthesis during gestation, actual milk secretion is inhibited until a few days before parturition by the high concentration of progesterone.

11–2.2 *Milk Secretion*

Hormonal changes that initiate parturition at the end of gestation also initiate secretion of milk *(lactogenesis)*. These changes include surges in both prolactin and the glucocorticoid cortisol (Figure 10–3), which are positive regulators of milk synthesis, and a drop in progesterone, which removes the negative influence. Of these hormones, prolactin appears to be the dominant factor. Prepartum milking of cows will override the negative effects of progesterone on lactogenesis and result in mammary secretions of normal composition several weeks before parturition. Prepartum milking mimics the suckling stimulus which causes release of prolactin and oxytocin. Therefore, the positive effect of prolactin on milk secretion and the role of oxytocin in facilitating removal of milk (Section 11–2.3) seem to be overriding factors in initiation and maintenance of milk secretion.

Maintenance of lactation *(galactopoiesis)* is regulated by several factors. Of these, the suckling stimulus (milking) and milk removal may be the most important, because failure to remove milk from the mammary gland will terminate lactation. If the pituitary gland is removed, milk production will decline precipitously. Milk yield can be restored by combined administration of prolactin, growth hormone, and triidothyronine (thyroid hormone). Prolactin appears to be dominant in maintaining early lactation. In cows, growth hormone is more dominant than prolactin in maintaining lactation after peak milk production is reached, approximately 2 months into the lactation. In research trials, injections of growth hormone have increased milk production in dairy cows by 10% to 40% (Figure 11–5). In individual trials the milk production response has been dose dependent. Growth hormone

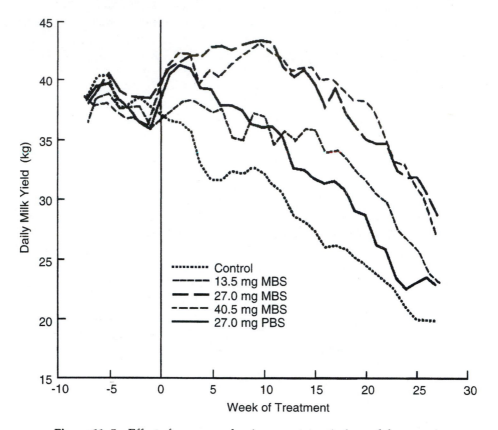

Figure 11–5   Effect of exogenous bovine somatotropin (growth hormone) on milk yield. Treatments commenced at week 0 (84 + 10 days postpartum) and continued for 27 weeks. Milk production data (unadjusted) represent weekly averages. Daily dose of methionyl bovine somatotropin (MBS) and pituitary bovine somatotropin (PBS) as indicated. (Bauman et al. *J. Dairy Sci.*, 68:1352, 1985.)

increases productive efficiency by partitioning nutrients for milk synthesis. As with prolactin, growth hormone is released by the suckling stimulus.

An adequate level of nutrition is necessary for the maintenance of lactation. However, during the first few weeks after parturition, lactation will proceed at the expense of the body reserves of the mother. This provides needed nutrients for the young but may extend postpartum anestrus well beyond the desired interval (Section 10–7.1). For optimum response from injected growth hormone, the feeding program must include adequate energy and protein. However, lactational efficiency is improved because growth hormone causes a diversion of nutrients from body tissues to milk production. This is potentially detrimental to reproduction, but further research is needed to clarify this area.

When milk is no longer removed from the mammary gland, milk synthesis will stop and involution of the mammary gland will begin. In cows, mammary gland involution will be complete in 3 to 4 weeks. With mammary involution, there will be degeneration of alveolar structures and loss of the epithelial cells involved in the synthesis of milk. However,

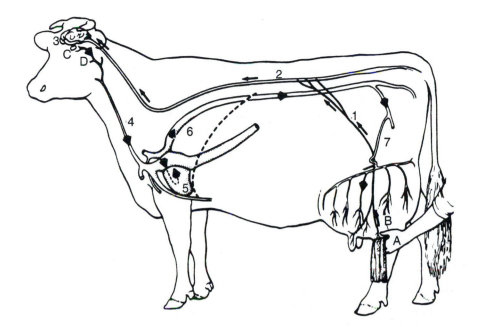

Figure 11–6   The neurohormonal reflex of milk ejection. The stimulus (A) that a cow associates with milking causes a nerve impulse (B) to travel via the inguinal nerve (1) to the spinal cord (2) and the brain (3). The brain causes the release of oxytocin (D) from the posterior pituitary (C). Oxytocin is released into a branch of the jugular vein (4) and travels to the heart (5) and is then transported to all parts of the body by the arterial blood. The oxytocin reaching the udder leaves the heart by the aorta (6) and enters the udder through the external pudic arteries (7). In the udder, it causes the myoepithelial cells to contract, resulting in milk ejection from the alveoli. (Schmidt. 1971. *Biology of Lactation.* W. H. Freeman and Co. Redrawn by permission of the author.)

lobes and lobules will retain their integrity. Redevelopment of the alveolar structures will begin 3 to 4 weeks before parturition in cows.

11–2.3 *Milk Ejection*

Milk ejection, often called "letdown" of milk, is physiologically a separate function from milk synthesis. Milk ejection is triggered by stimulation of sensory nerves in the teats, by either suckling the young or having the teats massaged (Figure 11–6). This stimulation results in the release of oxytocin from the posterior pituitary. Oxytocin reaches the mammary gland by way of arterial circulation. It stimulates the myoepithelial cells surrounding alveoli and small ducts, forcing the milk down into larger ducts, gland cisterns, and teats, where it can be readily removed. While stimulation of sensory nerves in teats will trigger this milk ejection reflex, milk ejection can become a conditioned response. The presence of young, even though physically separated from their mother, will sometimes cause milk ejection. A similar response is sometimes seen in cows waiting to be milked in a milking parlor. Sounds or odors associated with milking may trigger the release of oxytocin.

Excitement caused by a novel environment or abusive treatment will inhibit the milk ejection reflex. This may be caused by epinephrine, which is a vasoconstrictor of small arteries and veins. Therefore, epinephrine could prevent sufficient oxytocin from reaching the myoepithelial cells to cause ejection of milk. Another effect of epinephrine might be inhibition of the release of oxytocin from the posterior pituitary. It has been demonstrated that endogenous opioids released into the hypothalamus will inhibit release of oxytocin from axons in the posterior pituitary. Movement of animals to a new environment causes release of endogenous opioids. Although not clearly demonstrated, a relationship between epinephrine and opioid release is worthy of consideration.

11–3 COMPOSITION OF MILK

Even though milk is the sole nourishment for neonatal mammals, its composition varies among species. Fat is the most variable component, ranging from 1.3% in donkeys to 30% to 50% in sea mammals. Even in those species whose milk is sometimes used for human food, milk fat ranges from approximately 2% in mares to 7.5% in ewes (Table 11–2). Breed differences in milk composition are seen, also. Again, fat is the most variable component, with averages ranging from 3.6% in Holsteins to 4.9% in Jerseys. About 95% of the milk fat in cows is triglycerol, with the fatty acid portion of the molecule having carbon chain lengths of 4 to 18. About half of these fatty acids are synthesized within the mammary gland, with this *de novo* synthesis producing even–carbon numbered fatty acids ranging from 4 to 16. Precursers for this synthesis are acetate, which results from fermentation of carbohydrate in the rumen, and β-hydroxybutyrate, which is converted from butyrate (another rumen fermentation product) during absorption. Some 16-carbon and all 18-carbon fatty acids incorporated into the triglycerols are absorbed from feedstuffs via the digestive system or mobilized from fat reserves in the body. Phospholipids, cholesterol, diacylglycerols, monoacylglycerols, and free fatty acids make up about 5% of the total milk fat.

Protein content varies a good bit among farm species, ranging from 2.7% on a volume basis in mares to 7% in sheep. Protein content is lower in Holsteins than other breeds of dairy cows. The most important milk protein is casein, accounting for over 80% of the total milk protein. Whey proteins make up the other milk protein. Casein and the whey pro-

Table 11–2 *Species and breed differences in milk composition*

Species	Fat	Protein	Lactose	Ash
Horse	1.9	2.7	6.1	0.5%
Sheep	7.5	7.0	3.5	0.9%
Swine	5.4	5.4	4.7	0.9%
Goat	4.1	3.3	4.1	0.9%
Cattle				
Guernsey	4.7	3.6	4.8	0.7%
Holstein	3.6	3.1	4.6	0.7%
Jersey	4.9	3.7	4.8	0.7%
Shorthorn	3.6	3.3	4.5	0.8%

teins α-lactoalbumin and β-lactoglobulin are synthesized in the mammary gland. Blood-derived proteins found in milk in small quantities are immunoglobulins, lactoferrin, and serum albumin.

Lactose (milk sugar) is a disaccharide formed from the bonding of a glucose molecule and a galactose molecule. Of the major components of milk, it is the least variable in content because it regulates milk volume through its regulation of the amount of water in milk. If the concentration of lactose is high, as in the horse, then the concentration of protein and fat will be low because of the diluting effect of the water that lactose causes to come into the milk. Because the mammary gland synthesizes lactose from glucose and galactose (which is derived from glucose), blood glucose is the sole precurser for lactose. If lactose synthesis is limited because of low blood glucose, milk volume will be reduced.

Most minerals (ash) in milk are similar to that found in the blood because they are in a soluble form and are therefore in equilibrium with the same minerals in blood. Both calcium and phosphorus are much higher in milk than in blood. A fairly high percentage of the calcium and phosphorus in milk is bound in the casein micelle and therefore is not soluble. Only the soluble portion of these will be in equilibrium with the calcium and phosphorus in blood. Because of the high calcium and phosphorus concentrations, milk is the most important source of these minerals for bone growth in young animals and bone health in adult humans.

Marked differences are seen when comparing colostrum, the first milk secreted by the mammary gland near parturition, with normal milk that is produced through the rest of the lactation (Table 11–3). Most notable when comparing colostrum with normal milk is the much higher protein level in colostrum. Colostrum is especially higher in the gamma globulin fraction of protein, which is the immunoglobulin or antibody portion of milk. Colostrum is higher in vitamin A than is normal milk. The newborn is deficient in this vitamin. Colostrum is also higher in minerals.

Composition of milk during the lactation varies over a narrow range after the transition from colostrum to normal milk. During late lactation when a smaller volume is being produced, the fat percentage will be slightly higher. During milk removal, the first milk removed will be relatively low in fat, whereas that obtained by stripping the last of the milk from the mammary gland will be high in fat. Therefore, to get a true picture of its composition, milk should be removed from the gland as completely as possible and mixed before sampling.

Table 11–3 *Comparison of the composition of colostrum with that of normal milk*

Constituent	Cow		Sow		Mare	
	Colostrum	Milk	Colostrum	Milk	Colostrum	Milk
Total solids (%)	23.9	12.9	20.5	16.9	25.2	11.3
Fat (%)	6.7	4.0	5.8	5.4	0.7	2.0
Protein (%)	14.0	3.1	10.6	5.1	19.1	2.7
Lactose (%)	2.7	5.0	3.4	5.7	4.6	6.1
Ash (%)	1.11	0.74	0.73	0.71	0.72	0.50

From G. H. Schmidt. *Biology of Lactation.* W. H. Freeman. 1971. By permission of author.

SUGGESTED READING

AKERS, R. M. and A. V. CAPUCO. 2002. Lactation—Lactogenesis. *Encyclopedia of Dairy Sciences.* eds. H. Roginski, J. W. Fuquay, and P. F. Fox. Academic Press, an imprint of Elsevier Science.

BALDWIN, R. L. and T. PLUCINSKI. 1977. Mammary gland development and lactation. *Reproduction in Domestic Animals.* (3rd ed.) eds. H. H. Cole and P. T. Cupps. Academic Press.

BAUMAN, D. E., P. J. EPPARD, M. J. DEGEETER, and G. M. LANZA. 1985. Responses of high producing cows to long-term treatment with pituitary somatotropin and recombinant somatotropin. *J. Dairy Sci.,* 68:1352.

CAPUCO, A. V. and R. M. AKERS. 2002. Lactation—Galactopoiesis, effects of hormones and growth factors. *Encyclopedia of Dairy Sciences.* 14 eds. H. Roginski, J. W. Fuquay, and P. F. Fox. Academic Press, an imprint of Elsevier Science.

COLLIER, R. J., J. P. MCNAMARA, C. R. WALLACE, and M. H. DEHOFF. 1984. A review of endocrine regulation of metabolism during lactation. *J. Anim. Sci.,* 59:498.

COWIE, A. T. 1972. Lactation and its hormonal control. *Reproduction in Mammals. 3. Hormones of Reproduction.* eds. C. R. Austin and R. V. Short. Cambridge University Press.

HURLEY, W. F. and J. A. FORD, JR. 2002. Mammary gland anatomy—Growth, development, and involution. *Encyclopedia of Dairy Sciences.* eds. H. Roginski, J. W. Fuquay, and P. F. Fox. Academic Press, an imprint of Elsevier Science.

KENSINGER, R. S. and A. L. MAGLIARO. 2002. Lactation—Induced lactation. *Encyclopedia of Dairy Sciences.* eds. H. Roginski, J. W. Fuquay, and P. F. Fox. Academic Press, an imprint of Elsevier Science.

LARSON, B. L. and V. R. SMITH. 1974. *Lactation: A Comprehensive Treatise.* Vols. I, II, and III. Academic Press.

MCGUIRE, M. A. and D. E. BAUMAN. 2002. Milk biosynthesis and secretion—Milk fat. *Encyclopedia of Dairy Sciences.* eds. H. Roginski, J. W. Fuquay, and P. F. Fox. Academic Press, an imprint of Elsevier Science.

SCHMIDT, G. H. 1971. *Biology of Lactation.* W. H. Freeman and Co.

STELWEGEN, K. 2002. Milk biosynthesis and secretion—Protein. *Encyclopedia of Dairy Sciences.* eds. H. Roginski, J. W. Fuquay, and P. F. Fox. Academic Press, an imprint of Elsevier Science.

STELWEGEN, K. 2002. Milk biosynthesis and secretion—Lactose. *Encyclopedia of Dairy Sciences.* eds. H. Roginski, J. W. Fuquay, and P. F. Fox. Academic Press, an imprint of Elsevier Science.

Part 3

Artificial Insemination

Six chapters are included in this part, which will guide the student through the procedures that are required for successful artificial insemination. It is the first of three parts that emphasize application of basic concepts in management of reproduction. Artificial insemination is given special emphasis because of the worldwide impact that it has had on genetic improvement, especially in cattle. In spite of major advances in other reproductive technologies in recent years, artificial insemination remains the most practical and cost-effective method for genetic upgrading of cattle.

12

Introduction and History of Artificial Insemination

12–1 INTRODUCTION

Artificial insemination (AI) is the most valuable management practice available to the cattle producer. The procedure makes efficient use of the generous supply of sperm available from an individual male in a manner that greatly increases genetic progress as well as improving reproductive efficiency in many situations.

Many bulls are currently producing sufficient semen to provide enough sperm for 40,000 breeding units in one year. Using the long accepted standard of 10×10^6 motile sperm at the time of insemination with an average initial motility of 60% and a 33.3% loss of sperm during freezing and thawing, that number of breeding units would entail 1×10^{12} total sperm. By using thorough sexual stimulation and more frequent collections, twice that many sperm may be obtained from most bulls in a year without adversely affecting conception rate. Research has also shown that accepted diluents, freezing procedures, and thawing techniques, 10×10^6 total sperm per breeding unit will reduce conception only about one percentage unit. Using these parameters, a bull could produce 200,000 breeding units of semen per year. A bull is usually at least 4 years old when his genetic merit has been evaluated, and if he lived to be 10 years old, and retained his reproductive vigor, he could theoretically produce 2×10^6 breeding units of semen in his lifetime. Boar and buck semen can be frozen and utilized more efficiently, also. An average boar produces sufficient sperm to inseminate 1,500 to 2,000 sows per year. Artificial insemination is used only on a limited basis in sheep and horses.

Reproductive efficiency using AI is at least as good as using natural mating when no diseases are present and good management practices are employed. When certain diseases enter the picture, especially venereal diseases, AI becomes an important factor in their control.

AI is being used in farm species other than cattle and swine even though techniques for freezing and thawing are not perfected well enough for commercial use. Researchers have made some progress with freezing stallion semen, but little progress with ram semen. Procedures for identifying superior germ plasm in swine, sheep, and horses have not been developed as well as they have for cattle.

12–2 HISTORY

The first reported use of AI, although not documented, was in 1300 by some Arabian horse breeders. Rival chieftains reportedly stole stallion semen from one another to breed their own mares.

The first documented report of successful use of AI was by an Italian physiologist, L. Spallanzani, in 1780. After success with several amphibian animals, he decided to experiment with the dog. He used semen at body temperature to inseminate a bitch which had been confined to his own home. Sixty-two days later, she gave birth to three pups. In 1782, Spallanzani's experiment was successfully repeated by P. Rossi and a professor named Branchi.

Spallanzani later demonstrated that the fertilizing component of semen could be filtered out of the seminal fluid. The filtered fluid was sterile while the residue remaining on the filter was highly fertile. In 1803, Spallanzani reported that sperm cooled with snow were not killed but rendered motionless until exposed to heat, after which they were motile for several hours.

His investigations stimulated research of the sex cells and the process of fertilization, but no further reports on AI were recorded until near the end of the century. E. Milais, a dog breeder, inseminated 19 bitches between 1884 and 1887, with 15 becoming pregnant. W. Heape of England, writing about the work in 1897, concluded that AI was easy and that conception was as good as natural service. He also suggested that one ejaculate could be used to inseminate several bitches and that AI could be a tool to study genetic factors.

Scientists in Russia began studies with farm animals about 1900. E. I. Ivanoff started his work with horses but was the first to successfully artificially inseminate cattle and sheep. Ivanoff's success stimulated sufficient interest to have a physiological section established in the Ministry of Agriculture specifically to study physiology of fertility and to train veterinarians in the techniques of AI. Work with horses was initiated in Japan about 1913.

The first cooperative AI association was formed in Denmark in 1936. Aided by state support, the Danish breeders have continued to be leaders in the percentage of cows bred by AI. Professor E. J. Perry of Rutgers University was one of the pioneers in the United States. He organized the first AI cooperative in this country in 1938, with 102 members, which bred 1,050 cows the first year. Professor Perry visited the Denmark association (bull stud) and patterned the New Jersey association after it. Several other cooperatives were organized within the next 2 years. Artificial insemination had become a reality and was off with a running start.

A number of important discoveries are worth mentioning. Each raised the level of success of AI to a new plateau.

The first artificial vagina was used to collect dog semen by G. Amantea, a professor of human physiology at the University of Rome (Figure 12–1). Amantea began his research on dog sperm in 1914. Russian scientists patterned artificial vaginas suitable for the stallion, bull, and ram after Amantea's. The development of the artificial vagina suitable for the larger species may well be the most important single development in the history of AI, and the artificial vagina still is preferred where bulls, rams, bucks, and stallions are collected on a regular basis. The electroejaculator was developed in the late 1940s. It has been a useful innovation for collecting from reluctant or disabled bulls, rams, and bucks.

Artificial insemination was recognized by researchers and many breeders as a tremendous asset for genetic progress by the late 1930s. A limitation was that semen had to be used on the day of collection to give good results. When P.H. Phillips and H.A. Lardy, of the University of Wisconsin, discovered a buffered, nutrient medium for

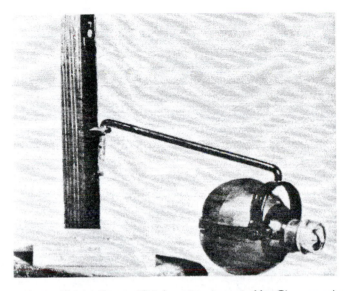

Figure 12–1   The earliest artificial vagina, invented by Giuseppe Amantea of the University of Rome, was used for the collection of dog semen. (From *The Artificial Insemination of Farm Animals*, 4th rev. ed., edited by Enos J. Perry. Copyright 1945, 1947, 1952, by the Trustees of Rutgers College in New Jersey. Copyright © 1968 by Rutgers University, the State University of New Jersey.)

diluting an ejaculate of semen, it was the first step in correcting the problem. They developed a yolk-phosphate diluter which protected sperm during cooling from body temperature to 5°C, provided a source of nutrients for sperm metabolism, and prevented pH change. With this diluter, sperm remained viable and capable of fertilizing ova for 3 to 4 days. G.W. Salisbury and coworkers improved the diluter by substituting sodium citrate for the phosphates used by Phillips and Lardy. The advantage of the yolk-citrate diluter was sperm visibility under the microscope, permitting more accurate determination of motility after dilution.

The problem of spreading reproductive disease still remained. Efforts were made to collect semen from healthy bulls, but several serious outbreaks of reproductive diseases occurred. The most commonly transmitted disease was vibriosis. Following World War II, penicillin and streptomycin became available for use by the livestock industry. J.O. Almquist, Pennsylvania State University, was the first to report the use of the "wonder drug" to control bacterial contaminants in bovine semen. It was adopted by the AI industry almost immediately, with marked improvements in conception rate.

Early inseminations were accomplished by simply depositing semen into the vagina of the female. The technique was later refined by using a speculum and a glass inseminating tube. The speculum was placed into the vagina, and with a light source (first a battery head lamp and later a pen size flashlight) the posterior of the cervix was visible. The inseminating tube was inserted into the opening and the semen deposited approximately 2 cm into the cervix. In 1937, Danish veterinarians developed the recto-vaginal (or cervical fixation) method of insemination for the cow. One hand was inserted into the rectum to manipulate the cervix while an insemination tube inserted through the vagina was passed into or through the cervix. The semen could then be deposited into the anterior cervix and/or the body of the uterus. This technique is still used today.

By the late 1940s, there were many AI organizations breeding cows all over the country. A fresh supply of semen had to be shipped to the technician or breeder every 2 or 3 days, but AI was being used with good results. Two Englishmen were responsible for the next important discovery. A.S. Parkes and C. Polge developed a successful method for freezing and storing sperm at very low temperatures. They discovered that glycerol would protect fowl sperm during the freezing and thawing process. At first, this method was not successful with mammalian sperm. Eventually, however, they found that allowing the sperm and glycerol mixture to stand overnight before freezing did work. This standing period is now called equilibration time in which the sperm cells absorb some glycerol to replace part of the free water in the cell. The glycerol acts as "antifreeze" to prevent water crystals from forming during freezing. These workers used dry ice as a refrigerant and stored the sperm at $-79°C$.

In 1957, the American Breeders Service pioneered the use of liquid nitrogen as a refrigerant for freezing and storing semen. Large stainless steel vacuum containers were developed by the Linde Corporation. This made it practical to transport semen long distances and store it on the farm. Containers now available need to be replenished with liquid nitrogen only every 60 to 90 days.

The Dairy Records Processing Center of the USDA began compiling and publishing sire summaries in 1961 that helped evaluate the genetic potential of sires. Prior to that date, some states and each bull stud had their own procedure of compiling genetic information. The absence of uniformity made it impossible to compare bulls owned by different studs. The USDA sire summaries provide a great deal more information than was previously available and the information is uniform nationwide. Both production and type information are provided.

The introduction of the straw, a small-diameter plastic tube, for packaging semen for freezing probably will not be the last chapter in the AI history book, but at present it is the latest major development. Sorensen introduced the use of straws for packaging semen in 1940. Reports of frozen semen in straws by Pares in 1953 and later by Friis Jakobson in 1956, with refinements by Adler in 1959 and 1961, created sufficient interest to keep researchers active.

The Cassouses of L'Aigle, France, a father-and-son team, are credited with the development of the straw to practical application in three stages. The first, in 1964, contained 1.2 ml of semen and showed an encouraging improvement in sperm survival when compared with the 1 ml glass ampule. Realizing that the coefficient of freezing surface was the main factor in determining survival, they changed to a straw with half the diameter of the original straw and a capacity of .5 ml. This straw gave excellent results and has been called the "medium straw." The medium straw is being used almost exclusively in the United States. The Cassous team developed a still smaller straw with a capacity of .25 ml in 1968 and claimed further improvements in the survival of sperm. This straw is called the "mini straw."

AI organizations and researchers in the United States began tests with the medium straw during the late 1960s. These organizations began switching from the glass ampules to the straw about 1972. All of the semen produced in the United States is packaged in straws. In addition to providing greater survival of sperm, the straw requires only about one-third the storage space as the ampule. This has led to the redesigning of liquid nitrogen storage tanks, particularly field units that require less nitrogen and have a longer holding time between recharges. Successful freezing of boar semen became a reality in 1975.

Even though penicillin and streptomycin served the AI industry well for 40 years by controlling known pathogen contaminants in semen, there was concern that mycoplasmas, ureaplasmas, *Haemophilus somnus,* and even *Campylobacter fetus venerealis* (due to changes in processing procedures) were not being adequately controlled. A new antibiotic combination and treatment procedure was developed and adopted in the late 1980s. Gentamicin, Tylosin, and Linco-Spectin are used in combination. More information can be found in Section 16–3.

12–3 ADVANTAGES AND DISADVANTAGES

The advantages of AI far outweigh the disadvantages. The major advantages are

1. Genetic improvement through more accurate evaluation of transmitting ability of males and greater use of superior germ plasm, even allowing its continued use after a bull's or boar's death
2. Control of venereal and other diseases
3. Improved record keeping on farms where used
4. More economical than natural service when genetic merit is considered
5. Safer by the elimination of dangerous bulls on the farm, especially for the dairy breeds

There are few disadvantages of AI. Perhaps the most noted one is that livestock managers must spend a great deal of time checking females for estrus. Some special facilities for corralling and inseminating are required and with beef cattle these need to be more elaborate. Trained personnel are required to perform the technique.

SUGGESTED READING

FOOTE, R. H. 1993. Harvesting and utilizing bull sperm power for maximal genetic progress through artificial insemination. *Reprod. Dom. Anim.,* 28:361–373.

FOOTE, R. H. 1998. *Artificial Insemination to Cloning.* Cornell University Resource Center.

FOOTE, R. H. 2002. Reproduction—Gamete and embryo technology—Artificial insemination. *Encyclopedia of Dairy Science.* eds. H. Roginski, J. W. Fuquay, and P. F. Fox. Academic Press, an imprint of Elsevier Science.

FOOTE, R. H. and M. T. KAPROTH. 1997. Sperm numbers inseminated in dairy cattle and nonreturn rates revisited. *J. Dairy Sci.,* 80:3072–3076.

HEAPE, W. 1897. The artificial insemination of mammals and subsequent possible fertilization or impregnation of their ova. *Proc. Roy. Soc. London,* 61:52.

MARDEN, W. G. R. 1954. New advances in the electro-ejaculation of the bull. *J. Dairy Sci.,* 37:556.

PERRY, E. J. 1968. *The Artificial Insemination of Farm Animals.* Rutgers University Press.

PHILLIPS, P. H. and H. A. LARDY. 1940. A yolk-buffer pabulum for the preservation of bull semen. *J. Dairy Sci.,* 23:399.

SPALLANZANI, L. 1803. *Tracts on the Natural History of Animals and Vegetables.* (Translated title) (2nd ed.) Edinburgh, Creech, and Constable.

WALTON, A. 1933. *The Technique of Artificial Insemination.* Edinburgh, Imperial Bureau of Animal Genetics.

13

Semen Collection

Semen collection is like harvesting any other farm crop. Effective harvest of semen involves obtaining the maximum number of sperm of highest possible quality in each ejaculate. The ultimate objective is to make maximum use of superior sires. This involves proper semen collection procedures used on males that are sexually stimulated and prepared. The initial quality of semen is determined by the male and cannot be improved even with superior handling and processing methods. However, semen quality can be lowered by improper collection and the processing techniques. Semen collection is a complex procedure involving coordinated efforts between the animal handler and the collector. See Table 13–1 for common characteristics of ejaculates for the farm species.

13–1 FACILITIES NEEDED FOR SEMEN COLLECTION

There are several essential features that must be considered in designing facilities for collecting semen. The most important consideration is the safety of the handler and the collector. This is especially true where bulls of the dairy breeds are being collected. Safety fences, usually constructed of 3-inch steel pipe with spaces large enough for a person to step through at 8-foot intervals, should be provided (Figure 13–1). The collection area must provide good footing to prevent slipping and injury to the male being collected. This is best provided by an earthen floor in the immediate collection area. Means to restrain the teaser animals to minimize lateral as well as forward movement must be provided. At the same time, easy access for semen collection must be maintained.

13–2 METHODS OF SEMEN COLLECTION

Several methods of collecting semen have been used since the inception of AI. The early procedures involved taking the semen from the vagina of the naturally mated female with a spoon or by other means. Later, a specially designed rubber breeding bag was placed in the vagina of the cow or mare to catch the ejaculate. The massage method, which involved massaging the vesicular glands and ampullae by way of the rectum, was reported as early as 1925. The quantity and quality of semen obtained by this method have severe limitations. The concept of the artificial vagina was presented by Amantea about 1914 and was adapted for use on the larger species by Russian scientists about 1933. A practical version of the electroejaculator was introduced in 1948.

160

Table 13–1 *Common characteristics of ejaculates for farm species*

	Volume (ml)	Motility (%)	Concentration (sperm/ml 10^6)
Dairy bulls			
Small breeds	5–6	50–80	1,000–1,500
Large breeds	7–8	50–80	1,000–1,500
Beef bulls	4–5	40–70	1,000–3,000
Rams and bucks	0.75–1.2	60–80	1,500–3,000
Boars	150–300	50–70	100–150
	*40–125	50–70	200–300
Stallions	75–100	40–70	100–150

*Gel-free fraction

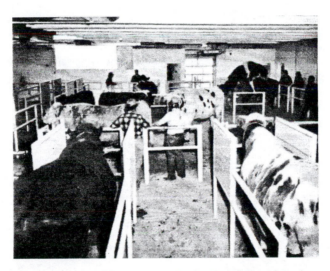

Figure 13–1 Semen collection area for bulls. Note safety fences over which bulls can be managed while protecting the handler. Earthen floor provides good footing for the bulls. (Courtesy of Select Sires, Inc., Plain City, Ohio.)

The remainder of this section will be devoted to the artificial vagina and the electroejaculation methods of collecting semen. Essentially, all semen used for AI is collected by these two methods except for boar semen.

13–2.1 *Sexual Stimulation Prior to Collection with the Artificial Vagina*

Sexual stimulation by exposing males to the normal courtship situations prior to semen collections increases the number of sperm per ejaculate for all species. However, the effect of sexual stimulation has not been as well defined for the boar, ram, and stallion as it has been for the bull. The remainder of this section will deal with the bull.

There are two reasons for providing adequate sexual stimulation: (1) to ensure that the male will mount and ejaculate in a reasonable period of time and (2) to ensure the collection of the maximum number of sperm with the highest possible quality per ejaculate. Except for the occasional male with low sex drive, the latter is the most important. Ejaculates with larger volume, higher concentration, and higher motility will have higher fertility in most cases and more breeding units can be prepared from an ejaculate, thus reducing the processing time and cost per breeding unit. In addition, the lifetime output of sperm by an individual male is increased.

Sexual stimulation is accomplished by exposing the bull to the teaser animal for several minutes. False mounts (allowing the bull to mount the teaser animal without ejaculation) enhances the degree of sexual excitement. The combination of a false mount, followed by a few minutes of teasing, plus one or two additional false mounts before collection seems to provide adequate preparation for most bulls. A period of 10 to 15 minutes of teasing without false mounts adequately stimulates most bulls. However, care must be taken to ensure that the bull is being stimulated, not just standing.

Bulls generally show a reduction in sex drive if handled in the same manner for a prolonged period of time. Some variations which will help maintain a high degree of sexual stimulus are

1. Introducing a new teaser animal, perhaps alternating between a cow and another bull
2. Moving the teaser animal to a different position at the same location or to a different location in the collection area
3. Presenting two teasers
4. Allowing the teaser or another bull to mount the bull to be collected
5. Bringing a new bull into the collection area
6. Collecting semen from the new bull
7. Avoiding distraction

Bulls that are on a high collection frequency tend to need more variation in stimulation procedure and may take longer to become sexually prepared than bulls on low collection frequency. Beef bulls tend to exhibit less sex drive than dairy bulls and therefore require more imagination on the part of the handler in getting them prepared for collection.

Sexual stimulus and preparation increase semen volume and sperm concentration of the ejaculates of all bulls. The increase is greater for some bulls than for others. An increase of 30% to 50% can be expected following adequate preparation. Refer to Table 13–2 for some average increases.

13–2.2 *Collecting Semen with the Artificial Vagina*

The artificial vagina (AV) method of collecting semen is the fastest and most sanitary of the various methods available. The AV provides a good imitation of the natural vagina. There are a number of modifications of the basic design along with different shapes and sizes for different species.

Table 13–2 *Characteristics of ejaculates from bulls with and without sexual stimulation*

	Volume (ml)	Motile (%)	Sperm per ejaculate (no. $\times 10^9$)	Motile sperm per ejaculate (no. $\times 10^9$)	Increase (%)	Usable ejaculates (%)
Unrestrained[*]	3.7	53	4.55	2.48		
1 false mount	4.3	56	6.19	3.62	46	
Unrestrained[†]	3.7	58	4.52	2.56		75.8
1 false mount	4.5	63	6.41	3.98	55	97.0
2 false mounts	4.9	61	6.37	3.89	52	93.9
Beef trial I[#, a]						
Unrestrained	5.6	54	11.82	6.41		
3 false mounts[c]	6.2	63	13.65	8.36	30	
Beef trial II[#, b]						
Unrestrained	4.6	60	9.93	6.06		
3 false mounts[c]	5.2	64	11.77	7.62	25	
Dairy[#, a]						
1 false mount	5.0	66	13.49	8.85		
3 false mounts[c]	6.2	68	18.23	12.26	38.5	

[*]From Collins, Bratton, and Henderson. *J. Dairy Sci.,* 34:224, 1951.

[†]From Branton et al. *J. Dairy Sci.,* 35:801, 1952.

[#]From Almquist. *J. Anim. Sci.,* 36:331, 1973.

[a]Figures represent total of two successive ejaculations taken on 1 day per week.

[b]Figures represent total of two successive ejaculations taken on 2 days per week.

[c]Three false mounts before each ejaculate with 2 min. restraint between first and second false mount.

13–2.2a Collecting from the Bull The basic design for the artificial vagina used to collect semen from the mature bull is shown in Figure 13–2. It consists of a rigid rubber casing 40 cm in length and 6.4 cm in diameter. The casing is fitted with a rough-textured latex inner liner. The ends of this liner are folded back over the outer ends of the casing and are secured with tight rubber bands. The space between the liner and the casing is filled with warm water to provide suitable temperature and pressure to evoke ejaculation. One end of the unit is fitted with a rubber funnel that is secured to the casing along with the turned back liner. A collection tube is attached to the small end of the funnel. Any tube with sufficient volume capacity for an ejaculate, either graduated or plain, can be used. Both 15-ml and 50-ml plastic tubes of uniform weight are used in the semen-processing industry.

In the most popular version of the AV, there is a hole 1 cm in diameter through the outer casing 10 cm from the end. A latex sleeve half the length of the casing is slipped over that end of the casing to cover the opening. Three functions are served:

1. The sleeve can be rolled back to expose the opening for filling the AV with water, and a small amount of air can be blown into the AV to provide additional pressure.
2. A rubber band can be rolled onto the end of the sleeve to hold it tightly, thus providing a chamber to hold displaced water when the penis enters the AV.
3. This expansion chamber allows the AV to be completely filled with water without danger of the folded inner liner slipping off the casing.

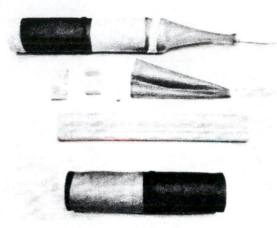

Figure 13–2   Artificial vagina used to collect semen from the bull. The completely assembled AV is shown at the top, with the component parts shown below. The protective covering for the funnel and collection tube is shown in Figure 13–5. Smaller versions are used for the ram and buck.

Even though it is necessary to use rubber bands on the ends of the liner to prevent the escape of water that could ruin the ejaculate, the bands must be counted after each collection to be sure that none remain on the penis. A tight rubber band left on the penis will obstruct blood flow and may amputate the penis.

It is important that the length of the outer casing, and to some degree its diameter, be gauged to fit the males being collected. Young bulls between 10 and 15 months of age should be started with casings 20 cm to 24 cm long and 5.1 cm in diameter. Casings of intermediate length and diameter need to be used on bulls between 15 months and 3 years of age. For reasons of sanitation, it is important that the end of the glans penis extend well into the collecting funnel at the time of ejaculation. Therefore, it is essential that the length of the AV properly correspond to the length of the penis.

The AV can be filled with water through an open end to within 3 cm to 4 cm of the top while holding the casing vertically. The inner liner is folded back over the end of the casing, being careful not to allow water to spill into the inner liner. The casing may also be filled through the expansion chamber opening (Figure 13–2). The casing cannot be filled as full if this method is used. Therefore, to obtain sufficient pressure on the inner liner, some air may need to be blown through the opening before the outer sleeve is rolled back over the opening.

The temperature of the water used to fill the AV casing needs to be high enough to bring the internal temperature of the unit to approximately 45°C. Internal temperatures from 38°C to 56°C have been used successfully. Most bulls will be stimulated to ejaculate at any temperature within this range. Some will not ejaculate unless the temperature is near 55°C, while others may not respond if the temperature is above 40°C. The initial temperature required to achieve an internal temperature of 45°C at the time of semen collection depends on the environmental temperature. In most cases, initial water temperature of 55°C to 60°C will be adequate. The internal temperature should be checked periodically with an accurate thermometer if collection is delayed or very low temperatures are experienced in the collection area. At least one bull stud fills the artificial vaginas the day before they are to be used and holds them overnight in a 49°C incubator. That is warm enough to allow for a small drop in temperature before the bulls serve them.

The collection funnel and tube must be maintained at near body temperature during collection. An insulated jacket which can be prewarmed should be attached to the end of the casing, covering the collection funnel and tube to provide protection from cold shock. A zippered opening is desirable so that the ejaculated sample can be examined. At the time of ejaculation, the glans penis of most bulls coils sufficiently to cause the collection funnel and tube to be twirled. The insulated jacket also protects the collection tube from possible breakage.

The AV must be lubricated before it is used to collect semen. The open end and one-third of the inner liner is lubricated with a water soluble surgical jelly on a sterile glass rod. The penis carries enough lubricant forward to lubricate the remainder of the liner. The jelly should be used sparingly, since an excessive quantity will contaminate the semen, causing clumping of sperm. At least one bull stud has an attendant use a gloved hand to lubricate the bulls' penises with surgical gel during one of the false mounts in the sexual stimulation exercise.

The frequency of ejaculation has increased through the years to the point that four to six ejaculates per week is the norm in the large bull studs. In some bulls, especially those collected six times per week, a tearing of the tissue where the prepuce attaches to the shaft of the penis has been observed. A suggested cause for this problem is that the 40-cm-long casing of the standard AV is long enough to accommodate the entire penile shaft and the pressure of water and added air pressure in the casing is sufficient to hold the penis securely during ejaculation. When the glans penis coils during ejaculation, stress is applied to the preputial attachment to the penile shaft. This stress eventually results in a tear and can result in the bull being taken out of service for a while. Some bull studs have found the problem to be more serious than others, and one person suggested that it may be genetically related.

One bull stud resolved the problem with a redesigned AV (Figure 13–3). A 19-cm (7.5-in.) length of 6.35-cm (2.5-in.) PVC schedule 40 pipe for the casing is used with two 1.5-cm holes drilled 2 cm from one end. A 36-cm-long inner liner of the same diameter with a very rough inside finish was used. When properly installed in the casing and secured at both ends, an expansion chamber approximately half the length of the casing is provided. A 40-cm collection funnel or cone allows plenty of room for the glans penis as well as a generous amount of the penile shaft. The portion of the penile shaft remaining in the casing is not held as rigidly, all of which prevents the tearing of the preputial tissue. In this version, a 50-ml collection tube is used.

Another stud is using a 30-cm standard casing with a regular liner to provide a chamber for the warm water. However, a one-piece inner liner and collection funnel, which is estimated to be about 55 cm in length, is used.

The AV method of collecting semen from the bull involves the use of properly restrained teaser-mount animals. Dummy mounts have been constructed but are seldom used. It is necessary for the bull to mount in order for him to serve the AV and ejaculate. The teaser-mount animal serves this purpose but in addition provides the sexual stimulus necessary to get the bull sexually prepared for ejaculation. Cows, bulls, or steers may be used as teaser-mounts.

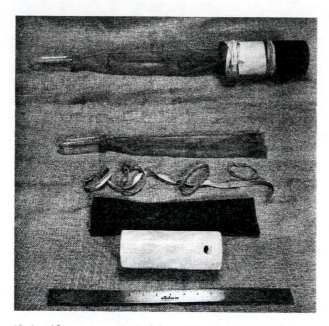

Figure 13–3   Alternate version of the artificial vagina. Note short casing, long collection funnel, and 50-ml collection tube. (Courtesy of Genex Co-operative, Inc., Ithaca, N.Y.)

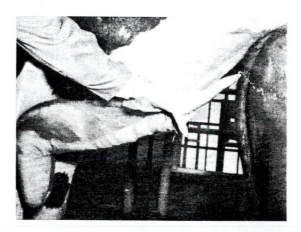

Figure 13–4   Grasping the bull's penis rather than the sheath may cause premature ejaculation. (Courtesy of Select Sires, Inc., Plain City, Ohio.)

When one is collecting from the right side of the bull, the AV should be balanced in the right hand with the palm up and held parallel to the expected path of the bull's penis. As the bull mounts and the penis is extended, the left hand is used to guide the penis to the side by grasping the sheath. The extended penis should not be touched by the hand because this results in either a retraction of the penis or ejaculation before the penis enters the AV (Figure 13–4).

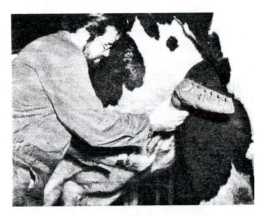

Figure 13–5 Semen collection from the bull using the artificial vagina. (Courtesy of Select Sires, Inc., Plain City, Ohio.)

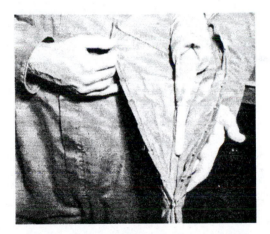

Figure 13–6 An ejaculate of bull semen. Note protective covering for the funnel and collection tube which prevents cold shock and tube breakage. (Courtesy of Select Sires, Inc., Plain City, Ohio.)

Best ejaculation results are obtained when the penis is covered by the AV on the upward movement as soon as the bull mounts. It is helpful for the attendant to place his or her left shoulder against the side of the bull as he mounts, so that their movements are in unison (Figure 13–5). Accurate timing is essential for best results. When the bull thrusts for ejaculation, the AV should be allowed to move with the thrust and maintained as near in line with the penis as possible. The AV should be held on the penis until the bull begins to dismount. Sharp bends of the penis which may cause discomfort, or even injury, should be avoided. An experienced semen collector soon learns individual differences between bulls and will alter the collection procedure accordingly. Figure 13–6 shows an ejaculate of bull semen in the protective covering.

Several precautions must be taken at the time of collection to ensure high-quality semen:

1. Cold shock is prevented by providing adequate protection for the collecting funnel and tube.
2. The collection tube must be protected from sunlight.
3. Contamination of semen by urine, water, or lubricating jelly must be avoided.
4. Microbial contamination is minimized by using a different sterile artificial vagina for each ejaculation.

A clean AV should be used even when a bull fails to ejaculate after the AV is placed over the penis. Second ejaculates collected with the same AV contain twice as many bacteria as first ejaculates. The number of bacteria also increases greatly with the number of insertions of the penis into the artificial vagina. Preputial hairs should be clipped as an aid to sanitation.

One study showed that as much as 20% of an ejaculate may be lost by semen adhering to the anterior end of the inner liner and the collecting funnel, especially with low-volume ejaculates. Moistening those parts with a compatible buffer solution before collection reduced those losses by more than 50%.

13–2.2b Collecting from the Ram and Buck
The AV used for the ram and buck is a smaller version of the one used for the bull. The recommended temperature and method for collection are the same as that for the bull. The collector must have quick reflexes, since these males mount and serve rapidly. The AV can be attached to a dummy with a sheep skin stretched over it. The ram mounts the dummy with little training. The AV is the preferred method for collecting ram and buck semen for use in AI.

13–2.2c Collecting from the Stallion
The AV for the stallion must be larger than that for the other farm species. The outer casing is usually made of leather or aluminum and is 75 cm to 80 cm in length (Figure 13–7). It must have a handle or strap to help the collector support its weight and to cope with the vigorous thrusting of the stallion. The inner liner and some version of the collection funnel and tube are also used. The AV is only partially filled with water to provide an internal temperature of 45°C. A valve designed

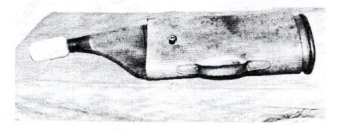

Figure 13–7   Artificial vagina used to collect semen from the stallion.

to relieve pressure as the penis enters is essential. Sufficient pressure and friction must be maintained to stimulate ejaculation. The penis should be washed with warm, soapy water and rinsed prior to ejaculation to remove smegma and other debris from its surface for first-time collections. For stallions being collected regularly, the washing should be omitted after the first collection, since experience has shown that repeated washings can result in a buildup of pathogenic organisms.

Steps to follow in collecting semen from a stallion include the following:

1. Tease him to get extension of his penis.
2. Wash his penis with water and a mild soap followed by complete rinsing (for stallions being collected for the first time).
3. Have stallion mount a dummy or the estrus mare from an angle.
4. Divert penis into the artificial vagina with a hand.
5. If he is mounting a mare, brace the artificial vagina against the thigh of the mare and hold it parallel to the direction of his thrust.

The outer end of the AV should be lowered sufficiently to allow semen to flow into the collection bottle. Ejaculation is complete in about 10 to 15 seconds.

13–2.2d Collecting from the Boar

Collecting semen from the boar requires an entirely different procedure. In natural service the boar ejaculates when the corkscrew-shaped glans penis is firmly engaged in the sow's cervix. Pressure of this engagement stimulates ejaculation. If an artificial vagina is used to collect semen from the boar, it must be designed so that the glans penis receives adequate pressure. Such artificial vaginas have been successfully used, but the AV is not the preferred method for collecting semen from boars.

The boar's ejaculate can be divided into at least three fractions. The first fraction consists of clear fluid and some gel-like substance. It is usually discarded as emitted. The second fraction is the sperm-rich portion (creamy white) but may also contain some gel. The final fraction contains clear fluid with a higher percentage of gel, and this, too, can be discarded. There may be some alternating phases of sperm-rich and sperm-free portions. The time required for ejaculation varies but usually lasts for 3 to 10 minutes.

Boars can be trained to mount estrual sows or dummy sows for semen collection (Figure 13–8). Sprinkling the dummy with semen, urine, or sheath fluids from another boar may be helpful in training boars to mount the dummy. After the boar mounts and starts thrusting, the glans penis should be grasped firmly enough to retain a grip with the hand (use of a rubber glove is preferred). The penis should be pulled from the sheath and pressure rapidly increased until the thrusting stops. Boars differ in the amount of pressure required to stimulate ejaculation. A prewarmed, widemouthed thermos covered with two layers of cheesecloth should be used to catch the semen. The cheesecloth will strain out the gel contained in the sperm-rich fraction.

13–2.2e Cleaning, Sterilizing, and Storing the AV

Washing and sterilizing the artificial vagina are extremely important. It should be completely disassembled, rinsed with tap water, and washed immediately. If washing cannot be accomplished

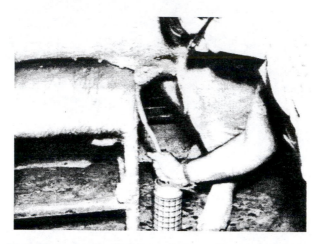

Figure 13–8 Semen collection from the boar. The gloved hand replaces the artificial vagina.

immediately, the parts should soak in lukewarm water until washing can be completed. The casings should be brushed with a stiff brush and water containing a detergent. They must be rinsed with tap water and allowed to air dry. Inner liners and funnels should be turned inside out and brushed thoroughly with the detergent water. They must be rinsed with tap water and then with distilled water prior to soaking for 5 minutes in 70% isopropyl or ethyl alcohol. Some prefer to boil the liners and funnels in distilled water for 15 minutes before rinsing with 70% alcohol. In the latter case, the alcohol serves primarily as a drying agent. After the alcohol rinse, the parts should be hung in a dust-free cabinet to dry. If used daily, they may remain in the cabinet; otherwise, each piece can be individually wrapped in clean paper towels for storage. Refrigerated storage of all rubber parts not used regularly will greatly extend useful life.

13–2.3 *Collecting Semen with the Electroejaculator*

This method of collecting semen is preferred to the AV method under certain conditions. It is used for dairy bulls that have become crippled, have low sexual activity due to age, or for other reasons are unable to serve the artificial vagina. It is extensively used with beef bulls, especially to check semen quality on bulls to be used in natural mating prior to the breeding season. Semen should not be collected and used from males that have not demonstrated normal sexual behavior or ability to ejaculate, as the cause may be genetic and transmitted to the offspring.

The equipment used for electroejaculating males consists of a bipolar electrode and a variable source of alternating current. The voltage ranges from 0 to 30, with a low amperage (0.5 to 1.0). The electrode may have either alternating positive and negative rings spaced 4 cm apart or four conductors, two positive and two negative, running longitudinally along the electrode. One model has three conductors, all on one side (Figure 13–9). The electrode is placed in the rectum immediately above the accessory glands so that the nerves of the reproductive system are stimulated.

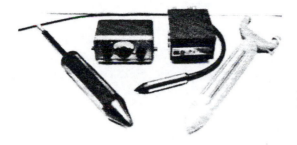

Figure 13–9 Electroejaculator used to collect semen from the bull and the ram. Small probe in the center is used on the ram.

13–2.3a Electroejaculation of the Bull

After removal of excess fecal material from the rectum, the lubricated electrode is inserted and positioned immediately over the accessory glands. Stimulation is begun with low voltage, which is gradually increased, a few volts at a time, alternated with 4-second rest periods in which the voltage is returned to 0. This rhythmic pattern is continued until the bull is stimulated to ejaculate. The secretion of bulbourethral fluid and penile erection should take place at the lower voltage, with ejaculation occurring at the higher voltage levels. Increasing the voltage too rapidly can result in ejaculation without erection, and the semen will be contaminated by the prepuce. Most bulls are stimulated to ejaculate in a period ranging from 2 to 5 minutes (Color Plate 17).

The nerves of the rear legs are also stimulated by the electrical current. This results in stiffening of the legs and in some cases the bull goes down. It is essential that the bull be restrained in a chute with good footing provided. In some cases, it is desirable to provide some support under the ribcage to help support the bull's weight.

Ejaculates obtained by the electroejaculation method are usually larger in volume but lower in concentration than those obtained with the artificial vagina. The total number of sperm and the fertilizing capacity are about equal for the two methods.

13–2.3b Electroejaculation of the Buck and Ram

The ram responds to a lower voltage and responds faster than does the bull. Ejaculation can be accomplished with the buck and ram either lying on a table or standing. Usually, three levels of voltage are required, with a peak of 8 volts. Some rams fail to respond, while others yield low-quality semen. Since the urethral orifice is continuous with the filiform appendage on the ram, it is necessary to direct the latter into the collection tube before ejaculation (Color Plate 18).

13–2.3c Electroejaculation of the Boar

The level of voltage required for ejaculation is greater in the boar than in either the bull or the ram. This is probably due to the insulating effect of the body fat. A probe designed for the boar that transmits a higher level of voltage to the reproductive tract is available. The high voltage results in considerable discomfort, making some type of anesthesia or tranquilization desirable. Sperm motility, fertility, and concentration of electroejaculated boar sperm are good, but the volume is usually low. The method is not satisfactory for routine collection of semen from boars.

SUGGESTED READING

ALMQUIST, J. O. 1973. Effects of sexual preparation on sperm output, semen characteristics and sexual activity of beef bulls with a comparison to dairy bulls. *J. Anim. Sci.,* 36:331.

ALMQUIST, J. O. 1978. Bull semen collection procedures to maximize output of semen. *Proc. 7th Tech. Conf. Artif. Insem. Reprod.,* p. 33. NAAB, Columbia, Mo.

BALL, L. 1978. Semen collection by electro-ejaculation and massage of the pelvic organs. *Proc. 7th Tech. Conf. Artif. Insem. Reprod.,* p. 57. NAAB, Columbia, Mo.

BRANTON, C., G. D'Arensbourg, and J. E. Johnston. 1952. Semen production, fructose content of semen and fertility of dairy bulls related to sexual excitement. *J. Dairy Sci.,* 35:801.

COLLINS, W. J., R. W. BRATTON, and C. R. HENDERSON. 1951. The relationship of semen production to sexual excitement of dairy cattle. *J. Dairy Sci.,* 34:224.

FOOTE, R. H. 1998. *Artificial Insemination to Cloning.* Cornell University Resource Center.

FOSTER, J., J. O. ALMQUIST, and R. C. MARTIG. 1970. Reproductive capacity of beef bulls. IV. Changes in sexual behavior and semen characteristics among successive ejaculates. *J. Anim. Sci.,* 30:245.

HERMAN, H. A. and F. W. MADDEN. 1972. *The Artificial Insemination of Dairy and Beef Cattle.* (4th ed.) Lucas Brothers Publishers.

McKINNON, A. O. and J. L. VOSS. 1993. *Equine Reproduction.* Lea and Febiger.

PICKETT, B. W. 1968. Collection and evaluation of stallion semen. *Proc. 2nd Tech. Conf. Artif. Insem. Reprod.,* p. 80. NAAB, Columbia, Mo.

Pork Industry Handbook. 1995. Current.

SALISBURY, G. W., N. L. VANDEMARK, and J. R. LODGE. 1978. *Physiology of Reproduction and Artificial Insemination of Cattle.* (2nd ed.) W. H. Freeman and Co.

14

Semen and Its Components

Semen is composed of spermatozoa and seminal plasma. Its sources are the epididymides and vasa deferentia, which supply the cellular components (spermatozoa), and the accessory glands, which provide most of the fluid portion (seminal plasma). The relative contribution, on a volume basis, is illustrated in Table 14–1 for the bull and boar. In terms of total volume, the contribution of the epididymides and vasa deferentia is relatively small. In bulls, the greatest contribution to the fluid volume of semen is from the vesicular glands, with minor contributions from the prostate gland and bulbourethral glands. In boars, there are greater contributions from the prostate and bulbourethral glands, with a smaller proportion from the vesicular glands. These differences are reflected in the chemical composition of semen, also (Table 14–2). Bull semen is higher in fructose and sorbitol, which comes from the vesicular glands, whereas boar semen is higher in most minerals, the major source of these being the prostate gland.

14–1 SPERMATOZOA

The concentration (no./ml) of spermatozoa in an ejaculate of semen is approximately 150 million for stallions, 200 million for boars, 1.2 billion for bulls, and 2 billion for rams (Table 14–3). Theoretically, 50% of the spermatozoa in a given ejaculate will contain X chromosomes and 50% Y chromosomes, which on a population basis would result in equal numbers of male and female offspring. Approximately 60% to 70% of the spermatozoa in semen are expected to be progressively motile, with an average speed of 6 mm per minute. In high-quality semen, 80% to 90% of the spermatozoa will have normal morphology. Concentration, motility percent, and morphology are all important criteria in the evaluation of semen before use in artificial insemination (Chapter 15). Spermatozoa of bulls have an overall length of 60μ to 70μ. The head is 8μ to 10μ long, with the tail accounting for the remainder. The head is flattened, about 4μ wide and 0.5μ thick. Both boars and rams have sperm of similar size, while sperm of stallions are smaller (about 50μ in length).

14–1.1 Normal Morphology

The normal spermatozoon is composed of a head and a tail that is divided into a mid-piece, main-piece, and end-piece (Figure 14–1).

Table 14–1   *Sources and relative contribution (volume %) to semen*

Species	Sources			
	Epididymides and vasa deferentia	Vesicular glands	Prostate gland	Bulbourethral glands
Bull	5–15	60–80	10	5
Boar	2–5	15–20	50–75	10–25

Table 14–2   *Average chemical composition of semen from different species (mg/100 ml)*

Constituent	Bull	Ram	Boar	Stallion
Fructose	530	250	13	2
Sorbitol	75	72	12	40
Glycerylphosphorylcholine	350	1,650	175	70
Inositol	35	12	530	30
Citric acid	720	140	130	26
Ergothionine	0	0	15	75
Plasmalogen	60	380	——	——
Sodium	230	190	650	70
Potassium	140	90	240	60
Chlorine	180	86	330	270
Calcium	44	11	5	20
Magnesium	9	8	11	3

Adapted from White, *Reproduction in Farm Animals*. (3rd ed.) ed. Hafez. Lea and Febiger, 1974.

Table 14–3   *Characteristics of semen from farm animals*

	Cattle		Sheep	Swine	Horses
	Dairy	Beef			
Volume (ml)	6	4	1	125*	60*
Sperm concentration (billion/ml)	1.2	1.0	2.0	0.2	0.15
Total sperm (billion)	7	4	3	45	9
Motile sperm (%)	70	65	75	60	70
Morphologically normal sperm (%)	80	80	90	60	70
pH	6.5–7.0	6.5–7.0	5.9–7.3	6.8–7.5	6.2–7.8

*Gel-free portion.

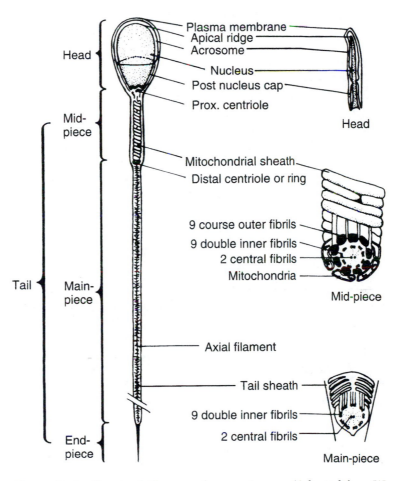

Figure 14–1 Structural diagram of spermatozoon. (Adapted from Wu. 1966. *AI Digest*, 14:7.)

The important components of the head include the *nucleus,* containing the genetic code, which is the sire's contribution to a new offspring, the *postnuclear cap,* covering the posterior portion of the nucleus, and the *acrosome.* The acrosome covers the anterior part of the nucleus and contains enzymes needed for penetration of the corona radiata and zona pellucida during fertilization (Chapter 8). If the acrosome is malformed, damaged, or missing, the spermatozoon will not be able to participate in fertilization. During aging, the acrosome becomes loosened from the nucleus starting at the apical ridge.

The point where the tail joins the head contains the *proximal centriole* and is called the implantation region. The head and tail become separated at this point during fertilization. Similar separation is sometimes seen in heat-damaged semen.

The mid-piece, a thickened portion of the tail some 8µ to 10µ long in bulls, is located just posterior to the proximal centriole. The *mitochondrial sheath,* which forms from the mitochondria of the spermatid, is a part of the mid-piece. The mitochondrial sheath contains enzymes which convert fructose and other energy substrates into high-energy compounds that can be used by spermatozoa.

The main-piece (40µ to 50µ long) and end-piece (3µ long) differ in that the end-piece does not have a protective sheath. A major feature of the tail is the *axial filament*. The axial filament is a small bundle of tiny fibrils that starts at the proximal centriole and runs through the entire tail. One center pair of small fibrils is surrounded by a circle of nine pair of small fibrils (Figure 14–1). Nine larger fibrils surround the circle of nine pair of small fibrils through much of the length of the tail. Contractions of these fibrils cause a lashing of the tail, which propels the spermatozoon forward. Contractions start at the proximal centriole proceeding sequentially around the perimeter fibrils and rhythmically down the tail. This results in an urn-shaped pattern of tail movement, causing a rotation of the entire spermatozoon as it moves progressively forward. This progressive motility can be observed under a light microscope.

14–1.2 *Abnormal Morphology*

Every ejaculate of semen will contain some morphologically abnormal spermatozoa. The expected range of 8% to 10% has no adverse effect on fertility. If the accumulated total abnormal spermatozoa exceed 25% of the total in an ejaculate, reduced fertility can be anticipated.

Abnormal sperm can be classified under abnormal heads (primary abnormalities), abnormal tails (tertiary abnormalities), and cytoplasmic droplets (secondary abnormalities) (Figure 14–2). Abnormal heads that have been observed include asymmetrical, tapering, pyriform, giant, micro, and double heads. Abnormal tails include enlarged, broken, bent, filiform, truncated, and double mid-pieces, along with coiled, looped, and double tails. Most spermatozoa with tail abnormalities will not be motile, and the remainder exhibit abnormal motility. Cytoplasmic droplets form on the neck of spermatozoa during spermiogenesis. As

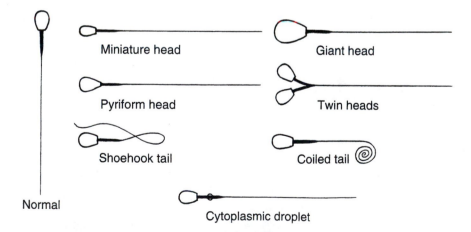

Figure 14–2 Morphological abnormalities of spermatozoa identified through examination of semen for quality.

discussed in Chapter 3, these are usually lost during maturation in the epididymis. If they are still present after spermatozoa are ejaculated, they are considered an abnormality and, as with other abnormalities, too high a percentage will reduce the fertility of the semen. Stress causes an increase in abnormal sperm. Abnormalities of all types increase, but the first to appear and the last to disappear are increases in cytoplasmic droplets. Cytoplasmic droplets on the tail of ejaculated sperm is an indication that the maturation process is not completed.

14–2 SEMINAL PLASMA

The fluid portion of semen is seminal plasma. The accessory glands contribute most of this, but a small amount of fluid is a part of the spermatozoa concentrate which comes from the epididymides and vasa deferentia. Seminal plasma serves as a buffered, nutrient medium which suspends and maintains the fertility of spermatozoa. Seminal plasma is slightly acidic in bulls and rams and slightly alkaline in boars and stallions. The osmotic pressure of seminal plasma is similar to blood (equivalent to physiological saline—0.9% sodium chloride). A number of organic and inorganic compounds are in solution in seminal plasma.

14–2.1 *Proteins*

Several proteins that have a relationship to fertility have been found in seminal plasma. The role of glycosaminoglycan (GAG)-binding proteins in capacitation has been discussed previously (Section 6–4). The binding affinity of ejaculated sperm for heparin and other glycosaminoglycans (via binding proteins) corresponds to fertility in bulls. These GAG-binding proteins are found in seminal plasma, as well as on the sperm membrane, with their source being the fluids of the vesicular glands. Studies of protein profiles in seminal plasma have revealed two proteins that were more prevalent in high fertility bulls and two other proteins that were more prevalent in low fertility bulls. In that the relative amounts of these fertility associated proteins remained constant in individual bulls over a period of 30 to 57 months, profiles of seminal proteins offer potential for predicting fertility of young, postpubertal bulls before they are proven and enter semen production. Based on profiles of seminal proteins, predicted fertility for individual bulls declined with successive ejaculates over a period of a few hours. This may or may not affect actual fertility, but it is a factor to consider in management of males that produce semen for artificial insemination.

14–2.2 *Inorganic Ions*

Sodium and chlorine are the principal inorganic ions in seminal plasma. Smaller quantities of calcium and magnesium are found, also. Potassium, which is present in substantial amounts in whole semen, is more concentrated in spermatozoa than in the fluid suspending the spermatozoa. Thus, when spermatozoa are concentrated, as in the epididymis, the potassium-to-sodium ratio is higher. These inorganic ions are important to the viability of spermatozoa, possibly through their effect on the integrity of the sperm cell membrane.

Along with the organic molecules in solution in seminal plasma, the inorganic ions help maintain an osmotic pressure that is optimum for the survival of spermatozoa.

14–2.3 *Buffering Agents*

In addition to inorganic ions, organic ions that serve as buffering agents are found in seminal plasma. The principal organic ion is bicarbonate. It is produced by the vesicular glands and functions as a buffering agent, guarding against changes in the pH of semen. Buffers are not found in sufficient quantities to prevent a reduction in pH when semen is maintained in storage. Therefore, good semen diluters must be used to provide sufficient buffering capacity for long-term storage (Chapter 16).

14–2.4 *Energy Substrates*

Several organic compounds that serve primarily as energy substrates for spermatozoa are found in seminal plasma. The principal ones are fructose, sorbitol, and glycerylphosphorylcholine (GPC). Fructose (a simple sugar) and sorbitol (a sugar alcohol) are produced by the vesicular glands, whereas GPC is produced in the epididymides. All are unique in that they are not found in substantial quantities elsewhere in the body.

Fructose can be used by spermatozoa as an energy substrate under the anaerobic (oxygenless) conditions of storage and the aerobic (oxygenated) conditions found in the female tract. Sorbitol and GPC can be utilized only aerobically. In addition, GPC must be acted on by an enzyme found in the female tract before it can be utilized. This enzyme splits the choline from the rest of the molecule, forming glycerylphosphate, which can be metabolized as an energy substrate. Lactic acid, a by-product of the anaerobic metabolism of fructose (Section 14–3), builds up in semen that is being stored and theoretically can be used as an energy substrate when placed in aerobic conditions.

Fructose is found in high concentrations in bull and ram semen but is much lower in both boar and stallion semen. The low concentration of fructose in boar and stallion semen may contribute to the problems of storing semen from these species.

14–2.5 *Other Organic Compounds*

Compounds found in seminal plasma in rather large concentrations but not used as energy substrates are inositol and citric acid. Both are produced by the accessory glands. Ergothionine is found in the semen of boars and stallions. These compounds are not found in substantial amounts elsewhere in the body.

14–3 ENERGY METABOLISM BY SPERMATOZOA

Energy metabolism is the means by which spermatozoa convert energy substrates into usable forms of energy. Enzymes for this conversion are in the mitochondrial sheath. In addition to fructose, sorbitol, and GPC, which are present in seminal plasma, plasmalogen, a lipid found within the spermatozoon is an energy reserve that can be used when other substrates are limiting.

Adenosine triphosphate (ATP), a high-energy compound, is the form of energy that can be used by spermatozoa. It is converted to ADP yielding 7,000 calories per mole of energy by the following reaction:

$$\text{'ATP} + H_2O \leftrightarrows ADP + H_3PO_4 + 7{,}000 \text{ calories/mole}$$

If there were no means of regenerating ATP, the spermatozoa would not survive due to lack of energy. Energy substrates provide a means by which ATP can be regenerated from ADP plus inorganic phosphorus. Fructose serves as a good example, since it can be utilized anaerobically and aerobically. The anaerobic reaction is as follows:

$$\text{Fructose} \overset{\text{No } O_2}{\leftrightarrows} 2 \text{ lactic acid} + 2 \text{ ATP (net yield)}$$

Fructose metabolized anaerobically yields a net of 2 ATP, or 14,000 calories. This reaction provides energy to maintain the viability of spermatozoa during storage. However, an end product of this metabolism is lactic acid. If steps are not taken to slow metabolism during storage, the buildup of lactic acid will soon lower the pH of the semen, adversely affecting the viability of spermatozoa.

Under aerobic conditions, the metabolism of fructose is

$$\text{Fructose} \overset{O_2}{\leftrightarrows} CO_2 + H_2O + 38 \text{ ATP (net yield)}$$

When oxygen is present, metabolism of fructose is 19 times more efficient in terms of energy yielded. The net energy from 38 ATP is 266,000 calories. When sufficient oxygen is present, the fructose molecule is metabolized completely to carbon dioxide and water. There is no buildup of lactic acid. In addition, sorbitol, plasmalogen, and, if in the female tract, GPC are available for metabolism and regeneration of ATP. Sorbitol and GPC are metabolized through the same biochemical pathways as fructose. Plasmalogen, a lipid rather than a carbohydrate, utilizes different metabolic pathways, but the needed enzymes are in the mitochondrial sheath.

14–4 FACTORS AFFECTING RATE OF METABOLISM

Rate of metabolism is the rate at which spermatozoa utilize their energy substrates. Under aerobic conditions, it can be monitored by measuring oxygen consumption, by measuring liberated carbon dioxide, or by methylene blue reduction. Under anaerobic conditions, the rate of reduction of pH or chemical determination of lactic acid buildup and/or fructose disappearance can be used as measures of metabolic rate. Control of metabolic rate is of interest because a reduction in metabolic rate is necessary to extend the storage life of semen. A number of factors contribute to reduced metabolic rate and extended life of spermatozoa in the epididymides (Chapter 3). In the epididymides, spermatozoa may remain fertile for up to 60 days. However, spermatozoa in a fresh ejaculate of semen will be fertile only for a few hours if steps are not taken to reduce their metabolic rate. The measures used must be reversible without injury to spermatozoa if they are to be practical for semen handling.

14–4.1 *Temperature*

Metabolic rate increases and the life span of spermatozoa decreases as the temperature of the semen rises. When the temperature rises above 50°C, spermatozoa suffer an irreversible loss of motility. If maintained at body temperature, spermatozoa will live for only a few hours due to exhaustion of available energy substrates, drop in pH due to buildup of lactic acid, or a combination of these factors. Reducing the temperature of the semen will slow metabolic rate and extend the fertile life of semen if precautions are taken to protect against *cold shock* and *freeze kill.*

Spermatozoa of all species studied are susceptible to cold shock if they are cooled too quickly. The most obvious indication of cold shock is an irreversible loss of motility. The most critical range for cold shock occurs when the semen temperature is being reduced from 15°C to 0°C. Cold shock protection is provided for bull, ram, and stallion semen by cooling slowly after addition of an egg yolk or a milk diluter. Both egg yolk and milk contain lecithin and lipoproteins, which protect against cold shock.

The second problem in reducing metabolic rate to extend the fertile life of semen is freeze kill. Spermatozoa may be killed during the freezing and/or thawing process, apparently by a disruption of the sperm cell membrane. Equilibration of bull semen in a diluter containing glycerol will give adequate protection. Some freeze kill will still occur, but fertility will not be affected if sufficient motile spermatozoa are placed into the semen unit before freezing. While there has been less success in freezing ram, buck, and stallion semen, glycerol is beneficial when freezing semen from these species. Excess glycerol is detrimental to boar and ram spermatozoa during freezing (Chapter 16).

Reducing the temperature of semen to lower its metabolic rate has been the most useful means of extending the fertile life of semen because it permits restoration of metabolic rate before insemination. Also, greater reduction of metabolic rate can be achieved without reducing fertility. When bull semen is frozen in liquid nitrogen at −196°C, its metabolic activity is reduced to less than 0.02% of the metabolic rate at body temperature. Further, fertility can be maintained in the semen for decades.

14–4.2 *pH*

A pH of about 7.0 (6.9 to 7.5 for different species) falls in the optimum activity range of most of the enzymes in spermatozoa. Therefore, a higher metabolic rate is expected when the pH of semen is maintained near neutrality (7.0). If the pH of semen deviates toward alkalinity or acidity, metabolic rate will be reduced. The practicability of altering the pH of semen to extend its life is limited by the narrow range over which pH can be altered without permanently reducing activity. Research in this area has established the importance of diluting semen in a buffered medium that resists changes in pH, so that maximum fertile life of the semen can be maintained.

14–4.3 *Osmotic Pressure*

Semen maintains maximum metabolic activity when diluted with an isotonic diluter. Either hypotonic or hypertonic diluters will reduce metabolic rate, but neither will extend the life of the semen. The spermatozoon membrane is a semipermeable membrane. Both hypotonic and hypertonic diluters will alter transfer of water through this membrane, disrupting the integrity of the cell. It is very important that only isotonic diluters be used. Spermatozoa remain motile longest when suspended in isotonic media.

14–4.4 *Concentration of Spermatozoa*

Increasing the concentration of spermatozoa above that found in the normal ejaculate will decrease metabolic rate. Potassium is the principal cation in the sperm cell, whereas sodium is the major cation in seminal plasma. Increasing the cellular concentration will increase the potassium-to-sodium ratio in the semen. Potassium is a natural metabolic inhibitor. Increasing its concentration will reduce the metabolic activity in the semen.

Generally, moderate dilution of semen in a buffered, isotonic medium containing fructose will not greatly alter metabolic rate but will extend the life of the semen. Dilution such as this is usually done before lowering the temperature of semen. Some caution must be observed. If dilution is excessive (> 1 to 1,000), motility and metabolic rate will be depressed.

14–4.5 *Hormones*

Testosterone and other androgens depress metabolic rate, but those concentrations found in the male system have no permanent effect. Fluids from the female tract increase the metabolic activity of spermatozoa. This is thought to be primarily an effect from estrogens, but other unidentified factors may be involved. The increased metabolic activity in the female tract likely increases motility, which increases the frequency of collisions between spermatozoa and the oocyte in the oviduct.

14–4.6 *Gases*

Low concentrations of carbon dioxide stimulate aerobic metabolism of spermatozoa. If the partial pressure of carbon dioxide exceeds 5% to 10%, metabolic rate is depressed. Carbon dioxide has been identified as a factor in regulating metabolic rate in the epididymides. Oxygen is necessary for aerobic metabolism. On the other hand, too high a level of oxygen is toxic and will depress metabolic rate. This is not likely to be a factor in the laboratory unless oxygen or air is being bubbled through the semen. Anaerobic metabolism can proceed under nitrogen, hydrogen, or helium gases with no effect on metabolic rate.

14–4.7 *Light*

Light intensities that are normally found in the laboratory can depress metabolic rate, motility, and fertility in spermatozoa. The harmful effect is observed only if semen is in contact with oxygen. The enzyme catalase will prevent the harmful effect of light, which suggests that light causes a photochemical reaction in the semen that results in the production of hydrogen peroxide. Semen should be protected from light and never exposed to direct sunlight.

14–4.8 *Antibacterial Agents*

Gentamicin, Tylosin, and Linco-Spectin (Section 16–3) are added to semen during processing to control bacterial growth. None have a demonstrated effect on metabolic rate. They sometimes increase fertility of semen from low fertility bulls. Also, these antibacterial agents may extend the fertile life of the semen by controlling bacteria, thus sparing energy substrates for spermatozoa.

SUGGESTED READING

FLIPSE, R. J. and W. R. ANDERSON. 1969. Metabolism of bovine semen. XIX. Products of fructose metabolism by washed spermatozoa. *J. Dairy Sci.,* 52:1070.

GRAVES, C. N. 1978. Semen and its components. *Physiology of Reproduction and Artificial Insemination of Cattle.* (2nd ed.) eds. G. W. Salisbury, N. L. VanDemark, and J. R. Lodge. W. H. Freeman and Co.

KILLIAN, G. J., D. A. CHAPMAN, and L. A. ROGOWSKI. 1993. Fertility associated proteins in Holstein bulls' seminal plasma. *Biol. Reprod.,* 49:1202.

MANN, T. 1964. *The Biochemistry of Semen and the Male Reproductive Tract.* Methuen and Co. Ltd.

SULLIVAN, J. J. 1978. Morphology and motility of spermatozoa. *Physiology of Reproduction and Artificial Insemination of Cattle.* (2nd ed.) eds. G. W. Salisbury, N. L. VanDemark, and J. R. Lodge. W. H. Freeman and Co.

THEIRIEN, I., G. BLEAU, and P. MANJUNATH. 1995. Phosphatidylcholine-binding proteins of bovine seminal plasma modulate capacitation of spermatozoa by heparin. *Biol. Reprod.,* 52:1372.

WHITE, I. G. 1973. Biochemical aspects of spermatozoa and their environment in the male reproductive tract. *J. Reprod. and Fert.* 18(Suppl.):225.

WHITE, I. G. 1974. Mammalian semen. *Reproduction in Farm Animals.* (3rd ed.) ed. E. S. E. Hafez. Lea and Febiger.

Semen Evaluation

The fertility level of an ejaculate is the ultimate evaluation. This can be accomplished only by inseminating females and waiting long enough to determine whether or not they return to estrus or until a pregnancy diagnosis can be made. Most AI organizations use a *nonreturn rate* as a measure of fertility for their bulls. Nonreturn rate is the percentage of females not reported as having had a second insemination within a given period of time. The earliest such information can be made available is about 35 days, and more reliable data are not available until 90 days after the semen is first used in the field. Even with frozen semen, a high percentage of an ejaculate may be used before any information is available on its actual conception rate.

It is imperative, therefore, that laboratory technicians learn as much about an ejaculate of semen as possible within the framework of economic feasibility. This chapter is devoted to several laboratory tests which, individually or in combination, give some indication of semen quality. The student should keep in mind that these tests are not actual measures of fertility and that an individual ejaculate that scores high on the laboratory tests may actually have a lower fertility rate than another sample that scores lower. However, the average conception rate of all ejaculates that score high on the laboratory tests will be higher than the average fertility rate for those that score low. The procedures for conducting each test will be described, and the value and limitations of each will be discussed.

15–1 GROSS EXAMINATION

Each ejaculate of semen is examined immediately for certain characteristics. The volume is determined not only for use in processing but also to establish a pattern for the individual male. Deviations from this pattern, particularly downward trends in volume, indicate a problem. The problem may be due to health factors, or it could be an indication that the collection procedures for that particular male need revision.

For many years, graduated 15-ml or 25-ml glass collection tubes were used and the volume was determined by visually reading the graduations on the tubes. Only one of the six large bull semen–producing businesses surveyed is still using the graduated tubes. The other five have implemented a procedure in which plastic tubes of uniform weights are being used as collection tubes. Three are using 15-ml tubes, while the other two are using 50-ml tubes. After collection, the tube with the ejaculate is weighed on a top-loading balance and the weight is converted to milliliters by a computer. Some bull semen–producing businesses are using a computer program to correct for the slight increase in weight

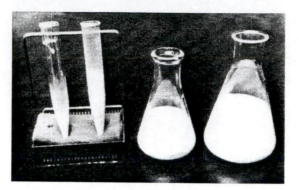

Figure 15–1   Freshly collected ejaculates of (*L to R*) ram, bull, stallion, and boar semen. Note differences in volume and density.

due to increased density of sperm, but others are overlooking that slight error. Weighing reduces errors by 10%, compared with visually reading tube graduations, especially when small volumes or bubbles are encountered.

The gross appearance of a normal ejaculate of bull semen is creamy white in color. When observed closely, swirls of movement can be seen. The layer along the glass tube may have a granular appearance due to sperm movement. Samples with low concentrations will appear watery or less opaque. Ram and buck semen, while lower in volume and higher in concentration, have a similar appearance to bull semen. Stallion and boar semen, being much less concentrated, will not have the dense appearance of bull, buck, and ram semen (Figure 15–1). Boar semen may have a pink tinge, indicating blood contamination or a slight yellow color indicating preputial fluid or urine contamination. Yellow samples usually have an offensive odor. All contaminated semen should be discarded.

A few minutes after collection the bottom of the collection tube or bottle should be examined for dirt or other debris. Presence of such contaminants indicates that the male has not been properly cleaned prior to collection or that careless collection techniques exist.

15–2   PROGRESSIVE MOTILITY

Motility of a sample of semen is expressed as the percentage of cells that are motile under their own power. A progressively motile sperm is one that is moving or progressing from one point to another in a more or less straight line. Most ejaculates will show other types of motility. These include both circular and reverse movement due to a tail abnormality and vibrating or rocking movement often associated with aging. Progressive motility is the most important individual quality test, because fertility is highly correlated with number of motile sperm inseminated. The percentage motility of semen ejaculates can range from 0% to 80%. The usual motility determination is a subjective measurement based on the judgment of the individual making the determination. Because of this, most laboratory personnel will use multiples of 10 in reporting progressive motility (that is, 40%, 50%, 60%, or 70%), feeling that this is as accurate as one can make the determination. Based on large numbers of ejaculates, there is little difference in the fertility level of ejaculates with initial motilities of 50% to 80% if the desired number of motile sperm are present at the time of insemination. Any difference is masked by the usual practice of adding additional sperm per breeding unit to bring the number of motile sperm to optimum. Samples with less than 40% initial motility are not suitable for use unless the ejaculate is from an exceptionally superior bull from which one would be willing to accept a low conception rate. It appears that the motile sperm present in these low motility samples have had their fertilizing capacity affected by the factor or factors that caused the low motility. Research has shown that dead or immotile sperm in a sample do not adversely affect the motility or livability *in vitro* of the motile sperm in the sample.

15–2.1 *Preparation of Slide*

Some precautionary measures should be taken prior to the preparation of the slide. If the sample has been standing for several minutes, it should be mixed by gently inverting the tube two or three times. Undiluted semen, particularly from the bull, buck, and ram, is too concentrated for accurate motility determinations. Small subsamples must be diluted with an *isotonic* solution (same free ion concentration as the semen) so that individual sperm can be observed. This requires a dilution rate of about 1 to 100 for bull, buck, and ram semen and 1 to 10 for boar and stallion semen.

Motility examinations must be made with the aid of the microscope and a suitable preparation on a microscope slide. A clean, dry slide should be placed in a stage incubator or on a heated microscope stage and allowed to warm to a temperature of 38°C. A small droplet of diluted semen is placed on the slide with a glass stirring rod or small pipette. It is important that uniform droplets be used in each preparation so that consistent determinations can be made. The droplet should be covered with a glass coverslip to spread to a uniform thickness and to prevent drying. The slide is now ready for microscopic examination.

15–2.2 *Use of Microscope*

When a stage incubator is used instead of a heated microscope stage, the prepared slide should remain in the stage incubator during examination to prevent changes in temperature (Figure 15–2). A magnification of approximately 400× is preferred. Several fields should be examined and an estimate made of the percentage of sperm that are progressively motile to the nearest 10%. For samples that are above 50% motile, it is easier to make the estimate from the percentage of sperm not progressively motile. Equipment is available that will display the microscopic image on a glass screen, making the determination easier and more accurate.

Motility determinations are made on diluted samples both before and after freezing in the same manner as described for fresh semen, except that it is not necessary to further dilute the samples before preparing the slide. It is important to remember that the diluted sample contains either egg yolk or milk and, in the case of frozen semen, glycerol. The viscosity contributed by these materials slows motility but does not alter the percentage of progressively motile sperm. Whole milk diluters and some others such as egg yolk with phosphate buffer make the individual sperm cells difficult to see. Motility percentage can be determined in these materials, but it is more difficult and less accurate.

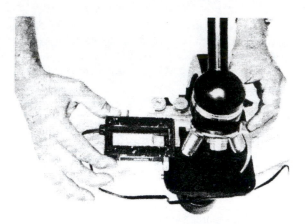

Figure 15–2 Stage incubator or heated microscope stage keeps semen smear warm while motility determination is made.

Circular and backwards motility are indications of either cold shock or contamination with water. *Hypotonic* (lower free ion concentration than semen) diluters due to error in preparation can also cause this problem. When this abnormal motility pattern is observed, check these three factors in the order listed. See Chapters 14 and 16 for additional information.

15–3 CONCENTRATION OF SPERM CELLS

Sperm cell concentrations are expressed as number of cells per ml and must be known for each ejaculate in order to make the maximum number of breeding units containing a given number of motile sperm per unit. A permanent record should be kept of the concentration of each ejaculate from each male. A downward trend in concentration for a particular male might indicate a serious problem. The problem could be related to insufficient sexual stimulation prior to collection, a collection schedule that is too strenuous, or an illness that occurred or began several weeks earlier. There is little relationship between concentration and fertility when the concentration is within the normal range. Again, some masking may occur due to compensating dilution rates. Ejaculates from bulls containing less than 500 million cells per ml should be used with caution because lowered fertility is likely. There is less information available on the other species, but caution is advised when the sperm cell concentration drops below 50% of normal.

15–3.1 *Direct Cell Count (Hemocytometer)*

The hemocytometer was designed for counting blood cells. It consists of a specially designed slide that contains two counting chambers and two dilution pipettes (Figure 15–3). The counting chambers are 0.1 mm in depth and have a ruled grid (Figure 15–4) on the bottom of the chamber that is 1.0 mm square. This grid is subdivided into 25 smaller squares.

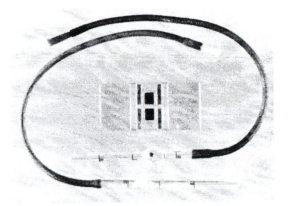

Figure 15–3 Standard hemocytometer slide and dilution pipettes. Large pipette is used for bull and ram semen, while small one is used for boar and stallion semen.

With a known depth and area, the number of sperm can be determined for a specific volume. One of the two pipettes is designated for counting red blood cells and is designed for dilution rates of 1:100 and 1:200. A dilution rate of 1:200 is normally used for bull, buck, and ram semen, while a dilution rate of 1:100 is preferable for gel-free boar and stallion semen. The smaller pipette, which was designed for counting white blood cells, may be preferred for use with boar and stallion semen of low concentration. The diluent used must kill the sperm so that counting can be accomplished. The authors have found that a 2% aqueous solution of eosin accomplishes this and has the additional advantage of staining the sperm heads so that they are easier to count. Semen is drawn into the capillary tube of the dilution pipette to the desired mark. The pipette tip is carefully wiped to remove semen clinging to the outside without drawing any from the capillary. The semen is pulled into the bulb of the pipette and the pipette is filled with the diluent. The contents of the pipette are mixed either with a mechanical shaker or by holding the ends of the pipette between the thumb and the index finger and shaking it vigorously in 100 back-and-forth 12-inch movements. The bulb of the pipette contains a small glass bead that makes thorough mixing possible. Sufficient diluted semen is blown from the dilution pipette to ensure that the diluent containing no sperm has been flushed from the capillary.

The coverslip is placed over the counting chambers and a small amount of semen is placed at the edge of the coverslip. Capillary action will draw the semen under the coverslip. Both chambers are thus filled with care being taken not to overfill. Overfilling results in semen running off the edge of the counting chamber, setting up currents which make counting difficult and inaccurate. The slide is placed under the microscope and the grid area of a counting chamber is located with the low-power objective (100×). The 1.0-mm square area is examined for uniform distribution of sperm. The high-power objective (400×) is used to count the number of sperm within the desired number of squares. With bull, buck, and ram semen, the corner and center squares are counted. With boar and stallion semen, it might be necessary to count all 25 squares. Both chambers can be counted for greater accuracy. When 25 squares are counted, the volume represented is 0.1 mm^3. If only 5 squares

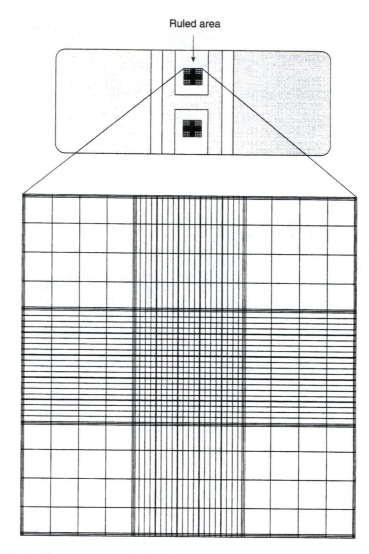

Figure 15–4 Hemocytometer slide with the grid of the counting chamber enlarged. Note the 25 squares that are further divided to facilitate counting of cells. (Campbell and Campbell. 1997. *Laboratory Mathematics— Medical and Biological Application*. Mosby.)

are counted, the number must be multiplied by 5 to obtain the number of sperm in 0.1 mm^3. The number of sperm/ml can be found by using the following formula:

No. sperm/ml = no. sperm in 0.1 mm^3 × 10 × dilution rate × 1,000

The hemocytometer is a time-consuming and tedious method of determining sperm concentration. It is also subject to considerable error for the inexperienced or careless tech-

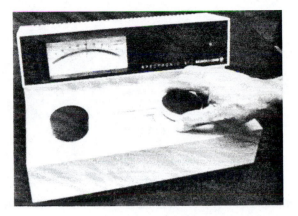

Figure 15–5   One model of a photoelectric colorimeter used to determine semen concentration.

nician. However, the conscientious individual with some experience can provide accurate information. The inexperienced person should make two dilutions of a sample and count two chambers from each dilution as a check on his or her technique. This should be continued until the two dilutions consistently agree within 5% of each other.

15–3.2 *Visible Spectrophotometry*

The visible spectrophotometry technology is used by all commercial cooperative and noncooperative semen-producing operations to determine preprocessing concentrations. A determination of sperm cell concentration can be made in approximately 1 minute. The procedure is based on light absorption by the sperm in the semen sample. The equipment consists of a light source, which passes through a series of lenses and filters and then through a diluted sample of semen. The light which passes through the semen is measured with a galvanometer (Figure 15–5). There are several makes and models of instruments suitable for use, but each must be calibrated by using samples of known concentration as determined by electronic particle counter, so that the galvanometer readings can be accurately converted to concentration figures.

A concentration determination is made by pipetting the required volume of 2.9% sodium citrate dihydrate solution into a vial especially designed for the instrument. To this is added the required amount of the ejaculate. The tube is mixed by inverting two or three times before inserting into the instrument. The instrument is turned on and allowed to warm up before use. A reading is taken from the galvanometer and referred to the calibration table for the concentration figure. Since the sodium citrate solution used to dilute the semen for this determination is a part of most semen diluters, this subsample may be added to the diluted ejaculate, provided that it has been handled properly and not allowed to become cold shocked.

15–3.3 *Electronic Particle Counter*

The electronic particle counter (EPC) can be used to accurately determine the number of sperm cells in an ejaculate (Figure 15–6). It is more accurate than either the hemocytometer or the photoelectric colorimeter. The instrument can be adjusted for particle size so that only

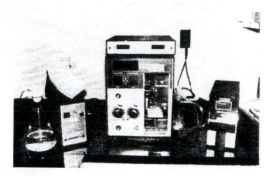

Figure 15–6 Electronic particle counters may be used to determine sperm cell concentration.

the sperm cells in a sample will be counted. A diluted sample of semen is passed through a capillary so that only one cell at a time can pass between two electrodes. The sperm head causes an abrupt increase in resistance, which is registered on a counter. The greatest disadvantage of this instrument is its cost. Four of the six large bull semen–producing businesses surveyed own an electronic particle counter and a fifth has easy access to one. Two of them use the instrument to determine the postthaw concentration of every ejaculate, while three use the EPC to randomly spot-check postthawed semen concentration as a check on their spectrophotometer. All of them use the EPC to calibrate their spectrophotometers.

15–4   Sperm Cell Morphology

Sperm cell morphology was covered in Chapter 14, and the student is referred to Figure 14–2 for the various sperm abnormalities. The abnormal sperm count is not conducted on every ejaculate of semen because of the time required. A count should be made monthly so that a trend in percentage of abnormal sperm can be charted on each male. Sudden increases in percentage of abnormals would indicate a problem which should be followed carefully. Semen ejaculates may show as few as 5% abnormal sperm, while others may approach 100%. Fertility is usually not affected until the level of abnormal sperm exceeds 20% to 25%. Any influence that may be contributed by the abnormal sperm up to the 25% level is probably masked by the usual practice of adding additional sperm per breeding unit to bring the number of motile sperm to optimum. Abnormal sperm do not show progressive motility. Therefore, as the percentage of abnormal sperm increases, the progressive motility percentage decreases. Many abnormal sperm can be detected while samples are examined for motility. This can be used as an indication of whether further morphological study is needed.

15–4.1 *Preparation of Slide*

It is essential that good technique be used in preparing the slides for morphological examination. Poor technique can result in damage to the tails, which could be interpreted as naturally occurring abnormalities. This can be quite serious, since a high percentage of the observed abnormalities involve the tail. If a freshly collected sample is to be examined, a small drop of 2.9% sodium citrate solution is placed on a warm microscope slide. A 3-mm

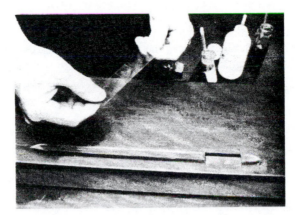

Figure 15–7 Slide preparation for sperm morphology determination. Semen and staining mixture are spread between two microscope slides. The slides are gently pulled apart and dried.

glass stirring rod is touched to the surface of the semen sample, and the sperm that adhere to the rod are transferred to the citrate solution on the slide. The semen is carefully mixed with the citrate solution and another warm slide is placed over the first, spreading the mixture evenly between them. The two slides are separated by pulling the ends in opposite directions with a smooth motion (Figure 15–7). Care must be taken to have sufficient fluid between the two slides to prevent pressure on the sperm. One of the slides should be placed flat on a warm surface and allowed to dry.

Slide preparations from diluted semen are made in the same manner, except the dilution rate of the semen must be considered. Samples that are diluted for maximum utilization usually do not need further dilution with sodium citrate solution. The objective of dilution is to disperse the sperm sufficiently so that individual sperm may be observed. If the sperm are too concentrated on the first slide, a second one can be made with the appropriate dilution.

15–4.2 *Staining Slides*

A large number of staining materials and techniques have been used. The principal objective of any staining technique is to make the cells easily observed so that abnormalities can be discerned. The easiest and most widely used techniques of staining incorporate the stains in the preparation of the slide. Eosin, along with a background stain such as nigrosin, opal blue, or fast green, works well (Section 15–5.1). Nigrosin is superior to opal blue and fast green for diluted samples containing egg yolk. Eosin does not stain the living sperm heads, but the background stain causes the unstained sperm heads to be clearly visible.

Other staining and counterstaining procedures have been used. Several variations using carbol fuchsin as a stain, with methylene blue or analine gentian violet as a counterstain, have been used successfully.

15–4.3 *Examination and Counting*

Several fields on each slide should be examined to determine whether a satisfactory slide has been prepared. The sperm should be dispersed so that the individual heads and tails can be observed clearly. A high percentage of bent or broken tails could indicate poor technique in slide preparation. When most of the abnormal tail bends are oriented in the same direction, one should suspect that abnormal pressure due to insufficient fluid between the two slides occurred during preparation. Should either of these problems be observed, another slide should be made with greater care. The slide should be examined with a magnification of approximately 400×.

One hundred sperm should be observed at random per slide and classified. Statistical studies have shown that little precision is gained by counting more than 100 sperm per slide. If more precision is desired, more than one slide should be made and counted on the same sample. (See Section 14–1 for the classification of morphologically abnormal sperm.)

15–5   DIFFERENTIAL STAINING OF LIVE AND DEAD SPERM

Eosin is referred to as a differential stain in that it cannot pass through living cell membranes but can pass through nonliving cell membranes. A background stain such as nigrosin, opal blue, or fast green helps make the unstained sperm heads visible. The percentage of live sperm in a sample of semen has been used as a verification of motility determinations. The student should keep in mind that the percentage of live sperm will always be somewhat higher than the percentage of motile sperm.

15–5.1   *Staining Techniques*

Several staining mixtures have given good results. All of them contain about 1% eosin plus one of the background stains. Preferred background stains are 2% fast green, 4% analine blue, or 5% nigrosin. Both eosin and the background stain are dissolved in 2.9% sodium citrate dihydrate buffer. The slides are prepared in the manner described in Section 15–4.1 with two exceptions: (1) the staining mixture is substituted for the sodium citrate buffer used to dilute the semen and (2) the slides must be dried quickly on a heated plate (55°C to 60°C) with a small electric fan directed across the plate (Figure 15–8). When slides are allowed to dry slowly, some of the sperm may die and be stained before the drying process is completed, thus giving a false indication of the percentage of live sperm.

15–5.2   *Counting Slides*

Several fields at random should be examined and counted. Between 300 and 500 total cells are usually counted in order to give accurate results. Partially stained sperm should be included with the totally stained sperm representing the number of dead sperm in the sample. The unstained sperm represent those that were alive in the sample.

15–6   SPEED OF SPERM

The rate of motility is defined as the speed at which sperm travel. Electronic equipment is available which can measure sperm speeds objectively, but the equipment is expensive and is not used in a routine semen-producing operation. The rate of motility is frequently as-

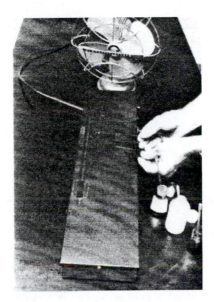

Figure 15–8 Slides for live-dead determination must be dried quickly using a heated plate and electric fan.

sessed subjectively on a scale of 1 to 5. This can be done about as accurately as the motility percentage but has little value in evaluating semen quality.

Individual bull sperm have been clocked at speeds of 21 mm per minute and, in samples of semen with excellent motility, several sperm have shown speeds averaging 15 mm per minute. When several sperm are checked from each of a large number of ejaculates, an average speed of 6 mm per minute can be expected.

15–7 EVALUATING FROZEN SEMEN

The previously described quality tests must be used to determine whether an ejaculate of semen is good enough to process. A second series of evaluations must be made following freezing. The freeze thaw survival rates of semen from different males and different ejaculates from the same male vary greatly. Since conception rate in AI depends greatly on an adequate number of motile sperm at the time of insemination, it is imperative that an accurate postthaw evaluation be made. Each ejaculate of frozen semen must be evaluated to determine whether it will provide that optimum number of motile sperm. Between 5% and 15% of the ejaculates from bulls meeting the standards for processing are discarded after freezing. Some of the variation in the percentage of ejaculates discarded seems to be related to season, with the highest rate in the summer.

15–7.1 *Photographic Method of Determining Progressive Motility*

Time-exposure photography as an objective method of determining motility has been reported. The procedure employs a dark-field microscope equipped with a camera. Semen should be diluted to 10 million sperm per ml and placed in a Petroff-Hausser counting

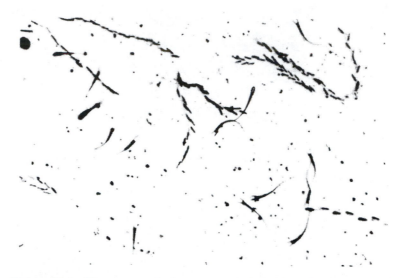

Figure 15–9 Time-exposed photomicrograph used to objectively measure progressive motility. Streaks represent motile sperm. (Courtesy of American Breeders Service, DeForest, Wis.)

chamber. This chamber has a depth of only 20 microns, compared with 100 microns of the hemocytometer chamber, and conforms better to the depth of focus on the microscope.

The filled chamber is warmed for 30 seconds on a 38°C warming plate before it is placed on the heated stage of the dark-field microscope. Six 2-second exposures are made at the periphery of the ruled area at the 1, 3, 5, 7, 9, and 11 o'clock positions. The desired magnification to the film is 75×. The developed film is projected on a white wall for further magnification and counting (Figure 15–9). Motile cell counts are made by counting the number of tracks on the film. Nonmotile cells must also be counted to determine percentage motility. The procedure gives highly repeatable results.

Motility can be determined photographically at any stage of processing. However, the procedure has been used primarily in determining postfreezing motility. This is probably due to the time and expense involved. An efficient laboratory technician can make 30 to 35 determinations in an 8-hour day. Only one of the six semen-producing businesses surveyed uses the procedure; however, it is used to check the freeze thaw survival rate on all ejaculates. The procedure does not work well when whole milk is used as a diluter.

15–7.2 *Changes in the Acrosome*

Researchers have reported that aging or an injury to sperm causes acrosomal cap deterioration. Changes are first noted at the apical ridge but progress to the point where the entire acrosome is gone. These changes were first noted with the electron microscope but can be seen with differential interference contrast and phase contrast optics. Differential interference contrast seems to be preferred (Figure 15–10).

The freezing and thawing of semen inflict injury to some sperm. The important point is to know accurately the percentage of injured sperm. Good-quality dairy bull semen will have about 90% intact acrosomes prior to freezing. After freezing, the percentage of intact

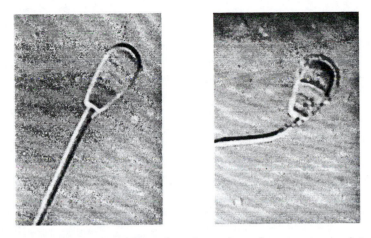

Figure 15–10 Photomicrographs of postthawed spermatozoa; intact acrosome *(left)* and damaged acrosome *(right).* (Courtesy of Select Sires, Inc., Plain City, Ohio.)

acrosomes drops to 60% to 65%. Most beef bulls will have 50% to 55% intact acrosomes in postthaw samples. Studies have shown higher correlations between intact acrosomes and nonreturns than between postthaw motility and nonreturns.

To determine damaged acrosomes, thawed semen is incubated in a 37°C water bath for 2 to 4 hours. A drop of incubated semen is placed on a warm slide and covered with a coverslip. Motility and acrosome integrity are evaluated by counting 100 sperm with the differential interference contrast microscope at 800×. If the first sample is substandard, a second smear should be made and examined. If it is also substandard, another sample may be thawed and examined the next day before a decision is made to discard the ejaculate.

There is no minimum percentage of intact acrosomes to use in discarding ejaculates. A profile must be developed for species, breeds within species, and then for individual males. When the percentage of intact acrosomes falls significantly below this profile for an ejaculate, it should be discarded.

The use of the intact acrosome procedure has been widely adopted in the AI industry. All of the six semen-producing businesses surveyed were using it to some degree. Two were using the procedure to evaluate all ejaculates after freezing and thawing, while the remainder were checking new bulls and problem bulls and spot-checking all other bulls. Again, the whole milk diluter causes problems.

15–8 Computer Automated Semen Analyzer

Several companies have developed technology and equipment for objectively analyzing semen samples for concentration, motility (including forward or progressive motility and circular motility), and morphology. The systems are referred to as computer automated semen analyzers (CASA). Developments in this area have been very rapid. In just a few years, the equipment is already in the second-and third-generation stages.

A problem that had to be solved with the first-and second-generation systems was eliminating debris from the medium. Such inanimate objects were not differentiated from immobile sperm. This required that the diluter be passed through a .2μ membrane filter system. A third generation system analyzes each object for a tail and if none is found it is not counted.

Another problem that needed to be overcome was the lack of visibility of sperm in milk diluters and other complex media. The employment of a stain (Hoechst 333420), which is adsorbed by the DNA in the sperm heads, and the use of ultraviolet strobe light enables the CASA to count immotile sperm and to track and analyze the motility pattern of the motile sperm even in the whole milk diluter. The motility of the stained sperm was compared with motility of unstained sperm of the same ejaculates and no adverse effect of the stain was noted.

Early research with these systems dealt with human semen, but considerable effort has been directed to semen from bulls and stallions. The objective of most of this research has been to improve the predictability of fertilizing capabilities of semen. This includes evaluating the postthaw survivability of sperm.

A very high correlation between the CASA and spectrophotometry methods for determination of concentration has given added confidence in the latter. Motility studies, however, showed that CASA provided a much more discriminating estimate of the percentage of motile sperm cells than did the subjective procedure, even when the latter was done by highly experienced technicians. A range of 30 percentage units was obtained with CASA, while the range for the subjective method was only 9 percentage units for 80 ejaculates evaluated in one study. Several characteristics of sperm movement have been studied, including various speeds of motility. When several of the variables were studied and collectively correlated with fertility, higher correlation coefficients were obtained. Further research with the CASA should determine which variables are most useful in estimating fertility of semen and should greatly enhance our ability to predict the fertility of an individual bull's semen. Of all semen characteristics of stallion semen studied with the CASA that are related to fertility, progressive motility had the highest correlation.

While the CASA systems are excellent research tools, it is doubtful that any will be used in the foreseeable future in a routine processing operation. Of the six semen-producing operations surveyed, only one owns a CASA and it is used only for in-house research. A second stud has a close working relationship with a university research team and felt their research needs were being met through cooperative efforts.

15–9 OTHER TESTS

Several other tests have been suggested and used in evaluating semen samples. Livability in storage was used extensively when semen was utilized in the liquid form. This involved daily motility determinations on the semen stored at 5°C. The freezing of semen has largely eliminated this procedure.

The resistance of sperm to cold shock has been used as a measure of quality. Several methods of measuring metabolic activity such as oxygen uptake, fructolysis, methylene blue reduction time, resazurin reduction time, and pH change all provide some information.

SUGGESTED READING

BLACK, E. L., R. P. AMMAN, R. A. BOWEN, and D. FRANTZ. 1989. Changes in quality of stallion spermatozoa during cryopreservation: Plasma membrane integrity and motion characteristics. *Theriogenology,* 31:283.

BLOM, E. 1950. A one-minute live-dead sperm stain by means of eosin-nigrosin. *Fert. and Ster.,* 1:176.

BUDWORTH, P. R., R. P. AMMAN, and P. L. CHAPMAN. 1988. Relationship between computerized measurements of motion of frozen-thawed bull spermatozoa and fertility. *J. Andrology,* 9:41.

ELLIOTT, F. I. 1978. Semen evaluation. *Physiology of Reproduction and Artificial Insemination of Cattle.* (2nd ed.) eds. G. W. Salisbury, N. L. VanDemark, and J. R. Lodge. W. H. Freeman Co.

FARRELL, P. B., G. A. PRESICCE, C. C. BROCKETT, and R. H. FOOTE. 1998. Quantification of bull semen characteristics measured by CASA and the relationship to fertility. *Theriogenology,* 49:871.

FOOTE, R. H. 1972. How to measure sperm cell concentration by turbidity. *Proc. 4th Tech. Conf. Artif. Insem. Reprod.,* p. 57. NAAB, Columbia, Mo.

JASKO, D. J., T. V. LITTLE, K. SMITH, D. H. LEIN, and R. H. FOOTE. 1988. Objective analysis of stallion sperm motility. *Theriogenology,* 30:1159.

MARSHALL, C. 1978. Use of differential interference contrast optics as a quality control and research tool. *Proc. 7th Tech. Conf. Artif. Insem. Reprod.,* p. 62. NAAB, Columbia, Mo.

MITCHELL, J., R. D. HANSON, and N. FLEMING. 1978. Utilizing differential interference contrast microscopy for evaluating abnormal spermatozoa. *Proc. 7th Tech. Conf. Artif. Insem. Reprod.,* p. 64. NAAB, Columbia, Mo.

SAACKE, R. G. 1972. Semen quality tests and their relationship to fertility. *Proc. 4th Tech. Conf. Artif. Insem. Reprod.,* p. 22. NAAB, Columbia, Mo.

SWANSON, E. W. and H. J. BEARDEN. 1951. An eosin-nigrosin stain for differentiating live and dead bovine spermatozoa. *J. Anim. Sci.,* 10:981.

TARDIF, A. L., P. B. FARRELL, V. TROUERN-TREND, M. E. SIMKIN, and R. H. FOOTE. 1998. Use of Hoechst 33342 stain to evaluate live fresh and frozen bull sperm by computer-assisted analysis. *L. Androl.,* 19:201.

VAN DELLEN, G. and F. I. ELLIOTT. 1978. Procedure for time exposure darkfield photomicrography to measure percentage progressively motile spermatozoa. *Proc. 7th Tech. Conf. Artif. Insem. Reprod.,* p. 55. NAAB, Columbia, Mo.

16

Semen Processing, Storage, and Handling

The processing of semen involves a great deal of responsibility. It not only includes the collection and evaluation of the semen, the procedures for which were covered in Chapters 13 and 15, but the processor also has the responsibility for preparing a satisfactory diluter that will maintain the viability of the sperm and ensure a disease-free product. Attention must also be given to semen dilution, dilution rate, method and rate of cooling, proper addition of a cryoprotectant, proper packaging, freezing method and rate, suitable storage, and shipping.

The U.S. AI industry realized the significance of the preceding responsibilities early and in 1946 organized the National Association of Animal Breeders (NAAB) to provide guidance and oversight. At the beginning, the association made recommendations to the member organization but compliance was voluntary. Each member organization has a proportionate number of delegates who have input in the development of policies and vote to elect a board of directors. The membership later realized that they needed an inspection and certification procedure so that those who purchase their semen stamped with a certification seal can be assured that it meets strict standards for quality, disease control, and genetic improvement claims. This led to the organization of Certified Semen Services (CSS) in 1976, which serves as an inspecting and certification arm of NAAB. This organization maintains an up-to-date document entitled *CSS Minimum Requirements for Disease Control of Semen Produced for AI,* which contains detailed procedures for (1) general sanitary conditions, (2) mount animal requirements, (3) preentry testing, (4) isolation and retesting, (5) resident herd testing, and (6) antibiotics and semen processing. An appendix also provides detailed instructions on the following:

1. Antibiotics/stock solutions
2. Neat semen treatment
3. Nonglycerol fraction of diluter
4. Glycerol-containing fraction of diluter
5. Final concentration of antibiotics
6. Required processing procedures
7. Deviation from required processing procedures
8. Tested and approved diluters

A CSS representative makes an on-site inspection of each member organization to review procedures and check all records to ensure compliance. All organizations that pass the inspection are allowed to use the CSS Certification Seal in their advertising and on their semen labels.

Also, NAAB sponsors and financially supports research related to AI and holds biennial technical conferences for the dissemination of research findings. Nonmember semen processors can obtain the certification services of CSS by paying the same fees paid by members and passing the annual inspection. About 97% of all bovine semen sold in the United States is certified by CSS. In 1998, CSS began discussing a possible certification program with the American Association of Swine Practitioners. At the same time, it was decided that equine AI programs were not adequately developed for CSS to offer a certification program.

For additional information about the services offered by NAAB or CSS, send inquiries to P.O. Box 1033, Columbia, MO 65205-1033.

The procedures outlined in this chapter are in line with the minimum standards of NAAB. The specific diseases, their symptoms, diagnostic procedures, and control measures are covered in Chapter 26.

16–1 IMPORTANCE AND PROPERTIES OF SEMEN DILUTERS

The success of AI, particularly in cattle, goats, and sheep, depended greatly on the development of satisfactory semen diluters. The AI industry has adopted the term "extender" to replace diluter. When AI was first being adopted, some felt that the use of the term "diluted semen" created a stigma, something that was not to be done, such as adding water to milk, so a switch to "extended semen" was made, but the authors prefer the original term, "diluter." A 6-ml ejaculate of semen from the bull may contain a sufficient number of motile sperm to inseminate 200 to 300 cows, but it would be virtually impossible to divide 6 ml into that many units. The AI pioneers also found that sperm in undiluted semen lived for only short periods of time and that cooling undiluted semen very slowly to 5°C caused the death of many sperm. It became obvious that a satisfactory semen diluter would have to do more than increase the volume of an ejaculate. The diluter would have to protect the sperm during cooling and extend the life of the sperm.

The following properties of a good semen diluter have been delineated along with examples of materials that satisfy these properties.

1. A diluter must be isotonic with semen (have the same free ion concentration)—2.9% sodium citrate dihydrate or 0.2 molar tris solution.
2. Buffering capacity must be provided (prevent pH change by neutralizing acid produced by sperm metabolism)—isotonic sodium citrate or tris solution or milk.
3. Diluters must protect the sperm from cold shock injury during the cooling from body temperature to 5°C—lecithin and lipoproteins from egg yolk or milk.
4. Nutrients must be provided for sperm metabolism—egg yolk, milk, and some simple sugars.
5. Microbial contaminants must be controlled—antibiotics such as Gentamicin, Tylosin, and Linco-Spectin.

6. Sperm must be protected from injury during freezing and thawing—glycerol.

7. The diluter must preserve the life of the sperm with a minimum drop in fertility—combination of known and unknown factors.

16–2   BUFFER SOLUTIONS USED IN SEMEN DILUTERS

The buffer solutions, which make up the major portion of semen diluters, serve a dual role. By neutralizing the lactic acid produced by the metabolic activity of the sperm, minute changes in pH are prevented. The proper concentration of the buffer salt provides an isotonic environment for the sperm. In addition, the salt used must not be toxic to the sperm at the level required for isotonicity. Of the many compounds and combinations of compounds available that satisfy at least one of the three criteria listed, only four buffer solutions have been found to be satisfactory for use in semen diluters.

16–2.1   *Phosphate Buffer Solution*

The phosphate buffer was a component of the first satisfactory semen diluter reported in 1939. It was composed of 2.0 g of $Na_2HPO_4 \cdot 12 H_2O$ and 0.2 g of KH_2PO_4 in sufficient distilled water to make 100 ml of solution. While just as satisfactory as other buffer solutions, phosphate buffer has not been used because it produces an opaque mixture when added to egg yolk, resulting in poor sperm visibility.

16–2.2   *Citrate Buffer Solution*

The suitability of sodium citrate dihydrate solution as a buffer for semen was discovered in 1941. It is composed of 2.9 g of sodium citrate dihydrate in sufficient distilled water to make 100 ml of solution. An alternate sodium citrate buffer can be made by mixing 2.12 g of sodium citrate dihydrate and 0.183 g citric acid monohydrate with sufficient distilled water to make 100 ml of buffer. The sodium citrate buffer soon replaced the phosphate buffer in preparing semen diluters. When mixed with egg yolk it leaves the mixture sufficiently transparent to give good visibility of the individual sperm.

16–2.3   *Tris Buffer Solution*

Tris (hydroxymethyl) aminomethane has been used as a buffered medium for bull and boar sperm since 1963. The tris buffer seems to have value in prolonging sperm life at ambient temperature, 5°C and −196°C. Various molarities and pH levels have been tested. A 0.2-M concentration and a pH of 6.5 plus 1% fructose gives best results for bull semen. To prepare the buffer, 3.028 g tris and 1.0 g fructose are placed in a 200-ml beaker and about 75 ml of distilled water is added. With the aid of a pH meter, enough 10% citric acid is added to lower the pH to 6.5. A magnetic stirring device is helpful. The mixture is poured into a 100-ml volumetric flask and brought to volume with distilled water. An alternate tris buffer can be made by mixing 2.42 g of tris (hydroxymethyl) aminomethane, 1.38 g of citric acid monohydrate, and 1 g of fructose with sufficient distilled water to make 100 ml of buffer.

16–2.4 *Milk*

Both whole milk and skim milk meet all three of the criteria for a satisfactory buffer when heated to 90°C to 95°C for 10 minutes, and they meet all other requirements of a satisfactory semen diluter.

16–3 ANTIMICROBIAL AGENTS FOR SEMEN DILUTERS

Attention was called to the problem of microbial contaminants in ejaculated bull semen as early as 1941. The number of organisms per ml can range from no detectable organisms to several million. The number of organisms can be reduced by properly cleaning the underline of the male prior to collection. All equipment used in semen collection, processing, and storing should be sterile and not contributors of other contaminants.

A wide variety of organisms has been isolated from semen. Many of these organisms are not pathogenic but do compete with the sperm for nutrients and do produce metabolic by-products that have an adverse effect on livability of the sperm. Fortunately, it has been the longtime goal of the commercial AI organizations to eliminate from their bulls the diseases that can be transmitted through the semen. (These specific diseases will be discussed in Chapter 26.) The possibility still exist that undiscovered pathogens may be ejaculated in the semen and unknown sources of extraneous contaminants may occur.

The beneficial effects of antibiotics added to semen diluters were discovered in 1946. Much of the increase in conception rate in those early years was the result of controlling the venereal disease, vibriosis (campylobacteriosis). Table 16–1 shows the effect of antibacterial agents on a group of low and a group of high fertility bulls. Even though the nonreturn rate was increased for the high fertility bulls, this increase was not nearly as dramatic as for the low fertility bulls. It was later determined that the primary difference in nonreturn rates for the two groups of bulls prior to the addition of antibacterial agents was due largely to *Campylobacter fetus venerealis (Vibrio fetus venerealis)* infection in the low fertility bulls. In the absence of specific infectious disease organisms, antibiotics are beneficial by reducing competition from other bacteria.

A vast array of antibiotics and fungicidal agents have been used experimentally. Many of the antibiotics and particularly some of the fungicidal agents are extremely

Table 16–1   *Fertility with antibacterial agents in 50% yolk-citrate: High and low fertility bulls*

	Increase in percentage of 60–90 day NR	
	Low bulls	High bulls
No antibiotic	58% base	65% base
Sulfanilamide	+3	+1
Penicillin	+10	+6
Streptomycin	+11	+4
Polymyxin	+3	+2
All combined	+15	+3

From Foote and Bratton. *J. Dairy Sci.,* 33:544, 1950.

toxic to sperm. At levels compatible with sperm, others are not very effective in controlling microbial contaminants.

For approximately 40 years, beginning in the late 1940s, penicillin (1,000 IU per ml of diluter) and streptomycin (1,000µg per ml of diluter) were used to control both pathogenic and nonpathogenic bacteria in semen. Polymyxin B was added later by most processors to broaden the spectrum of control and specifically to assist streptomycin in the control of *Campylobacter fetus venerealis* in frozen semen. As the years passed, concern increased that *Campylobacter fetus venerealis* may not be adequately controlled due to changes in processing procedures. There was also concern that microorganisms such as bovine mycoplasmas, ureaplasmas, and *Haemophilus somnus* were not being controlled by the traditional antibiotic treatment.

Researchers working with the AI industry evaluated selected antibiotics and developed a treatment protocol, including the combination and concentration of drugs that are effective in eliminating mycoplasmas, ureaplasmas, *C. fetus venerealis,* and *H. somnus,* as well as other contaminants. Further testing by the AI industry showed that the protocol did not adversely affect semen quality or fertility. It has been adopted by the National Association of Animal Breeders and the commercial semen processors, and it is recommended for all semen used to breed cows artificially.

The recommended antibiotics and their concentration per ml of neat (undiluted) semen and per ml of the nonglycerol portion of diluter are

500µg Gentamicin
100µg Tylosin
300/600µg Linco-Spectin (300µg Lincomycin and 600µg Spectinomycin)

Detailed directions for semen processing will be covered in Section 16–5.

16–4   EFFECTIVE DILUTERS FOR BULL SEMEN

16–4.1 *Yolk-Phosphate*

The yolk-phosphate diluter is prepared by mixing equal parts of the phosphate buffer solution and fresh egg yolk. The reaction of the phosphate ions on the fat globules of the egg yolk results in an opaque mixture, making it impossible to observe individual sperm in the mixture. Even though this diluter maintains good motility and fertility of bull sperm, it is not used.

16–4.2 *Yolk-Citrate*

The yolk-citrate diluter is prepared by adding fresh egg yolk to the citrate buffer solution. Prior to the adoption of frozen semen, the ratio of yolk to buffer solution was 1:1. Most of the reported research showed a slight decrease in nonreturn rate with lower percentages of egg yolk. When the semen is to be frozen, 20% yolk and 80% buffer solution gives best results. Antibiotics as prescribed in Section 16–3 should be added to the nonglycerol fraction of diluter (Table 16–2). The yolk-citrate diluter has become the standard against which all new and modified diluters have been compared.

Table 16–2   *Commonly used diluters for processing bull semen*[a]

Ingredients	Yolk-citrate		Yolk-tris		Homogenized milk
	1	2	1	2	
Buffer (g/100 ml unless otherwise noted)					
Sodium citrate, dihydrate	2.90	2.12			
Tris (hydroxymethyl) amino-methane			3.028	2.42	
Citric acid monohydrate		0.183	1.678	1.38	
Fructose			1.000	1.000	
Gentamicin (μg/ml)[b]	500	500	500	500	500
Tylosin (μg/ml)[b]	100	100	100	100	100
Linco-Spectin (μg/ml)[b]	300/600	300/600	300/600	300/600	300/600
Milk (ml)					100
Egg yolk (% v/v)	20	20	20	20	
Buffer (% v/v)	80	80	80	80	
Glycerol (% v/v)[c]	14	14	14	14	14

[a]From the literature.
[b]Added to only the nonglycerol portion.
[c]Added to only half of the diluter (glycerol portion). The glycerol portion is made without antibiotics.

16–4.3 *Yolk-Tris*

The yolk-tris diluter is prepared by adding 20% fresh egg yolk to the tris buffered solution. Antibiotics are added at the recommended level. Some processors have added 7% glycerol to the yolk-tris diluter prior to semen dilution but the recommended procedure is to glycerolate only half of the diluter. Section 16–5 has additional details (Table 16–2). Equilibration time may not be as critical with the yolk-tris diluter as with other diluters.

16–4.4 *Whole Homogenized Milk and Skim Milk*

Whole homogenized milk and skim milk satisfy the requirements of a good semen diluter. Milk heated to normal pasteurization temperature contains a material, *lactenin,* which is spermicidal. Heating the milk to 90°C to 95°C for 10 minutes inactivates lactenin. The only additions needed are the antibiotics to control microbial contaminants and glycerol if the semen is to be frozen (Table 16–2). Whole milk has the disadvantage of poor sperm visibility under the microscope. This problem is apparently caused by light refraction by the fat globules contained in the whole homogenized milk.

16–4.5 *Other Diluters*

The field of semen diluters has probably been more thoroughly researched since 1940 than any other research area of similar scope. The addition of many ingredients, such as simple sugars, amino acids, enzymes, and combinations of ingredients, has been tried.

Various concentrations of egg yolk and various mixtures of yolk-citrate and milk have been tried. Some of these combinations have been superior in some respects to the original yolk-citrate.

Of the six major semen-producing businesses surveyed, two were using yolk-citrate, two were using yolk-tris, and two were using heated whole milk as their diluter.

16–5 PROCESSING BULL SEMEN

The processing of semen starts with diluter preparation and involves semen collection, dilution, microbial control, cooling, packaging, freezing, and storage.

16–5.1 *Diluter Preparation*

After deciding which of the previously described diluters is to be used, a quantity that will meet the needs for the number of ejaculates to be collected should be prepared on the day preceding collection. The total quantity can then be divided into two equal parts and designated part A and part B. To part A, add 500μg Gentamicin, 100μg Tylosin, and 300/600μg Linco-Spectin for each ml of diluter. To part B, add 14% glycerol v/v for yolk-citrate, yolk-tris, and whole milk diluters. Both parts should be cooled and stored at 5°C until the day of collection.

16–5.2 *Semen Collection*

Well in advance of the actual semen collection, a small quantity (about 25 ml per ejaculate to be collected) of part A diluter should be measured into an Erlenmeyer flask and placed in a 35°C water bath and allowed to warm to that temperature before any semen is collected. Each collection tube must be labeled with the bull's ID number or code name. Each ejaculate of semen must be protected to prevent it from cooling below 35°C until it can be placed in the same water bath with the diluter. Antibiotics, as prescribed in Section 16–3, are added immediately. The semen must be allowed to remain in contact with the antibiotics for 3 to 5 minutes before any diluter is added. Quality tests (volume, motility, and concentration) should be conducted during that holding time.

16–5.3 *Semen Dilution*

The dilution of semen is carried out in two steps. The first step involves a predilution of the warm semen with three to four volumes of warm part A diluter for each volume of semen. The diluter used for predilution should contain no glycerol and be tempered in the 35°C water bath used to maintain the temperature of the semen. The diluter used in this manner provides lecithin and lipoproteins to protect the sperm from cold shock during the cooling process. These materials apparently prevent changes in cell wall permeability during cooling.

The cooling process is described in Section 16–5.5 and should take a minimum of 2 hours. This time interval also meets the CSS requirement that sperm must be in contact with the antibiotics in the part A diluter for a minimum of 2 hours in order for the antibiotics to act on any microorganisms present before any glycerol is introduced. The antibiotics in the prediluter apparently satisfy that requirement during the 2 hours required for cooling. The usual practice is to collect two (some studs collect three) ejaculates from a bull on each day of collection. Some processors collect the additional ejaculates as soon as the bull is adequately sexually stimulated. In that case, the first ejaculate may be partially prediluted and held in the 35°C water bath until one to three additional ejaculates are ready for predilution. All ejaculates may then be mixed before being cooled. Other processors wait an hour or two between ejaculate collections. In that case, each ejaculate is prediluted and cooled separately before being mixed for further processing. After the prediluted semen is cooled to 5°C, it is diluted to one-half the final volume with diluter which has been held at 5°C. The addition of glycerol will be discussed in a later paragraph.

16–5.4 *Dilution Rate*

The main objective in deciding what the dilution rate should be is to provide the optimum number of motile sperm per breeding unit that will be available at the time of insemination. It is generally accepted that 10 million motile sperm at the time of insemination will provide optimum conception rate. When semen was used in the liquid form, determining the dilution rate was fairly simple. One needed to know the initial motility and sperm concentration of the ejaculate. The number of breeding units was determined by dividing the total number of motile sperm by 10 million. The procedure is a bit more complicated with frozen semen. Not only do we need to take initial motility and concentration into account, but we need to have some idea of the survival rate of the individual bull being processed. This can be determined only by freezing several ejaculates from a bull and making postthaw evaluations on them. About 15 million motile sperm per breeding unit seems to be the minimum prefreeze concentration. Prefreeze concentrations of motile sperm as high as 30 million are not uncommon. Since the survival rate is greater for sperm frozen in straws than in ampules, fewer motile sperm are needed per straw unit. While 10 million motile sperm at the time of insemination is the accepted number, research indicates that this number can be reduced to 7 or 8 million for certain high fertility bulls without reducing conception rate. On the other hand, conception rate may be enhanced for certain low fertility bulls by increasing the number of motile sperm to perhaps 15 million at the time of insemination. Accurate postthaw evaluation is essential in determining the initial number of motile sperm required to obtain the desired number of motile sperm or percent intact acrosomes at time of insemination.

Currently, most processors are using the number of total sperm rather than motile sperm in calculating the dilution rate for ejaculates. They check the motility of each ejaculate to be sure it falls within a normal range before proceeding, however. The number of sperm used per breeding unit for most ejaculates is 20×10^6, but when postthaw evaluation and/or conception rate dictates, 30×10^6 or even 40×10^6 total sperm may be used per unit. As mentioned in Chapter 12, one research report indicated that under good conditions the total sperm per breeding unit can be reduced to 10×10^6 for most bulls with a reduction in nonreturn rate of about one percentage unit from maximum. Additional research in this area will no doubt be conducted.

The following is an example for calculating the number of breeding units that can be processed from an ejaculate of semen, including the amount of diluters and each antibiotic needed.

Given: 9-ml ejaculate, 60% motility, 1.25×10^9 total sperm (TS) concentration, and a goal to provide 10×10^6 motile sperm (MS) after thawing. Calculate: Number of 0.5 ml straws that can be filled, volume of part A and part B diluter needed, and the mg of each antibiotic needed. Solution: $1.25 \times 10^9 \times 9$ ml $= 11.25 \times 10^9$ TS $\times .60 = 6.75 \times 10^9$ MS divided by $15 \times 10^6 = 450$ straws (0.5 ml each) divided $2 = 225$ ml total volume of diluter divided by $2 = 112.5$, round to 113 ml of part A diluter and 112 ml of part B diluter. The 113 ml of part A diluter $+ 9$ ml of neat semen $= 122$ total ml to be treated with antibiotics. Multiply 122 by $500\mu g = 61{,}000\mu g$ or 61 mg of Gentamicin, 122 multiplied by $100\mu g = 12{,}200\mu g$ or 12.2 mg of Tylosin, 122 multiplied by $300 = 36{,}600\mu g$ or 36.6 mg of Lincomycin, and 122 multiplied by $600 = 73{,}200\mu g$ or 73.2 mg of Spectinomycin.

Note: A few ml of diluter and diluted semen will be lost due to adherence to glassware. That accounts for the 9 ml of neat semen not being considered in the calculation of amount of diluter needed. Also, Lincomycin and Spectinomycin are available in the 1:2 ratio needed (Linco-Spectin), so when the amount needed for one is calculated, the correct amount for the other is automatically obtained.

16–5.5 *Cooling Semen*

Cooling is accomplished by placing the prediluted 35°C semen container in a container of water at the same temperature (Figure 16–1). These are placed in a refrigerator and cooled to 5°C. The combined volume of prediluted semen and surrounding water should vary according to the desired cooling rate. There is disagreement as to what is the best rate of cooling for prediluted semen; however, the current procedure related to antibiotic treatment has brought some unity within the industry. As required by CSS, the sperm must be in contact with the antibiotics for a minimum of 2 hours before any glycerol is added. The antibiotics in the prediluter satisfy that requirement, so those organizations that were cooling in less than 2 hours extended their cooling time because they could not proceed with the processing until the 2 hours had lapsed, anyway. All of the studs contacted were cooling in 2 hours except one, which was cooling in 2½ hours. Livability studies more consistently support the slower cooling rates, and several authors have shown that postthaw motility favors slow

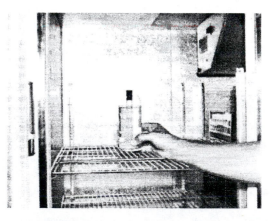

Figure 16–1   Prediluted samples of semen are placed in water at the same temperature. The volume of water should be sufficient to allow cooling to 5°C in 2 to 4 hours.

cooling over a 2- to 4-hour period. It is probable that experiments which have shown no difference between fast and slow cooling rates on fertility have involved excessive numbers of motile sperm which mask the adverse effects of fast cooling.

16–5.6 *Glycerolation and Equilibration*

Glycerol must be added to semen to protect it during freezing and thawing. Damage results from the selective freezing of free H_2O both inside and outside the cells. This results in concentration of other cell constituents and solutes outside the cell. In addition to upsetting vital cell components, changes in permeability of cell membranes may occur. Preferential leakage of solutes and pH changes in nonelectrolytes have been mentioned as contributing to sperm damage.

Glycerol binds water and decreases the freezing point of solutions. Less ice is formed in its presence at any temperature. Concentration of solutes is correspondingly decreased. Glycerol partially dehydrates the sperm cells, further reducing the selective freezing of water. Other cryoprotective materials have been compared with glycerol. Dimethyl sulfoxide has a salt-buffering capacity and enters the cells rapidly. It is most effective with slow freezing. Glycols and a number of saccharides have shown some cryopreservative effects.

The level of glycerol varies somewhat with the diluter ingredients. Yolk-citrate, whole milk, and yolk-tris diluters should contain 7% glycerol after final dilution. Skim milk diluter performs better with 10% glycerol. The part B fraction of diluter which has been cooled to 5°C is added to semen which has also been cooled to 5°C and diluted to one-half the final volume with part A diluter. Part B can be added to part A in a number of ways. Some processors pour the desired amount of part B diluter into a plastic bag that is suspended over the container of part A diluter plus semen. A small hole is made to allow part B to drip slowly into part A. Additional holes may be needed depending on the amount of diluter being transferred and the length of time desired for the process (Figure 16–2). Thirty minutes seems to be the minimum and an hour the maximum. Others divide the part B

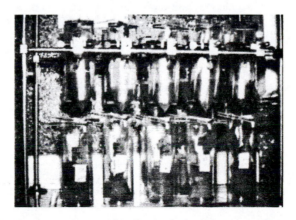

Figure 16–2 One technique for dripping the diluter containing glycerol into the portion containing no glycerol. (Courtesy of Select Sires, Inc., Plain City, Ohio.)

diluter into three equal portions and add stepwise at 10- or 15-minute intervals, or it may be divided into four volumes containing 10%, 20%, 30%, and 40% and added in order at 10- to 15-minute intervals.

The researchers that developed the yolk-tris diluter reported that glycerol can be added to all of the diluter when it is prepared with no harmful effects. However, it still is not an option for safe processing of semen because the glycerol can interfere with the action of the antibiotics on some microorganisms (Section 16–5.3).

Equilibration time is defined as the time required for the glycerol to reach equilibrium on both sides of the cell membrane. Several field trials indicate that semen can be safely frozen immediately after adding the glycerol, thus eliminating the equilibration time. That idea has not been adopted by the U.S. AI industry. There has always been disparity among processors relative to the optimum equilibration time and the final chapter still has not been written. Of the six processors contacted, two were using a minimum of 2 hours, one a minimum of 3 hours, one a minimum of 4 hours, and one a minimum of 10 hours. All of them indicated that longer equilibration times, even up to 20 hours, did not seem to be harmful. In fact, the longer times seemed to be beneficial for some problem bulls. The sixth processor did not respond to that question.

16–5.7 *Semen Packaging: Ampules and Straws*

Glass ampules with 0.5-ml, 0.8-ml, and 1.0-ml capacities were used almost exclusively for packaging from the onset of frozen semen until about 1970. The ampules were filled through a small opening and heat was used to melt the glass to form a seal (Figure 16–3). Six or eight ampules were clipped to an aluminum strip, called a cane, for storage in liquid nitrogen. The neck of the ampule was etched so that it could be broken to open the ampule.

The 0.5-ml plastic straw has been the package of preference since about 1970. Plastic straws with 0.25-ml and 0.3-ml capacities are used in Europe but are not popular in the United States (Figure 16–3). One end of the straw contains a three-part plug. A small amount of polyvinyl alcohol powder is placed between two small cotton plugs. The straws are filled by applying a vacuum to the end with the plugs. The powder allows air to pass

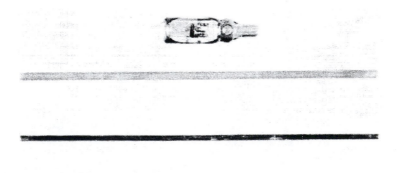

Figure 16–3   Semen for freezing is packaged in either ampules *(top)* or plastic straws *(bottom)*.

through as long as it remains dry, but when aqueous material (the semen) comes in contact with the powder it forms a seal which will not allow liquid or air to pass through. The opposite end of the straw is sealed ultrasonically after filling. One straw manufacturer provides a plastic bead that is forced into the filling end for sealing. Although the bead provides adequate sealing, the equipment provided was less than reliable; consequently, that sealing system has not been widely used in the United States. The 0.5-ml straw is 113 mm long and 2.8 mm in diameter. One major advantage of the straw over the ampule is the conservation of storage space. Up to three times as many straws can be stored in a field or storage unit as ampules. Most studies indicate that the straw offers the added advantage of increased sperm survival and a slight increase in conception rate over the ampule. Straws are placed in small plastic goblets which hold 5 or 10 straws each. Two goblets are attached to an aluminum cane for storage in field units. The goblets, when filled with liquid nitrogen (LN), provide protection to the straws while being transferred from unit to unit.

Both the ampule and the straw must be labeled to identify the donor bull and the semen-producing business. The full registration name and number of the bull plus his code number are printed on each unit. All semen-producing businesses are assigned a code number by the U.S. Department of Agriculture, and this number must also be printed on each unit.

Research involving the freezing of semen in pellets offers some promise. Small depressions are made in the surface of a block of dry ice using the procedure described for boars (Figure16–5). Semen containing about 10 times the usual number of motile sperm is placed in the depression to freeze. The usual volume is about 0.1 ml. After freezing, the pellets are transferred directly to liquid nitrogen for storage. For insemination, the pellets are thawed in enough warm diluter to provide adequate volume for insemination. Two major disadvantages of the pellet are identification of the individual pellet and microbial contamination incurred during handling. There is also some possibility of mixing sperm from different bulls from forceps used to handle the pellets.

16–5.8 *Freezing*

The standard procedure for freezing is to place a single layer of straws on a tray. The tray is placed about 5.5 cm above the liquid nitrogen level of a large storage unit. Ampules are attached to canes and set vertically into baskets, which are placed about 5.5 cm above the LN level. The cold nitrogen vapors in this area will freeze the semen at about the desired rate. Straws will reach the vapor temperature in about 2 minutes. The number of breeding units that can be frozen at one time and the number of batches that can be frozen during a working day depend a great deal on the size of the liquid nitrogen unit being used. The limitations on the number of batches that can be frozen in a day, and to some extent the size of the liquid nitrogen unit being used, have at least been partially eliminated by the technique of bubbling liquid nitrogen below the liquid level in a tank to force release of new vapor at a faster rate. With this technique, along with accurate thermocouples, one can maintain the desired temperature of the vapor area and thus a more precise freezing rate for the semen.

The reported research on rate of freezing indicates that there is a great deal of latitude. Table 16–3 summarizes some of these studies. It appears that semen can be frozen both too fast or too slowly. It would appear that rates between 126°C per minute down to

Table 16–3 *Freeze rates of semen in straws C/minute*

Mortimer et al. 1976 from 5 to −130	Robbins et al. 1976 from heat of fusion to −80	Almquist and Wiggins 1973		Rodriguez et al. 1975
		5 to −15	−15 to −60	
135[a]	126	82	43	
67	54	50	27	
38	30	43	25	38
19	15	32	23	(5 to −130)
11	7.5			11.9
7				(10 to −130)
				1.1
				(5 to −15)
				3.9
				(−15 to −79)

From Saacke. *Proceedings 7th Tech. Conf. on A.I. and Reprod.*, 1978.

[a]Dotted lines indicate freeze rates resulting in significantly depressed sperm viability postthaw.

7°C per minute will give satisfactory results. It is logical to assume that the optimum rate of freezing might be influenced by several factors. Among these would be the type of package, glycerol level, recommended rate of thaw, and diluter composition.

16–5.9 *Summary of Processing Procedures*

1. *Diluter preparation.* On the day preceding semen collection, prepare the needed amount of the diluter of choice. Divide it into two equal parts and label them as part A and part B. Add 500µg Gentamicin, 100µg Tylosin, and 300/600µg Linco-Spectin per ml of part A. Add 14% glycerol v/v to part B.

2. *Semen collection.* Transfer 25 ml of part A diluter from cold storage to 35°C thermostatic-controlled water bath in time for it to reach target temperature before collecting semen. The ejaculate should be maintained at 35°C while transferring from the collection area to the processing laboratory.

3. *Antibiotic treatment of neat semen.* Place the collection tube containing the ejaculate into the 35°C water bath. Add antibiotics to the neat semen as indicated for each ml of part A diluter and mix with semen by inverting tube. A 3 to 5 minute incubation time is allowed. Semen quality tests should be conducted during this period.

4. *Predilution.* To the semen, add a quantity up to half the desired final volume including semen of 35°C part A diluter. For ease of cooling, add 3 ml to 4 ml of diluter for each ml of neat semen. This diluter contains antibiotics as prescribed in item 3.

5. *Cooling.* Place the prediluted semen container in a container of 30°C to 35°C water, and transfer it to a 5°C environment. The quantity of water in the container should be sufficient to require a minimum of 2 hours to cool to 5°C.

6. *Final dilution.* If the prediluted sample is less than half the desired final volume, add additional cold part A diluter to reach that volume. Add an equal portion of part B diluter as described in Section 16–5.3.

7. *Equilibration time.* Allow a minimum of 4 hours for the glycerol to reach equilibrium through the cell membrane.

8. *Packaging.* While working in a 5°C environment, fill 0.5-ml polyvinylchloride straws with semen and seal them. The straws must be properly labeled. Packaging may be done during equilibration period.

9. *Freezing.* Place the sealed straws in a single layer in a shallow tray (screen mesh bottom) and transfer them to a liquid nitrogen container (a large storage unit or a unit designed for freezing straws) placed 5.5 cm above the liquid nitrogen level. About 2 minutes are required for semen to reach the temperature of the N_2 vapor.

10. *Storage.* Place the frozen straws in goblets that hold five straws each while working in the N_2 vapor. Place the goblets on aluminum canes, two per cane, and immerse them in the liquid nitrogen for storage.

16–5.10 *Protecting Sperm from Harmful Light Rays*

Considerable research has been conducted on the effects of various light rays on the livability and fertility of bull sperm. However, there is disagreement on what precautions should be taken during the collection and processing of semen to protect the sperm. Everyone seems to agree that semen should be protected from sunlight. The six large processors contacted were asked about what precautions they were taking in their processing rooms to protect sperm from light rays. Only one gave a positive response—they were using gold-colored fluorescent light tubes. Four were using standard fluorescent tubes and one failed to respond to the question.

16–6 STORAGE AND HANDLING OF BULL SEMEN

Semen that is going to be stored at above-freezing temperatures needs to be maintained at approximately 5°C. Frozen semen must be stored at a temperature below −75°C. The temperature of dry ice (−79°C) barely meets this requirement, and one study showed a decline in nonreturn (NR) rate of 13% between semen stored over 6 months, compared with semen stored 1 to 2 months at −79°C. In addition to being difficult to handle and transport, dry ice must be replenished frequently. The life span of bull semen stored in liquid nitrogen has not been determined. Experiments using split ejaculates have shown no decrease in the NR rate for semen stored up to 2 years. One study reported services at 6-month intervals from 6 months to 5 years with no decrease in NR rates. Some calves have been born from semen stored up to 20 years, but the number of services are too few to draw conclusions.

Liquid nitrogen with a temperature of −196°C is the refrigerant of choice. Double wall stainless steel or aluminum containers with a vacuum between the walls make highly satisfactory storage units. Figure 16–4 shows a large storage unit and a small field unit. This very popular field unit has a nitrogen capacity of 20 liters and will hold for 90 days between charges. It will hold approximately 1,200 straws of 0.5-ml capacity and approximately 600 ampules of 0.8-ml capacity. Most field units of this type are recharged at 60-day intervals to allow an adequate margin of safety.

Several precautions should be taken in handling semen. The packaged unit is very small, particularly the plastic straw, and when exposed to ambient temperatures of 25°C to 30°C the temperature rises very rapidly. Repeated changes in temperature, particularly of temperatures above −79°C can be detrimental to the survival of the sperm. The top of the

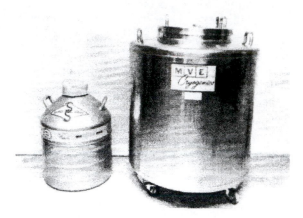

Figure 16–4   Liquid nitrogen tanks used for frozen semen. A field unit is shown on the left and a larger storage unit on the right.

canister, shown in Figure 17–5, should remain 3 cm to 5 cm below the top of the nitrogen tank when looking for semen from a particular bull. The top of the cane should be labeled with the code number of the bull so that the individual straws or ampules will not have to be examined. Semen from more than one bull should never be placed on the same cane. Once the cane is identified, it should be withdrawn from the canister just far enough so that the straw or ampule can be removed without exposing the remainder of the units to ambient temperature. Specially designed forceps are available for lifting straws from the goblets. When semen is being transferred from one unit to another, whole canes should be transferred insofar as possible so that the transfer can be made quickly.

It is a good idea to check the nitrogen level in field units about once a week. This can be done by inserting a ruler into the unit until it reaches bottom. Allow it to remain a few seconds before it is withdrawn and exposed to the atmosphere. Frost will form on the ruler, showing the exact depth of nitrogen in the unit.

16–7 WHAT DOES THE FUTURE HOLD FOR LIQUID BULL SEMEN?

The cattle AI industry in the United States and much of the rest of the world has relied almost exclusively on frozen semen for about 30 years. However, a few researchers have continued to look at alternatives. A revival of interest in the use of liquid bull semen has occurred in several countries and is beginning to be noticed in the United States. While frozen semen has made a tremendous contribution, there are several reasons for this renewed interest in liquid semen. The two most obvious reasons are improved reproductive results and faster genetic progress. Most field trials comparing conception rates for liquid and frozen semen (most of them were conducted in the 1960s) have shown an advantage for liquid semen. The question arises, will the same advantage hold with current technology for both frozen and liquid semen? Some large AI organizations are taking another look at that factor.

The rate of genetic progress is more important than conception rate and under certain circumstances liquid semen can more efficiently utilize the sperm produced by genetically superior bulls. The average prefreeze number of motile sperm being used per breeding unit of frozen semen is about 15×10^6. With liquid semen, even by 1960 standards, only 10×10^6 motile sperm are required for optimum conception. By utilizing liquid semen and a reduced number of motile sperm, an outstanding bull in Denmark has been used for 257,000 first services in 1 year. The AI industry in New Zealand is utilizing two innovations to increase the number of services possible from an ejaculate of semen. It developed and is using an ambient temperature diluter (LONG-LAST™ which contains 1% glycine, 0.3% glucose, 1.25% glycerol, and caproic acid) and a high dilution rate (2×10^6 sperm per unit). It is unknown how the conception rate for this product will compare with current frozen semen technology or a modern liquid semen program in the United States.

Other factors that relate to the renewed interest in liquid semen are delivery service and improved estrus synchronization. Overnight delivery service to any destination in the United States is available and is being utilized for shipping liquid swine semen. Synchronization of ovulation, which will allow pretimed insemination, will make it possible for breeders to special order liquid semen from a selected sire for a specified number of cows for a specific date.

Two AI organizations collaborated on a liquid semen trial. One diluted semen to 5×10^6 total sperm, while the other diluted semen to 10×10^6 total sperm and packaged both concentrations in 0.5-ml straws. Independent breeding trials were conducted. The lower concentrated semen was used on day 1 (day after collection), day 2, and day 3. The semen was delivered directly by car and was available for use on day 1. The nonreturn rates (NR) for each day's usage was compared with the pooled 3-day NR with the pooled frozen semen NR (processed for at least 10×10^6 motile sperm unit). Day 1 NR was 5.0% higher than the 3-day pooled NR and 3.5% higher than the frozen semen NR. Day 2 NR was 2.6% lower than the frozen semen NR, but the combined day 1 and day 2 NR was 0.7% higher than the frozen semen NR. The higher concentrated semen was used similarly, but some was used on day 0 (day of collection) and a small amount was used on day 4. The NR for days 0 and 1 were higher than the pooled frozen semen NR, but day 2 NR was about the same as for the frozen semen. The NR for days 3 and 4 were 3.5% and 3.6% lower, respectively, than for the frozen semen.

In another trial, semen was diluted to 1×10^5, 2.5×10^5, and 2.5×10^6 total sperm per 0.25-ml straw. The cooled semen was shipped overnight by commercial carrier from Lancaster, Pennsylvania, to Fort Collins, Colorado, and used to inseminate Holstein heifers in a large, privately owned herd that had been given two injections of $PGF_{2\alpha}$ at 12-day intervals to synchronize estrus. Ultrasound was used to determine the side of expected ovulation. Twenty-four hours following detected estrus, the heifers were inseminated deep in the horn on the side of expected ovulation with a side-opening embryo transfer straw gun. Pregnancy was determined by ultrasound 42 to 45 days postestrus. Pregnancy rates were 41%, 52%, and 62% for the 1×10^5, 2.5×10^5, and 2.5×10^6 sperm/insemination, respectively. While the two lower pregnancy rates are probably unacceptable for most situations and the numbers are small, this research opens the possibility for considering much greater use of semen from at least some genetically superior sires. Genetic progress could be increased proportional to the risk:reward ratio the bull owner and customer are willing to accept.

One should not expect liquid use to replace frozen semen, even though liquid semen continues to hold an advantage in conception rates and available diluters make it possible to dilute semen to 2.5×10^6 total sperm per unit. The fact that semen can be preserved indefinitely by freezing even during times of the year when semen demand is not great is an important advantage for frozen semen and compensates for much of its disadvantages. The logistics of two separate shipping systems appear to have prevented any of the semen-producing businesses surveyed from including liquid semen in their offerings.

16–8 PROCESSING BOAR SEMEN

Boars produce a large volume (40 ml to 125 ml gel-free) of semen that has a low concentration (200 to 300×10^6 per ml) of semen. These characteristics have caused problems in developing satisfactory procedures for freezing boar semen. While some frozen semen is available, liquid semen is utilized for most swine AI. Several commercial semen producers sell and ship liquid semen by overnight delivery to any destination in the United States. In addition, many vertically integrated operations have their own stud farms in connection with their sow operations, and some of these also sell semen. The percentage of pigs resulting from AI has increased markedly since 1995 and accounted for more than 50% of all pigs born in 1998. Sow operations that are too small to have a full-time staff for boar management, including semen collection and processing, are well advised to find a reliable commercial source of semen that meets their quality standards and costs parameters.

16–8.1 *Diluting Liquid Semen*

The preferred breeding unit of boar semen has a minimum of 3 billion motile sperm suspended in 80 ml to 100 ml of semen plus diluter. A minimum dilution rate of one part semen to one part diluter (1:1) is necessary to provide the proper environment for maintaining sperm life. Depending on ejaculate volume, concentration, and motility, dilution rates as high as 1:10 are possible. Commercial diluters are available in dry form that perform satisfactorily when mixed with the appropriate amount of distilled water (follow manufacturer's directions). Beltsville thaw solution is an excellent diluter for liquid boar semen (Table 16–4).

Table 16–4   *Composition of Beltsville F5 diluter and thawing solution for boar semen*

Ingredient	Diluter amount[*]	Thaw solution amount[†]
Tes-N-Tris (hydroxymethyl) methyl 2 aminoethane sulfonic acid	1.2 g	
Tris (hydroxymethyl) aminomethane	.2 g	
Dextrose, anhydrous	3.2 g	3.7 g
Egg yolk	20 ml	
Orvus ES paste	.5 ml	
Sodium citrate, dihydrate		.6 g
Sodium bicarbonate		.125 g
Sodium ethylenediaminetetraacetate		.125 g
Potassium chloride		.075 g

Pursel and Johnson. *J. Anim. Sci.,* 40:99, 1975.

[*]Brought to 100 ml with distilled water, centrifuged at 12,000 g for 10 min. diluter decanted.

[†]Ingredients dissolved and brought to 100 ml with distilled water.

16–8.2 *Semen Evaluation*

The freshly collected ejaculate should be visually checked for quality: volume, color—creamy white appearance, and smell—no offensive odor. If maximum utilization is to be made of an ejaculate, motility and concentration determinations need to be made so that the number of breeding units and thus the final dilution volume can be determined (or, alternately, the volume of diluter needed). The following formula may be helpful:

$$\text{volume (ml)} \times \text{concentration (no. sperm/ml)} \times \% \text{ motility} \div$$
$$3 \times 10^9 = \text{no. breeding units} \times 80 \text{ or } 100 = \text{final dilution volume (ml)} -$$
$$\text{ejaculate volume} = \text{volume of diluter (ml) needed}$$

16–8.3 *Processing Semen*

The semen should be maintained at near body temperature during the evaluation procedure. The diluter should be tempered to within 1°C of the semen. At this point, the ejaculate can be divided equally among the appropriate number of plastic inseminating squeeze bottles. Add sufficient diluter to each bottle by allowing the diluter to run down the inside of the bottle to bring the mixture to the desired volume (80 ml or 100 ml). If dilution rate is greater than 1:3, add half of the diluter and wait 10 minutes before adding the remaining half. Mix gently by swirling or inverting the bottles after each diluter addition. Label the semen bottle with boar identification, date, and time of collection. Alternately, the entire ejaculate can be diluted to the desired final volume in a large bottle or flask before transferring it to the plastic inseminating squeeze bottles. If the semen is to be stored, it should be allowed to cool to room temperature (22°C) for 2 hours in a dark area. Further cooling should be done at the rate of 1°C per 2 hours. With most diluters, the best storage temperature is 15°C to 18°C. Temperatures vary greatly among refrigerators, making it necessary to carefully check the intended storage area ahead of time to be sure proper temperature can be maintained. A commercial, thermostatically controlled liquid semen unit which maintains the desired temperature is available.

16–8.4 *Storing Liquid Semen*

Liquid semen can be stored up to 7 days. However, best fertility can be expected when used prior to the end of 3 days of storage. Semen bottles should be swirled carefully once or twice daily during storage. This resuspends sperm cells and prevents the heads from sticking together. Conception rates for AI using stored liquid boar semen have been equal or superior to natural mating, especially when two inseminations are made during the period of estrus using semen on day 1 or day 2 following collection.

16–8.5 *Processing Frozen Semen*

Researchers at Beltsville Agricultural Experiment Station developed a satisfactory procedure for freezing and thawing boar semen. Aliquots of ejaculates containing 6×10^9 spermatozoa were centrifuged for 10 minutes at $300 \times g$. The seminal plasma was poured off and the sperm were resuspended in 5 ml of Beltsville F5 (BF5) diluter (Table 16–4). The semen was cooled to 5°C over a 2-hour period. Five milliliters of BF5 diluter containing 2% glycerol was

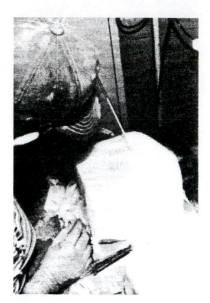

Figure 16–5 Boar semen is frozen in 0.10-ml to 0.15-ml pellets by pipetting the semen into small depressions in a block of dry ice. Pellets are placed in vials and stored in liquid nitrogen.

added and the semen was frozen immediately into pellets of 0.10 ml to 0.15 ml on dry ice (Figure 16–5). The pellets were transferred to liquid nitrogen for storage.

Success rates with frozen semen lag behind those obtained with liquid semen. On the average, conception rates have been 10% to 30% lower, and litter size has been one pig fewer for commercial frozen semen.

Outline for Freezing Boar Semen
Equilibrate at 20°C for 2 hours

Remove seminal plasma by centrifugation

Add BF5 diluter

Cool to 5°C (2 hours)

Add BF5 diluter + glycerol

Freeze 0.10-ml to 0.15-ml pellets on dry ice

Store in liquid nitrogen

Thawing was accomplished by removing 10 ml of pellets and holding them in a clean dry container for 3 minutes. The pellets were then placed in 25 ml of Beltsville thawing solution (BTS) (Table 16–4) at 50°C and swirled in the container until thawed. The thawed semen was poured into an inseminating bottle. The thaw container was rinsed with 15 ml of BTS and the rinse solution was added to the inseminating bottle. This quantity (50 ml) represented a breeding unit. Eighty-five percent of 28 gilts produced zygotes to two inseminations and 87% of the ova produced were fertilized. The gilts were slaughtered 24 to 120 hours after the second insemination. The zygotes were recovered and examined for cleavage.

With present technology, frozen boar semen is not likely to be used on a large-scale basis. The following problems still exist:

1. The large number of sperm required per breeding unit (6×10^9 compared to 3×10^9 for liquid use).
2. Laboratory evaluation of frozen boar semen has little value in predicting potential fertility.
3. Variation in freezing success of semen from different boars.
4. Processing procedure is complicated and time-consuming, compared with liquid semen.
5. Timing of insemination may be more critical with frozen semen.
6. Conception rates and litter size are lower with frozen semen than with liquid semen.

16–9 Processing Ram Semen

Contrary to what may be expected, ram semen does not react to processing and use as does bull semen. It is low in volume (0.75 ml to 1.5 ml) but extremely concentrated (1.5 to 3.0×10^9 sperm/ml). The recommended number of motile sperm per insemination depends on the method of insemination and site where sperm are deposited (Table 16–5). Some of the difference in sperm numbers between the ewe and cow for optimum conception is related to method of insemination. However, even when the semen is placed directly into the ewe's uterus, two to five times as many motile sperm are required. The recommended volume of a breeding unit of ram semen is only 0.2 ml to 0.5 ml. Conception is best for fresh semen (0 to 12 hours), but reasonable conception has been obtained with semen stored for 24 hours. Conception rates after 48 and 72 hours storage are unacceptable. Acceptable fertility has been reported with frozen ram semen when intrauterine deposition was used.

Some unpublished information indicates that ram seminal plasma, even though very low in volume, may adversely affect sperm livability. With a dilution rate of 1:1, it represents a high percentage of the total fluid. Because of the fragility of ram sperm cell membranes, washing and centrifugation may not be a viable means of removing the seminal fluid. Instead, a dialysis procedure may become the method of choice.

16–9.1 *Processing Semen for Liquid Use*

The sample diluters shown in Table 16–6 are satisfactory for diluting ram semen to the desired number of motile sperm suspended in an appropriate volume for each breeding unit. The diluter and equipment should be warmed to 37°C prior to semen collection. The appropriate

Table 16–5 *Number of motile ram sperm ($\times 10^6$) per breeding unit as affected by deposit site and processing*

Deposit site	Fresh	Chilled	Frozen
Vagina	200–300	300	500+
Cervix	150–200	200	300+
Intrauterine			
Laparoscopic	25–50	25–50	25–50
Transcervical	50–100	50–100	75–100

Table 16–6   *Sample diluters for liquid ram semen*

Yolk-tris-fructose		Yolk-glucose-citrate		Heated milk	
Tris (hydroxymethyl)		Na citrate (2H$_2$O)	2.37 g	Homo	100 ml
aminomethane	3.634 g	Glucose	.80 g	Skim	100 ml
Fructose	.50 g	Egg yolk	20 ml		
Citric acid (1H$_2$O)	1.99 g	Distilled H$_2$O to	100 ml		
Egg yolk	14 ml				
Distilled H$_2$O to	100 ml				

Add 1,000 IU sodium penicillin and 1 mg streptomycin sulfate or 300μg lincomycin and 600μg spectino-mycin per ml of each diluter.

amount of warmed diluter should be added to the freshly collected semen. The tube of diluted semen should be put in about 500 ml of 30°C water and place in a 5°C refrigerator. Cooling should be accomplished in not less than 2 hours. The semen should be protected from light during processing.

16–9.2 *Processing Frozen Semen*

Ram semen can be satisfactorily preserved at −196°C in liquid nitrogen indefinitely. Several protocols for freezing ram semen, including diluters, have been reported. A one-step method works well; semen is diluted to the final prefreeze volume (determined by intended method of insemination) at 30°C. It is then cooled to 5°C over a period of 2 hours. The diluter used has the cryoprotectant, glycerol, incorporated before the dilution is made.

The following diluter has given good results:

tris (hydroxymethyl) aminomethane	24.2 g
citric acid	13.6 g
fructose	10.0 g
glycerol	64.0 ml
egg yolk	200.0 ml
distilled water to 1 liter	

Several commercial diluters are available; use as recommended.

Plastic semen straws in 0.25-ml and 0.5-ml capacities have given good results. The straws are labeled, filled, sealed, and frozen as previously described for freezing bull semen. The frozen straws are stored in goblets in liquid nitrogen. The 2-hour cooling period in the presence of the glycerol allows adequate equilibration.

Ram semen can also be frozen in 0.2-ml pellets on dry ice and stored in liquid nitrogen as described for boar semen. The pellets are thawed in warm diluter.

16–10 PROCESSING STALLION SEMEN

The economic incentives continue to be very limited for stallion semen preservation in the United States. Most of the research being done is the result of academic interest. There has been some change in the attitudes of some of the major horse breed associations, but they still have a long way to go before the level of use approaches that of cattle and swine. The Jockey Club will not allow a foal that is the product of AI or embryo transfer (ET) to be registered under any condition. The American Quarter Horse Association will only register AI progeny resulting from semen used fresh or cooled. The cooled semen may be transported to other premises but must be used within 72 hours of collection, which, of course, rules out the use of frozen semen. Also, it will register foals that are products of ET but will only allow the registration of one foal per year from a donor mare, except in the case of twins resulting from a single ovum and single implantation. All AI and ET progeny must be identified by genetic testing. For a number of years, the U.S. Trotting Horse Association has allowed AI with use of liquid semen on the premise where the stallion is housed. Beginning in 1992, it began allowing AI with cooled semen, both on premises and transported, and, beginning with the 1997 breeding season, it approved the use of frozen semen. Genetic testing for identification is required. The American Paint Horse Association allows registration of foals resulting from use of fresh semen on the premises where it is collected, provided it is used within 24 hours of collection. Cooled (not frozen) semen may be transported and used on other premises, provided other association rules are met. Foals resulting from ET may be registered also if all rules are followed. Before using AI or ET with any registered horses, the respective breed association should be contacted for a complete set of rules.

16–10.1 *Processing Liquid Semen*

Semen should be mixed with a warm (37°C) diluter within 2 to 5 minutes after collection. A minimum dilution rate of 1:1 is recommended. If the semen is to be stored longer than 4 hours, it should be diluted to no more than 50×10^6 sperm/ml to maximize sperm survival *in vitro*. The seminal plasma in stallion semen adversely affects sperm livability in both liquid and frozen semen. Read Section 16–10.2 for the procedure for removing the seminal plasma by centrifugation. With the plasma removed, concentrations up to 100×10^9 sperm/ml can be used without harmful effects. Sample diluters for stallion semen are shown in Table 16–7. Typically, breeding units have contained 500×10^6 total sperm in 10 ml to 30 ml of diluted semen. Some researchers are now suggesting a minimum of 200×10^6 motile sperm at the time of insemination in a 5-ml breeding unit. The number of breeding units from an ejaculate will depend on its volume, sperm concentration, initial motility, and desired unit volume. If the seminal plasma is removed, the initial volume is not involved.

Table 16–7 *Sample diluters for liquid stallion semen*

Nonfat dry skim milk (NFDSM)–glucose		Cream gelatin[*]	
NFDSM	2.4 g	Knox gelatin, unflavored	1.3 g
Glucose	4.9 g	Distilled H_2O	10 ml
Penicillin	150,000 IU	Half & half cream	1 pint
Streptomycin	150,000µg	Penicillin	100,000 IU
Distilled H_2O	to 100 ml	Streptomycin	100,000µg

[*]Dissolve gelatin in water and sterilize. Heat cream to 90°C to 95°C in double boiler for 2 to 4 minutes. Mix 10-ml gelatine solution with 90 ml of heated cream and allow to cool. Add antibiotics.

Stallion semen retains motility and fertility best when properly cooled to 5°C following dilution. Good fertility usually is maintained for 48 hours, and acceptable fertility has been reported for semen stored at 5°C for 72 to 96 hours. Cooling from 37°C to 20°C can be accomplished rather rapidly, but cooling from 20°C to 5°C is critical and should be done at the rate of 0.05°C to 0.1°C/minute. Satisfactory cooling rate can be obtained with a commercially available unit designed for storage and transport of stallion semen.

16–10.2 *Processing Frozen Semen*

1. Collect semen, remove gel, and record volume, motility, and concentration.

2. Dilute semen 1:2 with centrifugation medium within 2 to 5 minutes after collection (Table 16–8). Transfer diluted semen to 50-ml centrifuge tubes. Allow 10 minutes for semen to equilibrate at room temperature (25°C). Centrifuge at 1,000 × g for 5 minutes (400 to 1,000 × g for 5 to 15 minutes have been reported). Remove supernatant with aspirator and resuspend the sperm pellets in 10 ml to 40 ml of cryopreservation diluter (Table 16–8). Actual amount depends on the number of sperm in combined pellets. Gently swirl tubes until sperm in the pellets are completely resuspended.

3. Determine total number of sperm in combined resuspended sample. Some sperm will be lost in the supernatant fluid after centrifugation. Divide total sperm number by 600×10^6 to determine the number of straws required and multiply that number by 5 to determine the total volume of diluted semen required. The 600×10^6 total sperm at this point should ensure having a minimum of 200×10^6 progressively motile sperm at the time of insemination. Add sufficient cryopreservation diluter to obtain that volume. Equilibrate extended semen, protected from light, for 20 minutes before beginning the freezing procedure.

4. Package semen by pipetting 5 ml into each five 280 mm (5 ml) polyvinylchloride straws that have been appropriately labeled. Seal each straw with a glass bead and cool to 5°C over a 2-hour period.

5. Position the air bubble in the center of the straw and freeze in a horizontal position in the liquid vapors precisely 1 cm above liquid nitrogen level for 20 minutes. Transfer straws to the liquid nitrogen storage tank and immerse them in the liquid nitrogen.

Table 16–8   *Sample diluters used in freezing stallion semen*

Centrifugation medium (Merck I diluter)		Cryopreservation medium	
D-Glucose	60.0 g	D-lactose sol (11%)	50.0 ml
Trisodium citrate (2H$_2$O)	3.7 g	Centrifugation med	25.0 ml
Disodium ethylenediamine-tetraacetic acid	3.7 g	Egg yolk	20.0 ml
Sodium bicarbonate	1.2 g	Glycerol	5.0 ml
Dihydrostreptomycin	0.8 g	Equex	0.8 ml
Sodium penicillin G	500,000 IU		
Distilled H$_2$O to	1,000 ml		

16–11 PROCESSING BUCK SEMEN

There is still considerable divergence of opinion among researchers concerning the freezing of buck semen. Like ram semen, it is low in volume and high in concentration. There seems to be agreement that the insemination dose must be low in volume (0.25 ml) and must contain a large number of motile sperm (100×10^6 or more).

There is strong evidence that buck seminal plasma contains an enzyme which may hinder sperm preservation. Further, researchers suggest an interaction between this enzyme and egg yolk which produces a toxin capable of killing sperm. It has been strongly suggested that diluters containing yolk should never be used unless the seminal fluid is carefully removed. Washing buck sperm with Ringer solution is recommended even when skim milk is used as a diluter. This is accomplished by adding 20 parts of Ringer solution (same temperature as semen) for each part of freshly collected buck semen, centrifuging 10 minutes at $1,000 \times g$ and pouring off the supernatant. After repeating this procedure, 1 ml of Ringer solution is used to resuspend the sperm before immediate further processing.

If skim milk is used as a diluter, it must be heated to 95°C for 10 minutes. Glycerol at a concentration of 7% is added to only half of the diluter, resulting in a concentration of 3.5% in the final dilution. Penicillin and streptomycin should be added to the nonglycerol portion at a rate of 2,000 to 4,000 units and micrograms respectively/ml. Semen is diluted to half desired final volume with diluter containing no glycerol and cooled slowly (2 hours). After the semen has reached 5°C, an equal volume of the glycerol-containing diluter (also 5°C) is added dropwise. The semen can then be packaged in 0.25-ml straws. Four hours should be allowed for equilibration before freezing.

The freezing rate suggested for buck semen is much slower than that used for bull semen. This necessitates the use of alcohol and dry ice, with the following rate of temperature change:

From 5°C to 0°C	30 minutes
From 0°C to −5°C	10 minutes ($\frac{1}{2}$°/min.)
From −5°C to −10°C	5 minutes (1°/min.)
From −10°C to −17°C	3 minutes (2°/min.)
From −17°C to −79°C	16 minutes (4°/min.)

Transfer to liquid nitrogen for storage

Conception rates reported for does inseminated with frozen semen have varied from 40% to 65%. Some of this variability has been due to processing and freezing procedures. However, insemination method and competence must be considered. Additional research is needed to standardize all areas.

SUGGESTED READING

AAMDAL, J. 1982. Artificial insemination in goats with frozen semen in Norway. *Proc. 3rd Int. Conf. on Goat Prod. and Disease,* Tucson, Ariz.

BARTLETT, F. D. and N. L. VANDEMARK. 1962. Effect of diluent composition on survival and fertility of bovine spermatozoa stored in carbonated diluents. *J. Dairy Sci.,* 45:360.

BUCKRELL, B. C., G. SPRONK, and F. RODRIGUEZ. 1994. Collection and processing of bovine semen for fresh or frozen semen insemination. *Theriogenology Handbook,* 03(8–94).

CORTEEL, J. M. 1974. Viability of goat spermatozoa deep frozen with or without seminal plasma: Glucose effect. *Ann. Biol. Anim. Bioch. Biophys.,* 14:741.

CORTEEL, J. M. 1977. Production, storage and insemination of goat semen. *Proc. Symp. Management of Reprod. in Sheep and Goats.* Univ. of Wisc., Madison.

FOOTE, R. H., L. C. GRAY, D. C. YOUNG, and H. O. DUNN. 1960. Fertility of bull semen stored up to four days at 5C in 20% egg yolk extenders. *J. Dairy Sci.,* 43:1330.

FOOTE, R. H. and M. T. KAPROTH. 1997. Sperm numbers inseminated in dairy cattle and nonreturn rates revisited. *J. Dairy Sci.,* 80:3072.

LEVIS, D. G. Current. *Artificial Insemination of Swine.* Nebraska Cooperative Extension EC 89–264–B.

LORTON, S. P., J. J. SULLIVAN, B. BEAN, M. KAPROTH, H. KELLGREN, and C. MARSHALL. 1988. A new antibiotic combination for frozen bovine semen. 2. Evaluation of seminal quality. *Theriogenology,* 29:593.

LORTON, S. P., J. J. SULLIVAN, B. BEAN, M. KAPROTH, H. KELLGREN, and C. MARSHALL. 1988. A new antibiotic combination for frozen bovine semen. 3. Evaluation of fertility. *Theriogenology,* 29:609.

MARSHALL, C., G. GILBERT, R. D. HANSON, M. KAPROTH, C. H. ALLEN, and G. E. SEIDEL. 1996. Field experiences and concerns with liquid semen (a panel discussion). *Proc. 16th Tech. Conf. Artif. Insem. Reprod.,* p. 40. NAAB, Columbia, Mo.

MITCHELL, J. 1997. CSS Minimum Requirements for Disease Control of Semen Produced for AI. Certified Semen Services, National Association of Animal Breeders. Columbia, Mo.

NEBEL, R. 1994. The AI and dairy industries in New Zealand. *Proc. 15th Tech. Conf. on AI and Repro.,* p.107. NAAB, Columbia, Mo.

PICKETT, B. W. and R. P. AMANN. 1993. Cryopreservation of semen. *Equine Reproduction.* Lea and Febiger.

PICKETT, B. W. and W. E. BERNDTSON. 1978. Principles and techniques of freezing spermatozoa. *Physiology of Reproduction and Artificial Insemination of Cattle.* (2nd ed.) eds. G. W. Salisbury, N. L. VanDemark, and J. R. Lodge. W. H. Freeman and Co.

PICKETT, B. W., L. D. BURWASH, J. L. VOSS, and D. G. BLACK. 1975. Effect of seminal extenders on equine fertility. *J. Anim. Sci.,* 40:1136.

POLGE, C. 1953. The storage of bull semen at low temperatures. *Vet. Rec.,* 65:557.

PURSEL, V. G. 1979. Advances in preservation of swine spermatozoa. *Beltsville Symposia in Agricultural Research 3., Animal Reproduction.* Ed. H. W. Hawk. Allanheld, Osmun and Co., Publisher; Halsted Press, a division of Wiley and Sons.

PURSEL, V. G. and L. A. JOHNSON. 1975. Freezing of boar spermatozoa: Freezing capacity with concentrated semen and a new thawing procedure. *J. Anim. Sci.,* 40:99.

SAACKE, R. G. 1978. Factors affecting spermatozoon viability from collection to use. *Proc. 7th Tech. Conf. Artif. Insem. Reprod.,* p. 3. NAAB, Columbia, Mo.

SENGER, P. L. 1980. Handling frozen Bovine semen—Factors which influence viability and fertility. *Theriogenology,* 13:52.

SHANNON, P., B. CURSON, and A. P. RHODES. 1984. Relationship between total spermatozoa per insemination and fertility of bovine semen stored in Caprogen at ambient temperature. *N. Z. J. Agri. Res.,* 27:35.

SHELTON, M. 1978. Reproduction and breeding of goats. *J. Dairy Sci.,* 61:994.

SHIN, S. J., D. H. LEIN, and V. H. PATTEN. 1988. A new antibiotic combination for frozen bovine semen. 1. Control of mycoplasmas, ureaplasmas, *Campylobacter fetus venerealis* and *Haemophilus somnus. Theriogenology,* 29:577.

STAFF. 1992. Back to the future. *Eastern A.I. Cooperator.*

17

Insemination Techniques

Successful AI culminates with the proper placement of high-quality semen in the female reproductive tract. The object of an insemination technique is to place the semen in the part of the reproductive tract that will give the best chances for conception. The insemination technique is different for each of the five farm species. This is due to the size of the females and to the anatomy of their reproductive systems.

17–1 INSEMINATION OF THE COW

Three basically different methods of inseminating the cow have evolved since the beginning of AI.

17–1.1 *Vaginal Insemination*

The earliest inseminations were accomplished by simply inserting a tube into the vagina and depositing semen at the mouth of the cervix. This procedure simulated a deposit of semen during natural mating and probably gave fair results when very large numbers of sperm were deposited. However, the environment of the vagina is not conducive to long life of sperm. Recent research with a limited number of services indicates that a modern breeding unit of semen containing approximately 10 million motile sperm will result in a very low conception rate when deposited in the vagina.

17–1.2 *Cervical Insemination*

Cervical insemination is accomplished by inserting a sterile speculum (2 cm to 3 cm in diameter and 35 cm to 40 cm long) into the vagina. With the use of a light source (pen light or head lamp), an inseminating instrument can be inserted into the opening of the cervix (Figure 17–1). Normally, the instrument can be inserted from 1 cm to 2 cm and the semen deposited at that point. This method is far superior to the vaginal method but usually gives 10 to 12 percentage units are lower conception rate than the recto-vaginal method (Section 17–1.3). Another disadvantage of this method is the amount of equipment that must be sterilized between inseminations.

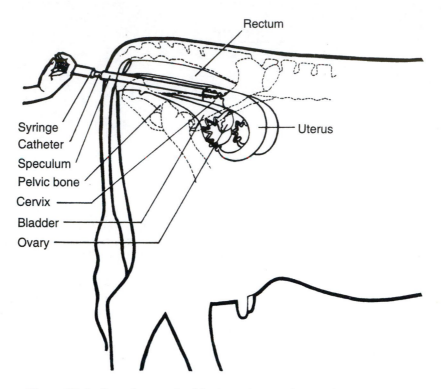

Figure 17–1   Speculum method for inseminating the cow. Similar method is used for the ewe.

17–1.3 *Recto-Vaginal Insemination*

The recto-vaginal insemination method is also referred to as the *cervical fixation* method. While this technique is not complicated, considerable practice with live cows is required to master it. The authors recommend that beginners take an academic course or a short course that provides hands-on practice. It is accomplished by inserting a gloved left hand, lubricated with a small amount of surgical jelly, into the rectum of the cow. The hand locates and grasps the cervix (Figure 17–2). The cervix can be distinguished from the vagina and uterus by its firm, thick walls. The inseminating instrument is inserted through the vulva into the vagina until it contacts the cervix and the left hand. The lips of the vulva should be spread slightly when inserting the inseminating instrument to prevent contamination by the outer surfaces of the vulva. The cervix should be held by its posterior end with index and middle fingers and thumb, leaving the other two fingers free to help guide the inseminating instrument (Figure 17–3). The instrument is guided into the opening of the cervix, and the left hand is used to thread the end of the instrument through the irregular cervical channel. The cervical folds make it necessary to manipulate the cervix in all directions in order to pass the instrument through the cervix. As the instrument progresses through the cervix, the fingers and thumb are moved forward so that the manipulation is taking place just forward to the end of the inseminating instrument. Progress of the instrument can be determined by the rigidity it gives to the cervix. The student is referred to Chapter 2, Section 2–4, for the

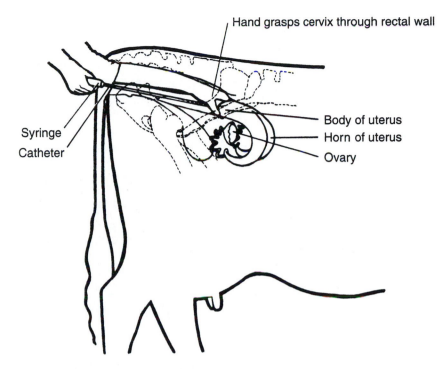

Figure 17–2 Recto-vaginal method for inseminating the cow.

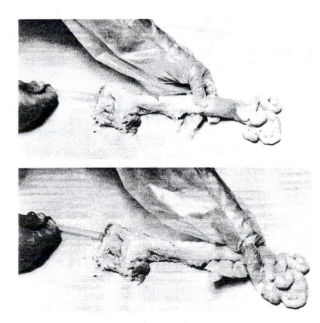

Figure 17–3 Right way (*top*) and wrong way (*bottom*) of holding the cervix for the recto-vaginal method of insemination.

anatomy of the cervix. The inseminating instrument should be stopped as soon as it reaches the anterior end of the cervix.

The inseminating instrument should not be removed from the vagina after insertion until insemination is completed. Extra passages through the lips of the vulva result in greater contamination. It is particularly important not to withdraw the instrument when the cow urinates. The opening would be pointed directly into the oncoming stream of urine, which is extremely detrimental to sperm.

The beginner should be aware of some problem situations.

1. The insemination instrument should be inserted into the vagina with the forward tip held higher than the other end. This will help prevent the insemination instrument from entering the suburethral diverticulum or the external urethral orifice.

2. Occasionally, muscular contractions will force the reproductive tract toward the anus, causing the vagina to become folded. This may make it seemingly impossible to bring the inseminating instrument into contact with the cervix. The cervix can be grasped with the left hand and pushed forward to straighten the vagina.

3. The cow will attempt to expel the left hand from the rectum with *peristaltic* muscular contractions. The contractions begin at the junction of the large intestine and the rectum and proceed toward the anus. When the contraction reaches the hand, its progress is stopped but the muscles continue to squeeze the hand. The hand will tire quickly if the contraction is fought. The cervix must be released and the hand pushed through the contraction. The rectum will relax so the cervix can be manipulated again.

4. The rectal muscles may contract, forming a large, hard-walled, tubular structure. The cervix cannot be felt or manipulated through this condition. This contraction can be overcome by reaching forward to the junction of the rectum and large intestine. The fingers can be cupped over the hardened rectal wall and the hand pulled toward the anus. This procedure usually causes the contracted rectal muscle to relax and soften so the cervix can be manipulated.

5. In practice situations, the vagina occasionally fills with air, making it difficult to grasp and manipulate the cervix. Firm pressure with the hand toward the vulva will dispel the air and restore favorable working conditions.

6. An extremely full bladder can make working with the cervix difficult. Manipulating the clitoris may cause urination.

The recto-vaginal method is more difficult to learn. However, its superior conception rate makes it the method of choice. Conception rates are lower for the beginner, but as the technique is mastered conception improves.

17–1.4 *Inseminating Equipment*

A plastic inseminating catheter fitted with a polypropylene bulb (poly bulb) or a 2-ml syringe attached to the catheter with a short rubber connecting tube must be used when liquid semen or semen frozen in ampules is being used (Figure 17–4). Care should be taken to draw all of the semen from the ampule, and this will require some practice when the poly bulb is used. Care must also be taken not to draw the semen into the syringe when one is

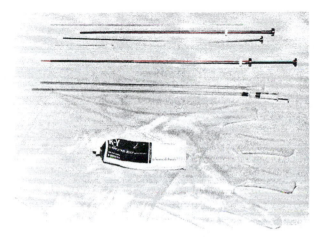

Figure 17–4 Equipment used to inseminate the cow. From the bottom: plastic glove and KY lubricating jelly; plastic catheters with 2-ml syringe and poly bulb; assembled 0.5-ml straw gun; unassembled straw gun (straw, plunger, barrel, and outer plastic sheath).

used. The semen should be discharged from the inseminating catheter slowly. If an attempt is made to expel the semen quickly, the surface tension between the semen and the inseminating catheter is such that the air will be forced through the semen column, leaving 25% to 50% of the semen in the catheter.

Insemination using semen packaged in the plastic straw requires specially designed equipment. The "straw gun" is a stainless steel tube with a small stainless steel rod to serve as a plunger (Figure 17–4). The lumen of the tube is the same diameter as the lumen of the straw except for a chamber in the anterior end, which is large enough to accommodate the external diameter of the straw. This chamber is 1 cm shorter than the straw so that the straw protrudes beyond the end of the gun. The straw is inserted with the plug seal going in first. The ultrasonically sealed end is cut perpendicular to the straw with surgical scissors or commercial straw cutter. A plastic sheath is slipped over the end of the straw and the gun. The posterior end of the gun tapers so that a plastic O-ring can be used to hold the sheath in place. The sheath is designed to fit tightly against the end of the straw, forming a seal to prevent the semen from being trapped between the straw and the sheath. The semen is expelled by pushing the stainless steel rod against the straw plug, which then acts as a plunger to deliver the semen to the site of insemination. This positive action ensures maximum delivery of sperm.

17–1.5 *Thawing Frozen Bull Semen*

The optimum thawing temperature for frozen semen appears to be related to the rate of freezing. Probably, there are other interactions such as glycerol level, equilibration time, and diluter composition. The effects of these interactions have not been worked out completely, but there is general agreement for thawing procedures.

17–1.5a Thawing Ampules The geometric configuration of the ampule results in a freezing rate somewhat slower than that for the plastic straw. An ice water bath provides the proper rate of heat exchange to thaw the ampule for maximum survival rate

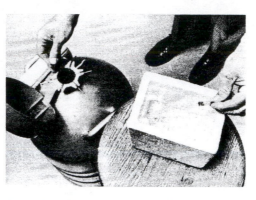

Figure 17–5   Ampules of frozen semen are thawed by transferring them to a container of ice water.

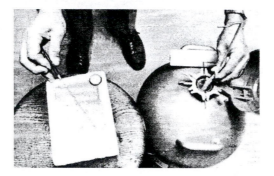

Figure 17–6   Straws of frozen semen are thawed by transferring them to a container of 32°C to 35°C water. Note thermometer in corner of thaw box.

(Figure 17–5). The ice water thaw is preferred to placing the ampule in the shirt pocket, allowing it to thaw at ambient temperature, or thawing in warm water.

Some precaution should be taken when thawing the ampule, since occasionally an ampule will be improperly sealed. While immersed in liquid nitrogen over a long period of time, the nitrogen seeps into and fills the air space above the frozen semen. When the ampule and liquid nitrogen are exposed to thawing temperatures, the nitrogen expands faster than it can escape through the tiny opening and the ampule explodes. Therefore, the ice water used to thaw ampules of frozen semen should be in an unbreakable container, such as a polystyrene thaw box or a soft plastic container.

17–1.5b Thawing Straws   Straws should be thawed in a 32°C to 35°C water bath (Figure 17–6). The actual thawing process will be completed in 12 to 15 seconds and the temperature of the semen will have reached approximately 5°C. One report involving 18,000 services showed a significantly higher 75-day nonreturn rate of 66.3% for straws thawed for 40 seconds, compared with 64.4% for those thawed for only 9 seconds. Even when semen was used with ambient temperature below freezing, the 40-second thaw time gave better results. Some semen-producing organizations recommend leaving the straw in the thaw bath for 45 to 60 seconds. Electrically heated, thermostatically controlled thawing equipment is available. The units are available with either a 12-volt (for use in automobiles) or 110-volt heating system.

17–1.5c Handling Semen After Thawing   Since most semen is now packaged in 0.5-ml plastic straws and the recommended thawing procedure raises the semen temperature to about 35°C, certain precautions are necessary to prevent sperm damage. This is particularly true when ambient temperature is below 5°C, since exposure of warm sperm to low temperatures will cause cold shock. The cow should be restrained and all equipment assembled before the semen is thawed. If possible, semen thawing and handling should be done in a heated area. The straw should be dried with a clean paper towel when it is removed from the thaw water. The barrel of the "straw gun" should be warmed to at least 25°C before the straw is inserted. If there is doubt, the tube can be warmed by rubbing it briskly for a few seconds with a paper towel. Wrap the loaded gun in clean paper towels and tuck inside the inseminator's clothing for protection until it is inserted into the cow's vagina. After the cow has been properly prepared, the gun can be slipped quickly from the towel sheath and inserted.

17–1.6 *Site of Semen Deposition*

Research conducted during the early 1950s indicated little or no difference in conception between inseminations when the semen was deposited in the middle to anterior cervix, body of the uterus, or deep in the uterine horns. This led to the practice of using the body of the uterus as the site of deposition, especially for first service. Additional research supporting this practice was reported in the 1960s, 1970s, and 1980s. Generally, the recommendation for repeat inseminations has been to deposit the semen in the anterior end of the cervix and not penetrate the uterus. Research on which the practice is based showed that inseminations in the cervix did not interrupt early pregnancies and did not significantly lower conception.

Two methods were reported for determining "after-the-fact" location of semen deposition (dye technique in the 1960s and radiographic technique in the 1980s). These procedures were viewed as being useful for training and for refresher training of individuals performing inseminations. Since earlier work had shown that conception was not affected by site of deposition from midcervix to deep uterine horn, these techniques may have limited value. A later research report has supported that concept. Deposition in the body of the uterus was compared with deposition of all of the semen in the ipsilateral horn (adjacent to ovary with follicle) or in the contralateral horn (opposite ovary with follicle). There were no differences between treatments. Granted, the numbers in that experiment were small but it does support a large amount of data already available.

Another recent report compared depositing all of the semen in the body of the uterus with depositing half in each uterine horn. These researchers reported a significant difference in favor of the uterine horn deposition. These results are in contrast to earlier studies and need further testing with acceptable control of semen sources, environment, and insemination. It should be tested with inseminators who may not be as skilled as those trained for the reported studies. The risk of damage to the endometrium is high with this technique, which could adversely affect fertility with insemination in the field.

The authors' recommendation on site of semen deposition remains unchanged. For first services, the semen should be placed in the body of the uterus. This is accomplished by placing the index finger of the positioning hand over the anterior end of the cervix when the inseminating instrument reaches that point. Hold the tip of the instrument lightly against the finger while expelling the semen. On repeat breedings, pass the inseminating instrument to within 1 cm to 2 cm of the anterior end of the cervix for semen deposition.

Research has shown that the conception rate of cows in which the semen was deposited in midcervix because the inseminator was unable to pass the insemination instrument beyond that point was about 15 percentage units lower than for cows in which the semen was deposited in the body of the uterus. This reduced fertility may have been due to irritation and swelling of the cervical mucosa or stress which prevented the semen from traversing the cervix.

17–1.7 *Restraining Facilities*

Cows must be adequately restrained during insemination to protect the inseminator and to allow proper placement of semen with a minimum of excitement and trauma to the cow. Many producers have work areas with lock-in stanchions that work well for inseminating dairy cows. Dairy heifers and beef cows may require more elaborate facilities. A chute narrow enough that cows or heifers cannot turn around can be used. The working end of the chute (the length of a cow) should be enclosed (sides and top) with plywood or similar material. The gate should be solid also and swing out to open. A piece of burlap or canvas can be fastened to the rear edge of the top and dropped down onto the cow's rump to provide as near total darkness as possible in the confinement area. The cow is driven in and held in place with a piece of pipe or a bar. The cow or heifer should be allowed to stand quietly for a few minutes before being inseminated. A narrow access gate (width of the chute) placed immediately behind the inseminating area is very helpful. This gate should open inward so that when it is open it closes the chute behind the inseminator, thus protecting him or her from cows waiting to be inseminated. Even the most excitable cows can usually be inseminated in this facility.

17–2 INSEMINATION OF THE EWE AND DOE

Because of the size of the ewe and doe, it is necessary to use either the vaginal or cervical method described for the cow. A small stainless steel spreading speculum is usually used. With the aid of a head light, the inseminating instrument is inserted into the mouth of the cervix, where the semen is deposited (Figure 17–7). The insemination unit contains 60×10^6 to 500×10^6 motile sperm in a small volume such as the 0.25-ml straw.

Two procedures have been described by which semen can be placed into the lumen of the ewe's uterus. In one procedure, a tubular perspex speculum and light described in the preceding paragraph are used to locate the external os. The end of an insemination catheter is fitted with a 10-cm-long, ball-tipped, 17-gauge needle, which is gently threaded through the cervix. Successful passage to the body of the uterus is possible in only about 50% to 60% of the estrous ewes. A second procedure, which is referred to as the Guelph System for Transcervical-AI, is similar but the cervix is stabilized by grasping the surrounding tissue with a pair of Bozman forceps. A fine (18G) stainless steel inseminating pipette (attached to a modified IMV inseminating gun) is introduced into the cervical opening. Gentle probing is used to ease the pipette past each cervical fold and into the lumen of the uterus.

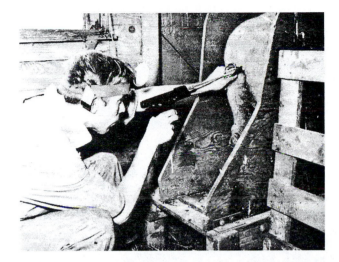

Figure 17–7 Inseminating the ewe. A stainless steel spreading speculum is used. (Courtesy of E. K. Inskeep. Division of Animal and Veterinary Sciences, West Virginia University.)

With either procedure, one can expect to pass the inseminating instrument all the way to the body of the uterus only 50% to 70% of the time. Inseminator skill accounts for part of the failures but the proper stage of the estrous period may be critical to successful passage. The cervix may change in the degree of dilation during estrus. Conception rates of about 70% have been reported in ewes in which the semen was deposited intrauterine but are much lower for those intracervically inseminated.

The invasive method of intrauterine insemination is accomplished by laparoscopy. Ewes to be inseminated are restrained in a laparoscopy cradle. A local anesthetic is used at the site of cannula insertion. The reproductive tract is located with the laparoscope and the semen is injected into the lumen of the uterus. Conception rates for this procedure are similar to those of successful transcervical inseminations.

The intrauterine insemination procedure for the doe differs from that described for the ewe in two respects. The doe seems to have a dorsal flap that at least partially covers the external os; it must be lifted or otherwise bypassed before entrance to the cervix can be gained. The insemination instrument preferred is the 0.25-ml straw gun. Once entrance to the cervix is gained, the gun can usually be passed to the uterine body.

17–3 INSEMINATION OF THE SOW

The anatomy of the cervix in the sow makes insemination easy. The inseminating tube can be inserted into the cervix without the aid of sight or cervical fixation. A commercially available inseminating tube with a design similar to the boar's glans penis has been developed for inseminating the sow (Figure 17–8). The anterior end is designed to fit into the cervix so that it simulates the locking of the boar's glans penis in the cervix during natural mating. A disposable clear plastic catheter with a simulated boar's glans penis is also available. It comes with

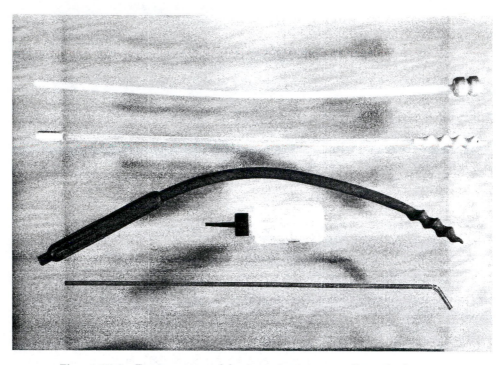

Figure 17–8   Equipment used for inseminating sows. From the bottom: plastic insemination catheter bent at a 30° angle 2 cm from the end; plastic squeeze insemination bottle; reusable rubber spirette; plastic disposable spirette; plastic disposable catheter with soft sponge end which seals into the mouth of the cervix.

matching squeeze bottle, which has a plastic nipple on the cap. This nipple has to be cut with scissors to form a connector for attaching to the catheter. A plastic disposable catheter with two rings of soft sponge, which seal the catheter into the mouth of the cervix, is also available.

Another technique involves heating a plastic inseminating tube to form a 30° bend about 2 cm from the end of the tube (Figure 17–8). This bent tube is inserted into the opening of the cervix and turned so that it threads its way into the corkscrew channel of the cervix. It also allows the end of the catheter to bypass the external urethral orifice without danger of entering the bladder instead of the cervix. A plastic squeeze bottle or large syringe is used to express about 80 ml to 90 ml of semen into the cervix.

Research has been reported that supports increasing the insemination time from 5 to 8 minutes per sow. The longer inseminations increased farrowing rates by 10 percentage units (75% to 85%) and an increase of 0.2 pig per litter. Regardless of sow herd size, those differences would more than pay for the extra time. The pressure of the insemination tool in the mouth of the cervix may increase and prolong the contractions of the uterine muscles, which in turn improve the sperm transport through the long uterine horns. A clamp that simulates the pressure of the boar's front legs on the sow's rib cage during natural mating has been reported to improve conception rates.

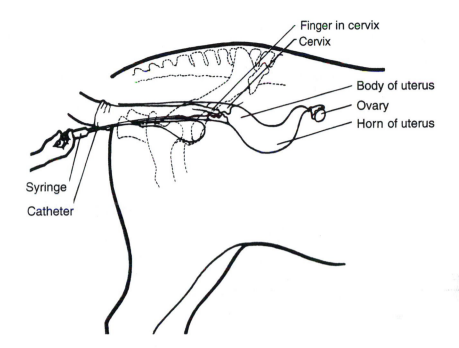

Figure 17–9   Method used to inseminate the mare.

17–4 INSEMINATION OF THE MARE

The method used for inseminating mares requires special emphasis on cleanliness, because the hand is placed in the vagina with a finger through the cervix. After confining the mare in a chute suitable to protect the technician, her tail is wrapped with cheesecloth and tied to one side. The vulva, anus, and surrounding area are then scrubbed with water and mild soap, with special emphasis on cleaning the creased areas on either side of the vulva. After rinsing with water, the area is dried with sterile gauze. A shoulder-length plastic glove is used by the technician with a sterile surgeon's glove worn over the plastic glove. A 50-ml syringe with a volume of semen containing 500×10^6 motile sperm is connected to a plastic inseminating catheter. The gloved hand is placed in the vagina with a finger through the cervix, the catheter is passed beside the hand and through the cervix, and the semen is deposited in the body of the uterus. It is easy to pass the catheter through the mare's cervix because it is dilated and softened during estrus (Figure 17–9). This procedure is used rather than the recto-vaginal method due to the mare's anatomy. The broad ligament is above the cervix and is more distinct than in the cow. Thus, the mare's cervix is more difficult to manipulate via the rectum. Additionally, the mare's rectum is more delicate, the mucosa is dryer than the cow's, and a tear is much more serious (usually resulting in death) in the mare.

SUGGESTED READING

AAMDAL, J. 1982. Artificial insemination in goats with frozen semen in Norway. *Proc. 3rd Int. Conf. on Goat Prod. and Disease,* Tucson, Ariz.

CORTEEL, J. M., C. GONZALEZ, and J. F. NUNES. 1982. Research and development in the control of reproduction. *Proc. 3rd Int. Conf. on Goat Prod. and Disease,* Tucson, Ariz.

FUKUI, Y. and E. M. ROBERTS. 1976. Studies of nonsurgical intrauterine insemination of frozen pelleted semen in the ewe. *VIIIth Int. Cong. on Anim. Reprod. and A.I.* p. 991.

HOLT, A. F. 1946. Comparison between intracervical and intrauterine methods of artificial insemination. *Vet. Rec.,* 58:309.

MOMONT, H. W., B. E. SEGUIN, G. SINGH, and E. STASIUKYNAS. 1989. Does intrauterine site of insemination in cattle really matter? *Theriogenology,* 32:19.

Pork Industry Handbook No. 64. 1995. Current.

SALAMON, S. and R. J. LIGHTFOOT. 1970. Fertility of ram spermatozoa frozen by the pellet method. III. The effects of insemination technique, oxytocin and relaxin on lambing. *J. Reprod. Fert.,* 22:409.

SALISBURY, G. W. and N. L. VANDEMARK. 1951. The effect of cervical, uterine and cornual insemination on fertility of the dairy cow. *J. Dairy Sci.,* 34:68.

SENGER, P. L., W. C. BECKER, S. T. DAVIDGE, J. K. HILLERS, and J. J. REEVES. 1988. Influence of cornual insemination on conception in dairy cattle. *J. Anim. Sci.,* 66:3010.

SULLIVAN, J. J., D. E. BARTLETT, F. I. ELLIOTT, J. R. BROVWER, and F. B. KLOCH. 1972. A comparison of recto-vaginal, vaginal, and speculum approaches for insemination of cows and heifers. *A. I. Digest,* 20:6.

WILCOX, C. J. and K. D. PFAV. 1958. Effect of two services during estrus on the conception rate of dairy cows. *J. Dairy Sci.,* 41:997.

WINDSOR, D. P. 1995. Factors influencing the success of transcervical insemination in marino ewes. *Theriogenology,* 43:1009.

WINDSOR, D. P., A. Z. SZELL, C. BUSCHBECK, A. Y. EDWARDS, J. T. B. MILTON, and B. C. BUCKRELL. 1994. Transcervical artificial insemination of Australian merino ewes with frozen-thawed semen. *Theriogenology,* 42:147.

Part 4

Management for Improved Reproduction

The next six chapters introduce a broad array of management techniques that improve reproductive efficiency through the manipulation of reproductive processes. These range from current methods for controlling reproductive cycles, inducing superovulation, and the practice of embryo transfer (Chapter 18) to descriptions of developing reproductive biotechnologies (Chapter 19) that may improve our reproductive management abilities even further. Other routine reproductive management practices (Chapter 20), methods for pregnancy diagnosis (Chapter 21), and the environmental (Chapter 22) and nutritional (Chapter 23) management of livestock are also presented, with reference to the physiological basis for the management procedures described. These chapters should help the student understand the complexity of the various factors that can be managed to improve reproductive efficiency.

18

Synchronization of Estrus and Superovulation with Embryo Transfer

A great deal of progress has been made during the past 30 years through better management of natural reproductive processes. However, livestock managers and researchers have recognized that certain natural reproductive processes can be altered artificially to the advantage of better management. This has included the use of various hormones and management practices that permit a greater control over the estrous cycle of the female and, thus, greater control over the timing of breeding and conception. To fully maximize the use of artificial insemination, discussed in detail in previous chapters, control of the estrous cycle becomes paramount as part of many reproductive management plans. In concert with artificial insemination, manipulation of the number of ova that can be ovulated during a given estrous cycle for embryo production has similarly greatly enhanced livestock management practices for animals of high genetic merit. This chapter will explore the current strategies for artificially managing the reproductive cycle of the female as a component of artificial insemination protocols, as a means for embryo production and transfer, and as a way of establishing different types of reproductive management plans for livestock.

18–1 SYNCHRONIZATION OF ESTRUS

Several advantages have been recognized in having a number of females in estrus during a very short period of time. It permits the manager to schedule livestock handling and breeding to fit into a work schedule. The time-consuming job of detecting estrus is reduced. The breeding season can be shortened because more females become pregnant during the first week of breeding. Animals can be grouped into desired parturition patterns so that intensive care may be provided for limited periods. Likewise, parturition season can be shifted to better coincide with the most favorable marketing patterns. In most cases, synchronization is a necessary part of the superovulation and embryo transfer procedure.

Synchronization of estrus would make AI much more attractive to commercial beef cattle managers by making it possible to get all of their cattle inseminated within 1 week. This is possible by handling the cows once for treatment and once for insemination. Having a high concentration of dairy heifers entering the milking string at one time has both advantages and disadvantages. Since heifers tend to have more difficulty calving than cows, having several calve during a short period would require less observation time. On the other hand, heifers require extra time and effort in the milking routine. Some dairy herd managers may not want to have a large number of heifers to "break in" at the same time.

18–1.1 *Synchronization of Estrus in Cows*

Cattle managers should be aware of some problem situations when considering synchronization of estrus. (1) Some cows or heifers may already be pregnant and $PGF_{2\alpha}$ will cause abortion when administered to pregnant females. This is especially a problem when bulls are kept on the same premises. Bulls on neighboring property will invariably breed an occasional female. (2) Synchronization should never be attempted until there is evidence that beef cows have passed the postpartum anestrus period. (3) Heifers must be checked to be sure they are not still in prepuberal anestrus. They can be observed for estrus (25% of a group should show estrus in a 5-day observation period) or palpated for the presence of corpora lutea on the ovaries.

The livestock manager should be fully aware that the synchronization of estrus is not a substitute for good herd management. Research conducted in privately owned herds has shown that synchronization can be highly successful in well-managed herds and a dismal failure in herds with only marginal management. Use only those drugs that have cleared FDA for specific classes and ages of livestock.

18–1.1a Prostaglandin Method   Prostaglandin $F_{2\alpha}$ administered as a single injection during days 5 through 17 of the estrous cycle will cause regression of the corpus luteum (CL) and subsequent return to estrus in 36 to 72 hours (Figure 18–1). Prior to day 5, the corpus luteum may not have sufficient receptor sites to respond to normal levels of $PGF_{2\alpha}$; however, response to very large doses has been observed. In addition, metabolic pathways may not have developed sufficiently at this point to allow complete response. After day 17, the corpus luteum usually is regressing.

Some studies indicate that the 5- to 7-day-old corpora lutea may be too young to respond at practical levels. The data in Table 18–1 show differences in progesterone level, response rate, and conception rate for cows injected at three stages of the estrous cycle. The 5- through 7-day group not only responded at an unacceptable rate, but those responding had a lower conception rate. The percentage (24.4%) of injected heifers conceiving is too low to be practical. As the age of the CL increases, both response rate and conception rate increase. These data indicate that some adjustment in synchronization procedures is needed to avoid injecting cows and heifers with $PGF_{2\alpha}$ until the eighth day of the cycle. Additional research is also needed to determine why the CL does not respond as readily during days 1 through 7 of the cycle.

When prostaglandin is injected intramuscularly (IM), a 25-mg dose is required to regress the CL. A 5-mg dose placed in the uterus will achieve the same results. When administered IM, the prostaglandin passes through the lungs, where a high percentage is deactivated prior to reaching the ovary. Prostaglandin placed in the uterus travels directly to the ovary by way of countercurrent circulation (Section 2–7), thus requiring a much smaller dosage. Only 0.5 mg of the prostaglandin analog (cloprostenol) injected intramuscularly is required to regress the CL. This material is not deactivated as readily as $PGF_{2\alpha}$.

Administration of $PGF_{2\alpha}$ or cloprostenol as described in the preceding paragraph between day 5 and day 17 of the estrous cycle has caused blood plasma progesterone levels to fall rapidly within 24 hours, followed by a rise in estrogen within 24 hours. A preovulatory peak of LH occurred on the average within 3 days and estrus occurred at about the time of the LH peak. Ovulation occurred about 24 hours after the onset of estrus.

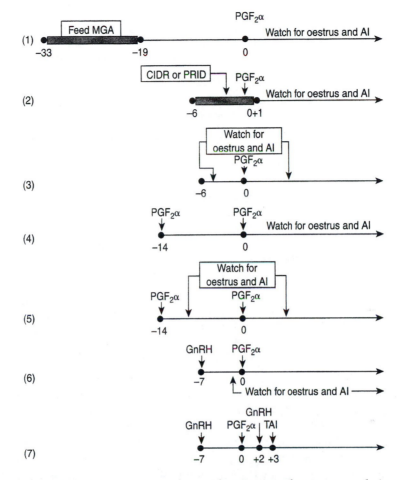

Figure 18–1 Seven programs for synchronization of estrus or ovulation in cattle are illustrated. *Program (1):* feeding melengestrol acetate (MGA) for 14 days and passing over the estrus expressed upon MGA withdrawal followed by an injection of $PGF_{2\alpha}$ given 17 to 19 days after MGA. *Program (2):* intravaginal insertion of a progesterone-releasing insert (CIDR or PRID) for 7 days with $PGF_{2\alpha}$ injection administered at or one day before insert removal. *Program (3):* visual detection of estrus for 6 days prior to injecting all noninseminated heifers or cows with $PGF_{2\alpha}$ on the 7th day. *Program (4):* two injections of $PGF_{2\alpha}$ given 14 days apart, with inseminations occurring after the second injection or *Program (5):* after both injections. *Program (6):* an injection of GnRH 7 days before an injection of $PGF_{2\alpha}$ (Select Synch) or *Program (7):* same as (6) but a second injection of GnRH is given 48 hours after $PGF_{2\alpha}$ with one timed-AI 12 to 20 hours later (OvSynch). *Source:* Reprinted from *Encyclopedia of Dairy Sciences*, 4, Stevenson, J. S., Breeding Standards and Pregnancy Management, p. 2428, 2002, with permission from Elsevier Science.

Table 18–1   *Plasma progesterone levels, response rate, and conception rate of dairy heifers injected with PGF$_{2\alpha}$ in early, middle, and late diestrus*

	Number of heifers injected	Mean progesterone level at injection ng/ml	Percentage of heifers responding	Percentage of responding heifers conceiving	Percentage of injected heifers conceiving
Early diestrus (days 5–7)	86	2.78 ± 1.19[a]	43.0[a]	56.8	24.4
Mid-diestrus (days 8–11)	104	5.18 ± 1.49[b]	83.7[b]	62.1	51.9
Late diestrus (days 12–15)	60	5.22 ± 1.28[b]	100.0[c]	78.3	78.3

Adapted from Watts, T. L., Master of Science Thesis, Mississippi State University, 1983.
[a,b,c]Values within a column with different superscript letters differ significantly (P < .001).

Since recycling of cows with prostaglandin is effective only when administered to cycling cows between day 5 and day 17 of the cycle, one can expect only about 60% to 65% of the cows to respond at any given time. The herd manager then is faced with four alternatives:

1. Rectally palpate all cows and inject only those that are judged to have corpora lutea that are 5 days or more in age. Treated cows may be time-inseminated 80 hours following treatment or inseminated during detected estrus. Again timed-insemination usually results in lower conception rate based on total cows bred. The remaining cows could be treated 12 days later and inseminated as the first group.

2. Treat all cows, inseminate those that come into estrus, and then treat all remaining cows 12 days following the first treatment. Cows treated the second time may be time-inseminated at 80 hours posttreatment or inseminated during detected estrus.

3. Check estrus for 5 days and inseminate those observed in estrus; treat remaining animals with PGF$_{2\alpha}$ on day 5 and inseminate at the ensuing estrus. This method has resulted in 65% to 70% conception rate.

4. Treat all cows, wait 12 days, then treat all cows again and either time-inseminate at 80 hours or inseminate during detected estrus. It must be remembered that only cycling cows will respond to prostaglandin treatment.

Beef cattle managers may prefer to combine synchronization of estrus and AI with cleanup natural mating. This would work with any of the four methods described. Inseminate the cows that respond during the 5 days following a selected treatment regimen and then put them with a cleanup bull. Method 2 can be used as described or the second treatment can be skipped, allowing the cleanup bull to breed those not responding plus those not conceiving to AI. Systems 1, 3, and 4 probably would result in a higher percentage of cows being artificially inseminated.

Variable results have been reported for timed-inseminations performed following synchronization of estrus with PGF$_{2\alpha}$. Pregnancy rates ranging from 40% to 70% are not unusual.

Table 18–2 *Distribution of estrus following 25 mg PGF$_{2\alpha}$ injected intramuscularly to Holstein heifers that had been observed for estrus for 5 days*

Hours after PGF$_{2\alpha}$	Mean progesterone levels at time of injection	Heifers responding[a]		Heifers responding[b]		Combined	
		No.	%	No.	%	No.	%
0–24	1.51	8	4.7	5	3.7	13	4.2
25–48	4.59	51	30.2	31	22.8	82	27.1
49–72	7.01	77	45.6	63	47.1	140	46.2
73–96	7.22	24	14.2	21	15.4	45	14.9
> 96	6.09	9	5.3	14	11.0	23	7.6
Total		169		134		303	

[a]Gonzales, L., Master of Science Thesis, Mississippi State University, 1982.

[b]Wahome, J. N., Master of Science Thesis, Mississippi State University, 1983.

Data in Table 18–2 show the distribution of estrus following PGF$_{2\alpha}$ injections. The heifers in the two trials involved had been checked for estrus for 5 days prior to a single injection of PGF$_{2\alpha}$. Some of them were in proestrus and demonstrated estrus during the first 24 to 36 hours. This is confirmed by the mean progesterone level at the time of injection. Those showing estrus within 24 hours after injection had a mean serum progesterone level of 1.51 ng/ml. Those coming into estrus in 25 to 48 hours postinjection had a mean serum progesterone level of 4.59 ng/ml, indicating that at least half of that group were in diestrus (earlier than the seventeenth day) at the time of injection. No single time could have been selected for timed-insemination that would have given more than 50% of the responding heifers an optimum chance to conceive. There was some variation in the distribution of estrus in the two studies, and even more could occur in other studies. This variation may account for the varied success with timed-insemination. Higher conception rates can be expected when inseminating at detected estrus. Some additional cows may be "picked up" by palpating those not detected in estrus by 80 hours and inseminating those showing symptoms of estrus (uterine tone or presence of a follicle). This will prevent wasting semen on those not responding.

Conception rates following prostaglandin treatments have generally been comparable to those obtained at naturally occurring estrus. A much higher percentage of cows become pregnant during the first 5 days of breeding whether synchronized with progestins or with prostaglandins than is possible with heat detection of unsynchronized cows. Unsynchronized cows have estrus distributed over a 21-day period. The advantage of synchronization is still significant at 25 days of breeding but disappears by day 45. Thus, synchronization reduces time required for detection of estrus, and artificially inseminating cows results in a higher percentage of the herd becoming pregnant early in the breeding season.

18–1.1b Progestin Method Early work demonstrated that injections of progesterone inhibited estrus and ovulation in sheep and cattle. The period of administration had to be sufficiently long to allow the corpora lutea to regress in order to obtain synchronization. The treatment period at the time was usually 16 days for cows; however, many current protocols are much shorter, with durations of 7 to 12 days. Exogenous progestins work by preventing the release of GnRH, which in turn results in reduced gonadotropins, which prevents estrus and ovulation from occurring until the progestin is withdrawn. Upon withdrawal of the progestin, the decreasing blood concentrations of progestins allows pulsatile releases of GnRH to return (i.e., removal of the progestin block), which results in release of gonadotropins and estrus occurring 2 to 6 days later, beginning around 48 hours after progestin withdrawal. This interval for the return to estrus following progestin withdrawal has been further refined by the addition of luteolytic hormones (e.g., $PGF_{2\alpha}$) as part of progestin-based synchronization protocols (Figure 18–1). As administration of these methods at any stage of the 21-day estrous cycle in the cow should result in synchrony, 80% to 90% of females generally respond and are synchronized. Progestins have been administered in feed or drinking water, as subcutaneous implants, by topical application, or as intravaginal progestin-releasing devices.

Some trials have shown conception rates from progestin-synchronized females to be the same as those bred based on natural detected estrus without synchronization, but overall the conception rates are at least 15% lower following progestin treatment. Breeding can be accomplished using timed-breeding for the entire synchronized herd at a specified interval after progestin withdrawal or following observations of estrus postsynchrony. Some researchers have reported that two properly timed-inseminations based on progestin withdrawal result in more cows pregnant than breeding at detected estrus. Some treated cows ovulate without showing overt signs of estrus and conceive to timed-inseminations which otherwise may have been missed if breeding solely by estrus detection was utilized. Nevertheless, over a large number of studies that have been conducted, conception rates are generally higher for cows bred during detected estrus. A more practical approach may be to combine detection of estrus with timed-insemination. All females not detected in estrus can be inseminated after a predetermined time. When expensive semen is being used, fewer units are required, and the quiet ovulators have a chance to conceive. Good managers may want to go a step further and palpate those cows not showing signs of estrus for uterine tone and the presence of a follicle, as well as checking for the presence of discharge of mucus before breeding. Conception rates have been very low (10% to 15%) for females not meeting any of these indications.

Norgestomet (Synthetic Progestin) Implants.   The need for more acceptable conception rates and better synchronization prompted progestin treatment to be combined with estrogen injections. An implant containing a synthetic progestin (*Norgestomet*), along with an estradiol valerate and progestin injection when inserting the implant (Figure 18–2 shows a Norgestomet implant being inserted), has resulted in synchronized estrus 2 to 3 days after removing the implant on the ninth day of treatment. The progestin treatment is shortened to 9 days because the estradiol injection speeds luteolysis and alters the ovarian follicular populations. For cycling cows in good body condition, conception rates have been equivalent to controls that were not synchronized when both were inseminated at detected estrus. Lower fertility occurs when cows synchronized in this manner are in poor body condition, likely due in part to inducement of estrus in cows that were not cycling. While cows at all stages of the estrous cycle can be synchronized with this method, a recent study demonstrated that synchronization with Norgestomet resulted in good fertility if the implant was inserted into cows with a corpus luteum present but fertility was lower if no corpus luteum was present at the time of insertion. The data in Table 18–3 show the conception rate of heifers time-inseminated following progestin (Norgestomet) treatment. One timed-insemination at 54 hours after implant removal gave results comparable to two timed-inseminations at 48 and 60 hours after implant removal. Seventy-two hours after implant removal is too late to inseminate and 48 hours may be too early. The advantages of this

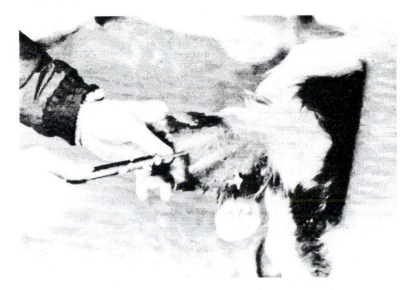

Figure 18–2 A progestin implant being inserted into a cow's ear. (Courtesy of W. Humphrey, Anim. Sci. Dept., Miss. State Univ.)

Table 18–3 *Effect of timing of insemination on the pregnancy rate of heifers treated with Norgestomet ear implants for 9 days*[*]

AI after implant removal	Number of heifers	Percent pregnant
48 & 60 hours	148	66.2
48 & 72 hours	145	62.1
54 hrs	137	65.7
Total	430	64.7

From Wishart and Drew. *Vet. Rec.*, 101:230, 1977.

[*]When the 6-mg implant was inserted, 5 mg of estradiol and 3 mg of Norgestomet were injected IM.

method (Norgestomet implant + estradiol valerate) are that (1) it will work on all cycling cows and heifers at various stages of the estrous cycle (2) it has an excellent ability to synchronize estrus, (3) it will not cause abortion in cattle that may already be pregnant and are synchronized without this knowledge, and (4) it traditionally has not required a prescription from a veterinarian, making it widely available to producers. A disadvantage is that it has not been approved for use in lactating dairy cows. The leading commercially available Norgestomet product was recently removed from the U.S. marketplace (at least temporarily); therefore, current availability and regulatory aspects for using this method should be investigated.

Intravaginal Progestin Inserts. Progestins have been incorporated into intravaginal implants that have the same effects as the Norgestomet ear implants for synchronizing estrus. These progestin-containing devices have been referred to as intravaginal CIDRs (Controlled Internal Drug Releasing), PRIDs (Progesterone-Releasing Intravaginal Devices), vaginal pessaries, and sponges. The progesterone-releasing CIDR has been used extensively throughout the world and in May 2002 was approved for use in the United States for beef and dairy heifers and beef cows (current regulations do not allow their use in lactating dairy cows in the United States). The CIDR is inserted into the vagina for a period of 7 days, with an injection of $PGF_{2\alpha}$ given 1 day prior to or at the day of CIDR removal (Figure 18–1). The CIDR inserts contain 1.38 g of progesterone, which is absorbed by the vaginal mucus from the surface of the insert, with progesterone deeper in the silicone rubber matrix of the implant continuously diffusing toward the reduced concentrations nearer the surface of the insert. The addition of $PGF_{2\alpha}$ toward the end of the CIDR insertion period assures that any progesterone-releasing luteal tissue on the ovaries is removed to prevent variability in the interval to estrus and improve synchrony. Research has shown that CIDRs are more effective in eliciting estrus, compared with a single injection of $PGF_{2\alpha}$. On average, 75% to 85% of dairy heifers show estrus within 3 days after CIDR removal. In one study using the PRID, 82% of treated animals exhibited estrus within 17 hours of PRID removal, 100% within 32 hours. Progestin treatment has also been shown to induce anestrous cows to start cycling earlier in the breeding season by priming the system, which is an added benefit when used in postpartum beef cows. As with the use of Norgestomet, recent research using estradiol benzoate injections at the time of CIDR insertion in addition to the use of $PGF_{2\alpha}$ at CIDR withdrawal suggests that pregnancy rates may be improved even further. These combination treatments (1) shorten the period of progestin treatment, possibly enhancing the chances of conception; (2) shorten the overall synchronization procedure; and (3) provide better synchronization.

Oral (Feeding) Progestins.   Steroid hormones, when ingested at the appropriate concentrations, are biologically active. A feed additive, melengestrol acetate (MGA), has been used to suppress estrus in feedlot heifers and has been adapted for use in the synchronization of estrus in beef and dairy heifers and beef cows (not for use in lactating dairy cows). As part of feeding MGA, the feed supplement to be used as a carrier is usually fed for 20 to 30 days to precondition the animals and to assure appropriate intake once the MGA is added. Animals that fail to consume the required amount of feed, and thus MGA, on a daily basis may prematurely return to estrus during the feeding period, which reduces the synchronization response. Therefore, adequate bunk space should be provided so that all animals can consume adequate portions of the feed. The MGA is fed with grain or a protein carrier and is either top-dressed onto the feed or batch-mixed for larger quantities of feed. The MGA is fed at a rate of 0.5 mg/animal/day for 14 days, which is enough time to produce corpora lutea in all cyclic animals, hold the corpus luteum in animals that may have begun MGA treatment during mid- to late diestrus, or maintain progesterone levels if luteolysis occurs at the beginning or during MGA treatment until the MGA is removed from the ration. Estrus is exhibited 2 to 5 days after withdrawal of the MGA; however, the estrus that occurs immediately after MGA feeding is a subfertile estrus, and females should not be inseminated based on this estrus. These females will ovulate an aged (and generally less fertile) oocyte and form a new CL. A single injection of $PGF_{2\alpha}$ is then administered 17 to 19 days after the MGA has been removed from the feeding program to regress the corpus luteum of the subsequent cycle following MGA treatment (Figure 18–1). After $PGF_{2\alpha}$, animals are inseminated at detected estrus until 72 hours; at 72 hours those not detected in estrus are inseminated in-mass.

18–1.1c   Ovulation Synchronization   A problem with the synchronization procedures described so far has been their lack of precision. This has meant that detec-

tion of estrus has been an essential part of most synchronization protocols for high fertility. Some research suggests that both the corpus luteum and follicular development must be controlled for precise synchrony of ovulation. Following the demonstration that GnRH would stimulate ovulation and the start of a new follicular wave, a program for synchronized ovulation was advanced. Since then, numerous GnRH-based synchronization protocols have been developed, including OvSynch, Select-Synch, and Co-Synch (Figure 18–1), among other variations. The OvSynch protocol begins with the administration of GnRH, which will start a new follicular wave by either ovulating a large dominant follicle (if present) and/or cause luteinization of smaller follicles. The first injection of GnRH is followed by an injection of $PGF_{2\alpha}$ 7 days later and a second injection of GnRH 36 to 48 hours after the $PGF_{2\alpha}$ injection. The outcome of this protocol is a synchronized ovulation 24 to 32 hours later. Artificial insemination is usually performed 16 hours after the second GnRH injection for best conception rates. In one study, ovulations among 40 lactating dairy cows were so well grouped that they all ovulated within 6 hours of one another. This procedure has worked well in cows but is less reliable in heifers, due to the differences in the follicular wave patterns between cows and heifers. Typically, mature cows have two follicular waves, while heifers have three follicular waves each cycle. A problem with the OvSynch system, less so for dairy cattle producers than beef producers, is the number of injections and working periods required to complete the synchronization protocols and breeding (four handling periods). The Co-Synch program eliminates the fourth restraint period by giving the second GnRH injection at the time of breeding (three working periods), while the Select-Synch program saves the cost of the second GnRH injection by simply breeding based on estrus detection after the administration of $PGF_{2\alpha}$ (three working periods). However, the Select-Synch requires more heat detection for a greater period of time, as opposed to the time breeding conducted with the OvSynch and Co-Synch systems. It is debatable which of the three ovulation synchronization methods works best and results are highly dependent on the management system and style employed. All three methods can provide good synchrony and good fertility.

18–1.1d Managed Breeding   A number of programs integrate estrous synchronization protocols into the routine management of the herd on a scheduled basis. Managed targeted breeding programs have evolved from standard estrous and ovulation synchronization programs using $PGF_{2\alpha}$ and GnRH and are being utilized in a number of dairy herds. One method employs a voluntary waiting period of 60 days postpartum to allow for uterine involution (Sections 10–7.2 and 20–2.4); then cows to be inseminated are injected with $PGF_{2\alpha}$. They are observed intensively for estrus for the next 4 to 5 days and inseminated after detection of estrus. Fourteen days later, those not inseminated plus any new cows that have cleared the voluntary waiting period are injected or reinjected with $PGF_{2\alpha}$, and this continues at 14-day intervals throughout the breeding season. Cows that recycle after insemination can be inseminated at the time of observation. Cows diagnosed as nonpregnant at any time are added to the next injection group. The major advantages of programs like these are the shortening of time needed for intensive observations of estrus, thus concentrating labor and estrus activity into a 4- or 5-day period. Managed breeding programs shorten calving intervals, as compared with breeding programs that do not control onset of estrus, which requires daily observations for estrus. In the latter case, frequently cows are not observed in estrus each cycle, which delays breeding. At an estimated cost of $1 to $3 per day for cows that remain nonpregnant more than 100 days postpartum, studies show that managed breeding programs are very cost-effective.

Modified targeted breeding programs are similar to so-called managed targeted breeding programs but use set-up shots or presynchronization to assure that cows are at the appropriate stage of the estrous cycle to respond to subsequent estrous synchronization efforts. Based on a voluntary waiting period of 60 days, $PGF_{2\alpha}$ is given around 36 days after calving, followed in 14 days with an injection of GnRH (around 50 days postpartum). A second injection of $PGF_{2\alpha}$ is given 7 days later (around day 57 postpartum) and then cows are observed for standing estrus and bred over the following 3 days. Any cows not observed in estrus are fixed-time inseminated between 72 and 80 hours after the $PGF_{2\alpha}$ injection. This protocol is basically a $PGF_{2\alpha}$ injection, followed 14 days later by the Select-Synch protocol but is timed to permit breedings to begin at 60 days postpartum to tighten calving intervals. These protocols are effective in well managed, healthy herds with a low incidence of postpartum diseases, good nutrition, or the absence of any other problems that may affect uterine involution and postpartum reproductive cyclicity. A variation of the modified targeted breeding concept and the use of set-up shots is the use of PreSynch, which is the administration of two injections of $PGF_{2\alpha}$ 14 days apart, starting around days 35 to 40 postpartum, with the second injection given 12 to 14 days before initiating OvSynch around days 60 to 65 postpartum. The $PGF_{2\alpha}$ injections induce estrus in about 30% to 40% of cows, with 60% to 80% expressing estrus after the second injection. PreSynch injections put cows in stages of the estrous cycle with corpus lutea at the time they start the OvSynch (days 5 to 12 of the cycle), so that a corpora luteum will be present when the $PGF_{2\alpha}$ is injected resulting in the appropriate timing for GnRH to be most effective on follicular growth patterns. The addition of the extra $PGF_{2\alpha}$ injection and use of the OvSynch program increases the number of cows that will respond to OvSynch at around 60 days postpartum. OvSynch is used for timed-insemination to reduce labor, which is required for estrus detection if a Select-Synch approach is utilized.

Recent studies have also shown that the timing of estrous or ovulation synchronization with other management-related activities on the dairy farm may further enhance conception rates. Treatment with bovine somatotropin (bST) at the beginning (around day 63 postpartum) or end (around day 73 postpartum) of the OvSynch protocol has resulted in greater pregnancy rates than for PreSynch + OvSynch cows inseminated at the same time but not treated with bST until 6 or 7 weeks later. Bovine somatotropin, or growth hormone, increases production efficiency in lactating dairy cows by partitioning nutrients for milk synthesis (Section 11–2.2). This coordinated treatment of bST appears to influence ovarian steroidogenesis and follicular development for improved fertility when timed appropriately with the OvSynch program, although more investigations are needed in this area.

18–1.2 *Synchronization of Estrus in Mares*

Prostaglandin $F_{2\alpha}$ has been effective in synchronizing estrus in mares starting on day 6 postovulation through day 18 of the cycle. After treatment, they return to estrus in 4 to 5 days and ovulate 10 to 12 days postinjection. When injected on day 6, 80% to 90% of the mares respond. It is necessary to know the status of the ovary with respect to an active corpus luteum or a follicle before treatment. Palpation or an ultrasonograph is helpful in determining presence of luteal tissue.

A synthetic oral progestin, altrenogest, has also been approved for use in synchronizing estrus in mares. The recommended amount (0.044 mg altrenogest/kg bodyweight) given orally directly into the mouth or top-dressed on feed is usually administered for 14 to

15 days. Estrus will occur in 2 to 4 days, with ovulation occurring 6 to 7 days after withdrawal. The manufacturer recommends timed-insemination on day 5 postwithdrawal. Some synchronization protocols have shortened the duration of progestin treatment to 7 to 8 days, with the addition of $PGF_{2\alpha}$ given on day 8.

To assist in the timing of ovulation after $PGF_{2\alpha}$ or progestin-based synchronization, hCG (2,000 to 3,300 IU) has been administered 48 hours after the onset of estrus and is effective for inducing ovulation provided a 30 mm to 40 mm follicle is present on the ovary. Human chorionic gonadotrophin will stimulate the follicle to ovulate within 24 to 48 hours after treatment. However, repeated use of hCG in the mare has been associated with anti-hCG antibody formation, which can lead to a decreased responsiveness when used in subsequent estrous cycles. A GnRH analogue, deslorelin implant, has also been used for induction of ovulation in cycling and transitional mares. As with hCG use, a follicle greater than 30 mm must be present for GnRH analogue treatment to be effective. The smaller molecular weight of GnRH compared with hCG makes it less antigenic, allowing for multiple administrations of GnRH to be feasible within the same breeding season or alternated with hCG until conception occurs. Return to estrus has been reported to be delayed in 10% to 20% of mares that do not conceive following ovulation induction using GnRH, which may affect subsequent attempts at estrous cycle manipulation. If ovulation does not occur within 48 hours of hCG or GnRH administration, breeding practices are continued based on observations of estrus and routine reproductive management procedures.

18–1.3 *Synchronization of Estrus in Sows and Gilts*

Synchronization of estrus in sows with $PGF_{2\alpha}$ is not practical, because the sow's CL will not respond until day 12 of the cycle. The short response period makes it difficult to get a group of sows synchronized.

The early oral progestins were not satisfactory for use in synchronizing estrus in sows; however, some of the more recently released materials are providing good results. Altrenogest, when fed for 14 to 18 days, (15 to 20 mg/pig/day), will bring 90% to 95% of a group of sows into estrus within 6 days after withdrawal. Conception rates for synchronized sows have been equal to conception rates for nonsynchronized sows in the same herd.

For acyclic gilts nearing puberty or sows immediately postweaning, combinations of PMSG (400 IU) and hCG (200 IU) have been used for induction of follicle growth and ovulation. Acyclic gilts and anestrus sows usually show estrus within 3 to 6 days after treatment. Conception rates and litter sizes are comparable to animals with naturally occurring estrous cycles. In some herds, gilts are bred on the second or third postpubertal estrus to maximize the number of ovulations and increase potential litter size. Therefore, the use of PMSG/hCG in prepubertal gilts can be used to synchronize a group for subsequent breeding at the second or third heat after treatment. The use of PMSG/hCG for induction or synchronization of estrous cycles in swine is not effective in animals with corpora lutea that have already commenced ovarian activity.

18–1.4 *Synchronization of Estrus in Ewes*

Some adverse effects of exogenous hormones used in synchronization of estrus have been reported in the ewe. Increased fertilization failure, embryonic mortality, and effects on sperm transport in the female have been reported for ewes synchronized both in and out of the breeding season and have been attributed in some cases to the synchronization method. Nevertheless, there are several methods for estrous synchronization in the ewe that have been developed to facilitate artificial insemination, embryo transfer, and managed breeding programs for sheep.

Prostaglandin $F_{2\alpha}$ can be used in cyclic ewes to induce luteolysis of the corpus luteum. A single injection will induce 60% to 70% of the flock to express estrus within 36 to 48 hours, while a second injection 9 days following the first injection will provide greater synchrony in the entire flock. Prostaglandin $F_{2\alpha}$ can also be used during or immediately following progestin treatment to tighten synchrony after progestin withdrawal. Progestin-based synchronization methods in the ewe include implants (Norgestomet), vaginal pessaries (CIDR, PRID, sponges), and oral administration via the feed (MGA). Progestin implants or pessaries are inserted for 12 to 14 days. An injection of PMSG (400 to 750 IU) or a combination of PMSG (400 IU) and hCG (200 IU) is often administered at progestin withdrawal to improve estrous synchrony and ovulation. Artificial insemination is performed 50 to 60 hours after progestin withdrawal. Use of Norgestomet ear implants or CIDR/PRID vaginal pessaries have also been successful for inducing out-of-season breeding in ewes, although lower fertility rates are expected than achieved during the normal breeding season. Feeding MGA (0.25 to 0.30 mg/ewe/day; often fed as 0.125 to 0.15 mg/ewe twice daily) has also been used in sheep with variable success and is generally done for 12 to 15 days, followed by a PMSG injection around 5 to 10 hours after the last MGA feeding. As the timing for AI is difficult to predict in sheep after MGA withdrawal, natural mating is suggested, with rams introduced to the ewes 48 hours after MGA withdrawal. Many of these synchronization methods use products designed for cattle and other species; therefore, their use in sheep is considered "off-label" and should be done in consultation with a veterinarian or with knowledge of the appropriate regulatory guidelines.

18–1.5 *Synchronization of Estrus in Does*

The primary method that has been used in the doe goat involves the use of intravaginal sponges containing 40 to 50 mg of synthetic progesterone, flurogestone acetate. The sponges are placed in the vagina for 17 to 22 days, and 300 to 500 IU of PMSG is injected at removal of the sponges. Goats generally come into estrus 12 to 36 hours after sponge removal. Good synchrony and good conception rates have been reported. Note that the doe requires a longer intravaginal progestin treatment than is used in the ewe and requires a higher progestin dose. Sponges with less hormone, like those marketed for sheep, have resulted in lower conception rates in the doe. Progestin ear implants (Norgestomet) have also been used in the doe and, unlike the longer duration of intravaginal sponges, are inserted for approximately 14 days with PMSG administered around the time of implant removal. Studies have indicated that the implant dose provided for cattle (6 mg Norgestomet) can be reduced to 2 to 3 mg by cutting the implant. Following synchronization, does come into estrus within 72 hours. Feeding MGA can also be used for the induction and synchronization of estrus in does in conjunction with PMSG administration, as with sheep; however, more research is needed as to its efficacy and the appropriate protocols for administration. Prostaglandin $F_{2\alpha}$ is also suitable for synchronization during the breeding season, which generally produces a more synchronized estrus than that obtained with a progestin-PMSG treatment, but subsequent fertility has been reported to be somewhat reduced. As stated previously for the ewe, many of these synchronization methods use products designed for cattle and other species; therefore, their use in the doe goat is considered an "off-label" use and should be used in consultation with a veterinarian or with knowledge of the appropriate regulatory guidelines.

18–2 SUPEROVULATION AND EMBRYO TRANSFER

Artificial insemination makes it possible to utilize the sperm produced by the male reasonably efficiently. The potential ova contained in the ovary of the female have not been utilized effectively. Superovulation is a procedure in which the female is treated with hormones to cause her to produce several ova instead of the one that she normally produces at each estrus (Figure 18–3). In the ewe, doe, or cow, an average of 12 ovulations can be expected. In one study with 40 donor cows, an average of 7.9 embryos were collected nonsurgically. From 60% to 70% of superovulated ova form normal embryos. Reliable superovulation has not yet been achieved in the mare because ovulation occurs at one site on the ovary, the ovarian fossa.

Superovulation in calves has been accomplished and when made practical could shorten the generation interval by a year or more. Superior germ plasm could be identified earlier and utilized more efficiently. To date, the response has been variable and fertilization rates have been very low.

18–2.1 *Techniques of Superovulation*

The cow normally produces only 1 ovum per estrous period, the doe and ewe 1 to 3 ova (depending on breed), and the sow 12 to 20 ova per estrous period. The object of superovulation

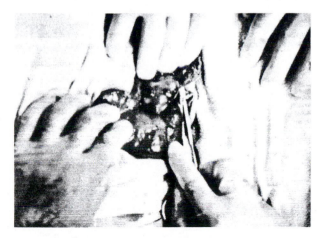

Figure 18–3 Multiple ovulation sites can be seen on this superovulated ovary, which has been exposed by surgery. (Courtesy, of Codding Embryological Services, Foraker, Okla.)

is to cause the female to produce a large number of ova that after fertilization and sufficient development can be transferred to other females.

Theoretically, superovulation can be accomplished at intervals equal to the length of the estrous cycle. With midluteal initiation of treatment, the interval may be shortened. Extreme variation between animals and diminished response with repeated treatments are some problems that still need to be solved. With current technology, donor cows are superovulated at 60-day intervals for an average of three ovulations. Some cows continue to respond for 10 treatments, but most become refractory much sooner. Allowing them to go through a pregnancy helps restore responsiveness. The reduced response may be due to an immune reaction in which antibodies are produced in response to the injections of the foreign proteins used on the donor to induce a superovulatory response. It may not be solved easily. Assuming that these problems can be overcome, up to 5 embryos from a cow might be obtained every 15 days. This would mean 120 or more embryos from one cow in a 12-month period.

18–2.1a Cows

For a number of years, superovulation in cows was accomplished using FSHp, an extract obtained from the anterior pituitaries of pigs that had been recovered from slaughter plants. This hormone was injected twice daily for 4 to 5 consecutive days. A problem encountered when using FSHp was the variable response to a standard treatment. While some of this variability was due to responsiveness of the donor animal, a great deal of it was attributed to the purity of the FSHp. As an extract from the anterior pituitary, it contained varying amounts of LH and evidence was reported that ovulation rate decreased as the LH in the extract increased.

When this was confirmed, research was initiated to produce a FSH preparation with low LH activity by purifying the FSH extracted from the anterior pituitaries of pigs. This preparation of FSH with low LH:FSH activity has yielded a more consistent superovulation response than was previously possible with FSHp. A vial contains the FSH equivalent of 400 mg. Injections of FSH are started on day 8 to 10 following observed or induced estrus, and 50 mg are administered intramuscularly twice daily for 4 days (a total of eight injections of FSH).

Superovulation regimens can be started on any day of the estrous cycle between day 6 and day 15. However, one report indicated a poor response when started on day 11. For sake of superovulation response and ability to control the onset of estrus in the donor, most recommendations call for starting FSH on day 8, 9, or 10. If started on day 8, 9, or 10, the donor will have a corpus luteum to respond when $PGF_{2\alpha}$ is given at the time of the sixth FSH injection. With estrus in the donor controlled, recipients can be synchronized with the donors more easily. Progestin-based synchronization can be used in combination with a superovulation protocol, with injections of FSH traditionally started 5 or 6 days after progestin device insertion and $PGF_{2\alpha}$ given the day before or the day of progestin withdrawal. A summary of the steps used in superovulation of the donor using unpurified FSH extracts leading up to embryo transfer procedures appears in Table 18–4.

Some embryo transfer technicians prefer a regimen of descending doses of FSH during the 4-day injection period. For example, they might inject 60 mg twice on day 1, 50 mg per injection on day 2, 40 mg per injection on day 3, and 30 mg per injection on day 4. If a donor is not in estrus on day 5, 20-mg doses would be given. Three artificial inseminations have been recommended at 12-hour intervals starting at onset of estrus, when using the extracted FSH product containing LH. This was needed to provide adequate capacitated sperm at the site of fertilization to ensure maximum fertilization since sperm transport was impaired.

Table 18–4 *Summary of events in superovulation and embryo transfer in the cow using unpurified FSH extracts*

Day of cycle	Action
9	Inject FSH at 7 A.M. and at 7 P.M.
10	Inject FSH at 7A.M. and at 7 P.M.
10	Inject recipients with 25 mg $PGF_{2\alpha}$ at 7 P.M.
11	Inject FSH at 7 A.M. and at 7 P.M.
11	Inject donor with 25 mg $PGF_{2\alpha}$ at 7 P.M.
12	Inject FSH at 7 A.M. and at 7 P.M.
13 (if not in estrus)	Inject FSH at 7 A.M. and at 7 P.M.
13–15	Estrus
Onset of Estrus	Inseminate
Onset of Estrus + 12 hours	Inseminate
Onset of Estrus + 24 hours	Inseminate
7 new cycle	Collect and evaluate embryos
7	Match embryos (stage of dev.) with recipients' day of cycle and transfer embryos into uterine horns of recipients
7	Inject $PGF_{2\alpha}$ into donor after the flush

The recent availability of recombinant FSH preparations for use in human-assisted reproduction has led to some investigations of such agents for use in cattle superovulation. However, studies suggest that heifers stimulated with recombinant human FSH, which possesses no LH bioactivity, in fact, require some LH activity in addition to FSH for normal preovulatory follicular development. Therefore, while low LH:FSH ratios are called for, exposure to both gonadotropins appears requisite.

Pregnant mare serum gonadotropin (PMSG) can also be used for superovulation in cattle and is given as a single dose of 2,000 IU to 2,500 IU. This is followed by a luteolytic dose of $PGF_{2\alpha}$ 2 to 3 days later. A second injection of $PGF_{2\alpha}$ is occasionally given 12 to 24 hours after the first and seems to improve embryo production in some cases. Experience has dictated that each batch (lot) of PMSG be tested for potency before it is used to superovulate a valuable donor cow. This may be done by injecting a grade cow with 2,000 IU as a starting point and adjusting the dose depending on the response. Use of FSH has surpassed that of PMSG as the primary method of superovulation in cattle. In most studies comparing the two procedures, the FSH treatment has resulted in slightly higher numbers of transferable embryos.

Dose level should be scaled to the size of the cow. If the dose level for a Holstein (700 kg) is 360 mg to 400 mg, the dose level for a Jersey (500 kg) should be only 300 mg to 340 mg. Rectal examination of ovaries during the injection period is recommended so that dose level can be reduced if overstimulation of ovaries is detected. Overstimulated ovaries may reach a diameter of 10 cm, while the desired size is 4 cm to 5 cm.

Donors selected for embryo transfer are cows that with special mating will produce offspring of high value. For good success, they should be less than 10 years old. Also, they should be cycling normally and be in good general and reproductive health. They should be in good body condition but not obese (Sections 23–3.1 and 23–3.2). With respect to other species of bovids, superovulation protocols for water buffalo are similar to the procedures described using FSH and PMSG, however some reports suggest that the buffalo's ovarian response to FSH and PMSG are weak, compared with that domestic cows. Another major problem with superovulation in the water buffalo is the difficulty in detecting estrus for both donors and recipients (Section 7–2).

18–2.1b Sows and Gilts   Because sows and cycling gilts normally ovulate 10 to 25 ova each cycle, superovulation in swine has not been essential for embryo production. However, evidence suggests that differences in ovulation rates of donors may affect pregnancy rates after transfer, with greater success from those with higher ovulation rates. In sows, 750 to 1,500 IU of PMSG (dose varies with size) should be injected subcutaneously on day 15 of the cycle. At the onset of estrus, 500 IU of hCG is injected subcutaneously. In cycling animals, PMSG can also be administered after synchronization of estrus with oral progestin (altrenogest) treatment. In a recent review of 12 studies using superovulation in gilts, some studies reported responses as high as 32 embryos collected; in some cases, no improvement in superovulatory response was observed, attesting to the highly variable superovulatory responses that may be seen even in animals of the same age, breed, and weight.

18–2.1c Ewes   Although most ewes respond to superovulatory regimens, embryo recovery rates vary between approximately 30% to 60%. Six hundred to 1,000 IU of PMSG injected subcutaneously on day 12 or 13 of the cycle has been effective for increasing the number of ova ovulated in ewes. When used in combination with an estrous synchronization protocol, 1,000 IU of PMSG are injected 1 to 2 days prior to intravaginal progestin sponge removal. While the level of LH released from the ewe's pituitary gland may be adequate to cause ovulation of the induced follicles, 750 IU of hCG are usually given the day after progestin withdrawal to assure ovulation of all the follicles. In a recent study of St. Croix White ewes synchronized and superovulated with this protocol, control ewes that were only synchronized averaged 2.7 ovulations, while superovulated ewes averaged 6.7 ovulations. The administration of FSHp at the end of progestin treatment in decreasing doses has also yielded some success in the ewe, during both the breeding and nonbreeding (anestrus) seasons; however, further research is needed as to the appropriate protocols.

18–2.1d Does   The superovulatory response in the doe is lower and more variable with PMSG than in a FSH-induced superovulation. Problems associated with PMSG-induced superovulation in the doe are an increased number of nonovulated follicles and short, irregular estrous cycles. PMSG is usually given as a single injection of 1,500 to 2,000 IU at the end of a progestin treatment. In contrast, FSH is administered in decreasing doses of 1 to 5 mg, injected at 12-hour intervals, over a 3- to 5-day period around the time of progestin withdrawal. Ovulation rates in does following FSH superovulation protocols can be as high as 10 to 25 ova, but the number of viable embryos may be significantly lower.

18–2.2 *Embryo Collection and Evaluation*

The history of embryo transfer began in 1890, when Walter Heape transferred embryos from an Angora rabbit to recipient Belgian rabbits. This experiment not only was the first successful embryo transfer but also demonstrated that the recipients' genetics would not unduly influence the transferred embryos' genetic makeup or developmental processes. In 1930, the first embryo was collected from a cow, but it was not until 1951 that the first embryo transfer in the bovine was conducted using surgical means, and, in 1964, the first nonsurgical method of embryo collection was successful in cattle. Embryo transfers in sheep and goats were first reported in 1949; for the pig, in 1951. Offspring from frozen mouse embryos were produced in 1972, and the following year the production of offspring from frozen cow embryos were reported.

Early collection techniques involved either slaughtering the females and excising the oviducts or surgically removing the oviducts from the live females at 72 hours postovulation so that the embryos could be recovered by flushing. This defeated the primary purpose of superovulation, so other methods were developed. A surgical method was developed first and is accomplished by performing a *laparotomy* (flank or midline abdominal incision) to expose the reproductive tract (Figure 18–4). A clamp or the thumb and forefinger can be used to block the distal one-third of the uterine horn so that fluid injected into that segment can be forced through the oviduct with a gentle milking action and collected at the infundibulum. An alternate procedure is to occlude the uterine horn at the body of the uterus, with culture medium being introduced through a puncture at the uterotubal junction or through the oviduct until the uterus is turgid. The uterus is then punctured with a blunt needle attached to a flexible catheter. The pressure will cause the medium to gush through the catheter with enough turbulence to carry the embryos into a collection tube. These procedures allow for the recovery of a high percentage of embryos, but because of the surgical trauma and resulting adhesions it can be repeated only a few times. The adhesions make it difficult, if not impossible, to expose the reproductive tract repeatedly.

Nonsurgical techniques of recovery have been developed for the cow and mare that give results essentially equal to surgical methods. They involve the use of a size 18 to 24 French Foley catheter (two-way flow catheter), which allows flushing fluids to pass into the uterus and at the same time allows fluids to be returned from the uterus to a collecting

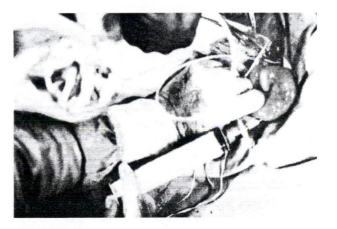

Figure 18–4 A surgical procedure is being used to flush embryos from the oviduct. (Courtesy of Codding Embryological Services, Foraker, Okla.)

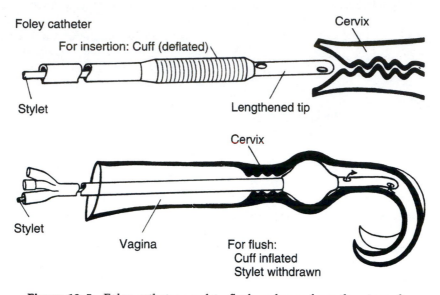

Figure 18–5 Foley catheter used to flush embryos from the uterus by nonsurgical means.

receptacle (Figure 18–5). A small balloon near the end of the catheter, which can be inflated just inside the uterine horn to prevent the flushing fluid from escaping through the cervix, is also a feature. The Foley catheter is larger in diameter than the usual insemination instrument. As embryo collections are conducted during early diestrus (days 6 to 8 after breeding), when the cervical lumen is constricted and lubricating mucus like that present during estrus is absent, the Foley catheter often cannot be passed through the cervix without the aid of a cervical dilator to physically open the cervical canal.

In sheep and goats, embryo collection and transfer has been hampered by the difficulty of introducing a catheter through the cervix and the inability to perform rectal manipulation of the reproductive tract. This has led to the use of predominately surgical means of embryo recovery in the past. Laparoscopic means, which results in fewer adhesions than traditional surgical techniques, have produced some success in the ewe and doe. One study investigating repeated embryo recoveries in subsequent estrous cycles in the ewe achieved embryo recovery rates ranging from 35% to 76% using laparoscopic approaches. With the development of improved catheters specifically for sheep and goats, some success has been achieved using nonsurgical, transcervical approaches. In does, studies have shown nonsurgical embryo recovery rates to be similar to those of surgical approaches, with one study demonstrating a 78% total embryo recovery rate and 62% transferable embryo recovery rate. These studies, and others, indicate that less invasive and nonsurgical means are feasible in small ruminants for embryo collection and transfer.

With nonsurgical collection methods, it is difficult to determine how many ovulation sites are present on the ovary, so it is not possible to determine when all of the embryos have been collected. In controlled experiments, about 50% of embryos resulting from superovulation were recovered by either surgical or nonsurgical procedures. Embryos are recovered from donor animals in the morula or early blastocyst stage. In the cow, ewe and doe, best results are obtained when embryos are recovered between days 6 and 8 (day 0 equals estrus). Conception rates of recipients following transfer of embryos collected on day 6 or 7 can produce conception rates of 70% to 80%, whereas embryos collected and transferred on day 4 or 5 have lower conception rates of 50% to 60%. Embryos can be recovered earlier when they are still in the oviducts of the donor at around the eight-cell stage. These embryos need to be transferred into the oviducts of synchronized recipients or are cultured *in vitro* to the blastocyst stage (Section 19–12) when they can be transferred into the recipient's uterus.

The fluids for flushing must be compatible with the embryos. A number of fluids have been successfully used, but the ideal medium is yet to be discovered. Autoserum (from the same species) alone or with an equal volume of 0.9% saline solution has been recommended for ewes. All sera used for flushing or culture of embryo of any species must be heated to 55°C for 30 minutes to deactivate factors detrimental to embryos. For most, if not all species, Modified Dulbecco's phosphate-buffered medium can be used (Table 18–5). Antibiotics are added to protect the embryos from bacterial contaminants acquired during flushing and to avoid transferring pathogens to the recipient. The donor cows are usually treated with large doses of antibiotics after flushing. Injection of $PGF_{2\alpha}$ is recommended to speed recovery of the ovaries and to prevent pregnancy, if viable embryos are not dislodged by the flush. In addition, an injection of $PGF_{2\alpha}$ is given to speed recovery of the ovaries and to prevent pregnancy in the donor in the event viable embryos were left behind.

The success rate for embryo transfer depends a great deal on an accurate evaluation of the embryos recovered. Experience has shown that certain deviations from normal development in 6- to 8-day embryos can be detected with the light microscope. Some characteristics which should be observed in an evaluation process are (1) compactness of the

Table 18–5   *Modified Dulbecco's phosphate-buffered medium*

Ingredients	Amount for 10 liters g
Part I	
NaCl	80.0
KCl	2.0
Na_2HPO_4	11.5
KH_2PO_4	2.0
Glucose	10.0
Streptomycin sulphate	.5
Na pyruvate	.36
Na penicillin G	1,000,000 units
Part II	
$CaCl_2\ 2H_2O$	1.32
$MgSO_4\ 7H_2O$	1.21

1. Dissolve part I in 8 liters of deionized, distilled water.
2. Dissolve part II in 2 liters of deionized, distilled water.
3. Add part II to part I slowly with constant stirring to prevent precipitation.
4. Add heat-treated autoserum immediately prior to use: 1% for flushing and 20% for culture.
5. Sterilize by passing through millipore filters with 0.22µ pores.

Adapted from Seidel et al. General Series 975. Colorado State Univ., Exp. Sta. and Animal Reprod. Lab. 1980.

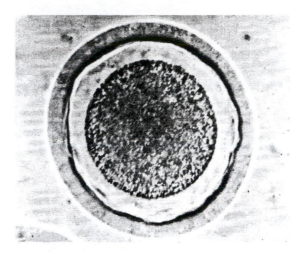

Figure 18–6   An unfertilized sheep ovum.

cells—a normal embryo is compact rather than a loose mass of cells; (2) regularity of shape—spherical is preferable to oval, etc.; (3) variation in cell size— blastomeres of similar size; (4) color and texture of cytoplasm—should be neither very light nor very dark; (5) presence of vesicles—cytoplasm should not be granular or unevenly distributed and should contain some moderate-sized vesicles; (6) presence of extruded cells—there should be no disassociated cells; (7) normal embryo size; (8) regularity of the zona pellucida— perivitelline space should be empty and of regular diameter, and the zona pellucida even (neither wrinkled nor collapsed); (9) presence of cellular debris—no cell fragments should be visible around the blastomeres. Using these subjective criteria, embryos are classified as Grade 1: excellent or good; Grade 2: fair; Grade 3: poor; or Grade 4: dead or degenerating. Embryos are also evaluated for their stage of development as follows: Stage 1: unfertilized (Figure 18–6); Stage 2: 2 to 12 cells; Stage 3: early morula; Stage 4: morula; Stage 5: early blastocyst; Stage 6: blastocyst; Stage 7: expanded blastocyst; Stage 8: hatched blastocyst; and Stage 9: expanded hatched blastocyst. Figure 9–1 shows embryos at different stages of development. In a recent study of beef and dairy cows composed of 15 different breeds, 58% of all embryos collected were considered transferable, 31% were unfertilized, and 11% were degenerated.

18–2.3 *Selection of Recipients and Transfer of Embryos*

Another important factor in successful embryo transfer is selection of recipients. Recipients should be young, reproductively sound, and cycling normally. If heifers are used, they should meet size standards for breeding (Section 20–2.1) because small heifers will increase incidence of dystocia and neonatal loss (Section 10–5). Good body condition and good general health are important. Their cycles should be synchronized with that of the donor and they should have a well-formed corpus luteum at the time of transfer. Failure to provide recipients that meet these criteria is a frequent shortcoming in countries that do not have an established embryo transfer program. Some report that *Bos indicus* (Zebu) cattle have lower embryo survival after transfer than *Bos taurus* or *Bos indicus/Bos taurus* crosses.

Embryos must be transferred to recipients that have their estrous cycles synchronized with that of the donor. Recipients that are 2 days ahead or 2 days behind the day of the cycle of the donor when embryos are collected and transferred can reduce pregnancy rates by 20% to 50% in sheep and cattle. Techniques for estrous synchronization were discussed in an earlier section of this chapter (Section 18–1.1). When recipients are synchronized with $PGF_{2\alpha}$, they should be injected three days before the anticipated estrus of the donor or 12 hours before injecting the donor with $PGF_{2\alpha}$. This optimizes the probability that the recipient will be at the same stage of the estrous cycle as the donor when the transfer is performed. If using a progestin implant, removal should be 2 days before the donor's estrus is expected. Both surgical and nonsurgical techniques have been used for transferring embryos. The surgical procedure involves a laparotomy to expose the reproductive tract. The normal embryo, depending on stage of development, is placed in either the oviduct or the uterus of the recipient. A small syringe fitted with a 21-gauge needle is used to make the transfer. When the embryo is placed in the uterus, the needle is carefully inserted through the wall of the uterine horn adjacent to the ovary which contains the corpus luteum. When the embryo is placed in the oviduct, the needle is carefully inserted through the infundibulum into the ampulla where the embryo is deposited.

Two nonsurgical procedures for transferring embryos to recipients have been described and used in the cow and mare. In one procedure, a long hypodermic needle is inserted into the vagina and used to bypass the cervix and puncture the uterine horn so that the embryo can be deposited into the lumen of the uterus. Currently, the most common procedure is to place the embryo in a 0.25-ml plastic straw which has been described for packaging semen. This straw is then placed in the stainless steel embryo transfer gun, which is passed through the cervix for the deposit of the embryo into the uterus. The straw gun is carefully passed into the uterine horn adjacent to the ovary with the functional CL. Extreme caution should be taken to prevent injury to the endometrium. Nonsurgical transfers have a success rate somewhat lower than surgical methods; however, most commercial embryo transfers are made by nonsurgical means. A summary of the steps used in superovulation and embryo transfer in the cow using unpurified FSH extract appeared in Table 18–4.

18–2.4 *Storage, Freezing and Thawing Embryos*

Embryos can be maintained at near body temperature in the media used for flushing during the period between recovery and transfer to the recipients. If embryos are to be held longer than 2 hours before transfer, media containing 20% heat-treated serum should be used. The embryos should be transferred to fresh, sterile medium every 2 hours to help control bacterial contaminants. If embryos are cooled to 5°C (refrigerator temperature), they can be maintained for 2 to 4 days. Holding temperatures should be maintained and not allowed to fluctuate.

Embryos may be held in 20% heat-treated serum up to 10 hours without a reduction in survival. Lower temperature must be used if embryos are to be retained for longer periods of time. Sheep embryos held at 10°C have retained viability up to 72 hours. Embryos from cows and ewes may be frozen and stored in liquid nitrogen, but a 15 to 20 percentage units reduction in pregnancy rate should be expected.

Technology for freezing and thawing of bovine embryos has improved greatly in recent years. As with semen, cryoprotectants are needed for acceptable survival. Until recently, glycerol was the cryoprotectant used most frequently for freezing embryos.

Equilibration of the embryo in a holding medium containing glycerol permitted glycerol to replace water within the embryo. As ice crystals started forming, the salts in the liquid-holding medium became more concentrated, with the resulting change in osmotic pressure drawing more water out of the embryo as glycerol moved in. The problem came after thawing. The embryo requires rehydration before being placed into a recipient. Since water diffuses through cell membranes more quickly than glycerol can diffuse out, rehydration had to be done in a stepwise manner. Otherwise, excessive swelling frequently damaged cell membranes, destroying the embryo. Rehydration was accomplished by transferring the embryo through several holding media, each with a lower concentration of glycerol, until sufficient rehydration had occurred. Adding sucrose to the media as an osmotic buffer permitted more direct rehydration but was not accepted well by the industry.

More recently, ethylene glycol has been used as a cryoprotectant when freezing embryos. Since ethylene glycol diffuses rapidly through cell membranes, as does water, direct rehydration of embryos within straws is possible. To accomplish this, the embryo is placed in 1.5 M ethylene glycol in the center column of a 0.25-ml straw with a column of phosphobuffered saline on either end of the straw. The columns are separated by an air bubble. The recommended ratio of ethylene glycol to phosphobuffered saline in the straw is 1:3. Freezing follows a stepwise procedure. The prepared straw is placed directly into an alcohol bath freezer ($-7°C$). The straw is then seeded by touching a metal rod, cooled by immersion in liquid nitrogen, to the straw at a location away from the embryo. After a 5-minute hold, the prepared straw is cooled at 0.5°C per minute to $-35°C$, held for 15 minutes, and then plunged into liquid nitrogen. Straws are thawed in a 30°C water bath and then transferred directly to recipients. Rehydration occurs during the transfer. Pregnancy rates of about 50% are equivalent to that achieved by other accepted methods. Only top-quality embryos freeze well. Therefore, lower-quality but acceptable embryos should be transferred as fresh embryos only.

The advances in this technology have made international shipment of embryos more practical and competitive with shipment of live animals. Advantages of shipping frozen embryos over shipping live animals include availability of better genetics, elimination of disease transmission with proper processing of embryos, and opportunity for savings in costs, especially when the comparative genetics are considered. A concern in a number of countries is the availability of suitable recipients (Section 18–2.3).

18–2.5 *Promoting Twinning*

Transfer of two embryos to each of a group of recipients will increase the twinning rates in that group of females and has become the method of choice to accomplish that goal. Modifications of the superovulation treatment discussed in Section 18–2.1 have been employed to induce twinning in cattle and in sheep. While the number of offspring per pregnancy can be increased, it is not possible to limit the number of ovulations to only two. When the treatment produces several ova, space limitations in the uterus usually result in embryonic mortality to reduce the number of fetuses to one, two, or three. Unfortunately, it does not always occur this way; instead, too many implantations frequently occur and later result in abortions.

While twinning is desirable in sheep, the disadvantages outweigh the advantages for twinning in cattle. Some of these are (1) short gestations accompanied by small, weak calves; (2) high incidence of retained placentae; (3) freemartins result from heterosexual twins; (4) more stress on the cows—dairy cows produce 10% less milk in the lactation following the delivery of twins; (5) increased reproductive problems—one study reported that 50% of the cows producing twins failed to calve the next year; (6) increased incidence of cystic ovaries—anytime exogenous FSH, particularly in the form of PMSG, is used, one must expect an increase in the incidence of cystic ovaries; and (7) most beef cows do not produce enough milk for two calves. Based on work with sheep, a considerably higher level of nutrition is needed during late gestation to support fetal growth.

SUGGESTED READING

ARMSTRONG, D. T. and M. A. OPAVSKY. 1986. Biological characterization of pituitary FSH preparation with reduced LH activity. *Theriogenology,* 25:135.

BOLAND, M. P. 2002. Gamete and embryo technology—Multiple ovulation and embryo transfer. *Encyclopedia of Dairy Sciences.* eds. H. ROGINSKI, J. W. FUQUAY, and P. F. FOX. Academic Press, an imprint of Elsevier Science.

DONALDSON, L. E., D. N. WARD, and S. D. GLENN. 1986. Use of porcine follicle stimulating hormone after chromatographic purification in superovulation of cattle. *Theriogenology,* 25:747.

DROST, M., J. M. WRIGHT, JR., W. S. CRIPE, and A. R. RICHTER. 1983. Embryo transfer in water buffalo *(Bubalus bubalis). Theriogenology,* 20:579.

FOOTE, R. H. 1978. General principles and basic techniques involved in synchronization of estrus in cattle. *Proc. 7th Tech. Conf. Artif. Insem. Reprod.,* p. 74. NAAB, Columbia, Mo.

HANSEL, W. and W. E. BEAL. 1979. Ovulation control in cattle. *Beltsville Symposia in Agricultural Research. 3. Animal Reproduction.* p. 91. ed. H. W. HAWK. Allanheld, Osmun and Co., Publisher; Halsted Press, a division of Wiley and Sons.

HIXON, D. L., D. J. KESLER, T. R. TROXEL, D. L. VINCENT, and B. S. WISEMAN. 1981. Reproductive hormone secretions and first service conception rate subsequent to ovulation control with synchromate B. *Theriogenology,* 16:219.

KAFI, M. and M. R. MCGOWAN. 1997. Factors associated with variations in the superovulatory response of cattle. *Anim. Reprod. Sci.* 48:137.

LEIBO, S. P. 1984. A one-step method for direct nonsurgical transfer of frozen-thawed bovine embryos. *Theriogenology,* 21:767.

LUCY, M. C., H. J. BILLINGS, W. R. BUTLER, L. R. EHNIS, M. J. FIELDS, D. J. KESLER, J. E. KINDER, R. C. MATTOS, R. E. SHORT, W. W. THATCHER, R. P. WETTEMAN, J. V. YELICH, and H. D. HAFS. 2001. Efficacy of an intravaginal progesterone insert and an injection of PGF_2 for synchronizing estrus and shortening the interval to pregnancy in postpartum beef cows, peripubertal beef heifers, and dairy heifers. *J. Anim. Sci.,* 79:982.

MARTIN, J. C., E. KLUG, H. MERKT, V. HIMMLER, and W. JOCHLE. 1981. Luteolysis and cycle synchronization with a new prostaglandin analog for artificial insemination in the mare. *Theriogenology,* 16:433.

MCKELVEY, W. A. C., J. J. ROBINSON, R. P. AITKEN, and I. S. ROBERTSON. 1986. Repeated recoveries of embryos from ewes by laparoscopy. *Theriogenology,* 25:855.

MOMCILOVIC, D., L. F. ARCHBALD, A. WALTERS, T. TRAN, D. KELBERT, C. RISCO, and W. W. THATCHER. 1998. Reproductive performance of lactating dairy cows treated with gonadotrophin-releasing hormone (GnRH) and/or prostaglandins F_2 ($PGF_{2\alpha}$) for synchronization of estrus and ovulation. *Theriogenology,* 50:1131.

PATTERSON, D. J., G. H. KIRACOFE, J. S. STEVENSON, and L. R. CORAH. 1989. Control of the bovine estrous cycle with melengestrol acetate (MGA): A review. *J. Anim. Sci.* 67:1895.

PEREIRA, R. J., B. SOHNREY, and W. HOLTZ. 1998. Nonsurgical embryo transfer in goats treated with prostaglandin F_2 and oxytocin. *J. Anim. Sci.,* 76:360.

PURSLEY, J. R., M. R. KOSOROK, and M. C. WILTBANK. 1997. Reproductive management of lactating dairy cows using synchronization of ovulation. *J. Dairy Sci.,* 80:301.

PURSLEY, J. R., M. C. WILTBANK, J. S. STEVENSON, J. S. OTTOBRE, H. A. GARVERICK, and L. L. ANDERSON. 1997. Pregnancy rates per artificial insemination for cows and heifers inseminated at a synchronized ovulation or synchronized estrus. *J. Dairy Sci.,* 80:295.

SEIDEL, G. E. JR. 1979. Application of embryo preservation and transfer. *Beltsville Symposia in Agricultural Research. 3. Animal Reproduction,* p. 195. ed. H. W. HAWK. Allanheld, Osmun and Co., Publisher; Halsted Press, a division of Wiley and Sons.

SEIDEL, G. E., JR., and R. P. ELSDEN. 1989. *Embryo transfer in dairy cattle.* W. D. Hoard & Sons Company.

SMITH, R. D., A. J. POMERANTZ, W. E. BEAL, J. P. McCANN, T. E. PILBEAM, and W. HANSEL. 1984. Insemination of Holstein heifers at a preset time after estrous cycle synchronization using progesterone and prostaglandin. *J. Anim. Sci.,* 58:792.

SREENAN, J. M. 1978. Non-surgical embryo transfer in the cow. *Theriogenology,* 9:69.

STEVENSON, J. S. 2002. Replacement management, cattle—Breeding standards and pregnancy management. *Encyclopedia of Dairy Sciences.* eds. H. ROGINSKI, J. W. FUQUAY, AND P. F. FOX. Academic Press, an imprint of Elsevier Science.

THATCHER, W. W. 2002. Oestrous cycles, control—Synchronization of ovulation. *Encyclopedia of Dairy Sciences.* eds. H. ROGINSKI, J. W. FUQUAY, AND P. F. FOX. Academic Press, an imprint of Elsevier Science.

TWAGIRAMUNGU, H., L. A. GUIBAULT, and J. J. DUFOUR. 1995. Synchronization of ovarian follicular waves with a gonadotropin-releasing hormone agonist to increase precision of estrus in cattle: A review. *J. Anim. Sci.,* 73:3141.

VOELKEL, S. A. and Y. X. HU. 1992. Direct transfer of frozen-thawed bovine embryos. *Theriogenology,* 37:23.

WILTBANK, J. N. and E. GONZALEZ-PADILLA. 1975. Synchronization and induction of estrus in heifers with a progestogen and an estrogen. *Ann. Bio. Anim. Bioch. Biophys.,* 15:255.

XU, Z. Z. 2002. Oestrous cycles, control—Synchronization of oestrous. *Encyclopedia of Dairy Sciences.* eds. H. ROGINSKI, J. W. FUQUAY, AND P. F. FOX. Academic Press, an imprint of Elsevier Science.

19

Reproductive Biotechnology

One definition of biotechnology is the application of scientific knowledge to transfer beneficial genetic traits from one species to another to enhance or protect an organism. Thus, the technologies explored in previous chapters of this book, artificial insemination, estrus synchronization, superovulation, embryo transfer, and so on, were all at one time considered "cutting-edge" biotechnologies directed toward the genetic improvement of livestock. Today, most of the transfer of these technologies has taken place, with these reproductive management techniques now commonplace within our livestock industries. Currently, reproductive biotechnologies are taking scientists into new levels of understanding with respect to gaining control of an organism's developmental functions. Research at the molecular level has assisted in the harnessing of specific traits within an animal's genetic code, and the applications of technologies such as cloning and transgenics may prove revolutionary in their applications to livestock production and human medicine. This chapter will provide an overview of the development and practice of new reproductive biotechnologies currently in use, as well as the current status of technologies that are still in the early stages of development, with specific references to their potential use in livestock production.

19–1 ASSISTED REPRODUCTIVE TECHNOLOGIES

Assisted reproductive technologies (ART) is a name applied today primarily to human infertility and the use of *in vitro* techniques to assist couples incapable of conceiving by natural means. However, these techniques were first developed in livestock and laboratory animals and include means with which to combine sperm and oocyte for fertilization and initial embryo development to occur *in vitro,* outside of the oviduct and uterus. These techniques have led to the development of more advanced ART, such a intracytoplasmic sperm injection (ICSI), and have become an important part of biotechnological procedures associated with cloning (Section 19–3) and the production of transgenic livestock (Section 19–4).

19–1.1 In Vitro *Separation and Capacitation of Spermatozoa*

Scientists worked for many years trying to perfect *in vitro* fertilization (IVF; Section 19–1.3) techniques before it was recognized that sperm must undergo capacitation before fertilization is possible. Capacitation of spermatozoa is the cellular changes that must occur before the acrosome reaction and penetration of the oocyte can occur (Section 6–4). During this period, factors from seminal plasma which have coated the sperm surface are removed, and this removal triggers the parallel molecular processes necessary for fertilization to take place. Early investigations used various biological fluids to capacitate spermatozoa (e.g., oviductal fluid, follicular fluid, blood serum); however, the complexity of these fluids did not permit the factors that were inducing or suppressing capacitation to be determined. Some success with a chemically defined medium (DM) for *in vitro* capacitation of bovine sperm was accomplished by incubating spermatozoa in a high ionic strength medium at 38°C for 5 minutes, then centrifuging at 330 xg for 5 minutes. The supernatant liquid was discarded and the sperm cells resuspended in 1.0 ml of DM for an additional 5 to 23 hours of incubation. Following this, the sperm were then ready for incubation with the oocytes for IVF. Table 19–1 gives the composition of DM and high ionic strength medium. Today, commercially prepared media (modified Tyrode's and Krebs-Ringer's solutions) supplemented with appropriate energy sources (glucose, lactate and pyruvate) and albumin are often utilized, as well as various types of tissue culture media supplemented with blood serum. However, no single medium has been found to work well for all species to achieve optimal conditions for *in vitro* capacitation and IVF procedures.

The finding that the glycosaminoglycan (GAG) heparin can be used to capacitate sperm has been a major advancement in the IVF of bovine oocytes and has produced high and repeatable bovine IVF with frozen-thawed semen. Spermatozoa are first prepared using the swim-up motility enhancement procedure to purify or separate motile spermatozoa from dead sperm and other debris. Using this procedure, the motile sperm swim up out of the extender they are frozen in and into the incubation medium. The dead or nonmotile sperm do not move into the medium. The top portion of the medium is then collected, and the sperm from this layer are used for IVF after determining the concentration of sperm. One method for accomplishing this uses TALP (Tyrode's Albumin Lactate Pyruvate) nutrient buffered media, in which 1 ml is layered over each of four 0.25-ml semen aliquots. Af-

Table 19–1   *Defined medium (DM) for* in vitro *fertilization*[a]

Components	g
NaCl	6.550
KCl	0.300
CaCl 2H$_2$O	0.330
NaH$_2$PO$_4$ H$_2$O	0.113
MgCl 6H$_2$O	0.106
NaHCO$_3$	3.104
Glucose	2.500
Anhydrous Na pyruvate	0.137
Crystalline bovine albumin	3.000
Penicillin, Na salt	0.031
Distilled H$_2$O to 1,000 ml	

High ionic strength medium is prepared by adding 34 mg of enzyme grade NaCl to 10 ml of above medium. Also add 100 IU penicillin and 100 μ g streptomycin/ml.[b]

[a]Brackett and Oliphant. *Biol. Reprod.,* 12:260, 1975.

[b]Brackett et al. *Biol. Reprod.,* 27:147, 1982.

ter a 1-hour incubation period (39°C) to permit time for sperm swim-up, the top 0.85 ml of media from each semen aliquot is then pooled and taken through a series of centrifugation (200 × g) and wash steps using TALP media. These washings remove the diluter in which the sperm were frozen, as well as minute quantities of seminal fluid, the latter of which may contain substances that inhibit capacitation. The final sperm pellet is then resuspended to 100 × 10⁶ sperm/ml and incubated (39°C in 5% CO_2 in air) with the GAG heparin (10 μg/ml) at a ratio of 1 μl heparin in TALP per 50 μl sperm for 15 minutes (final sperm concentration with heparin-TALP addition is 25 × 10⁶/ml). Capacitation can be accomplished independently and prior to IVF; however, some researchers prefer to add the heparin to the IVF medium and accomplish both processes simultaneously. Penicillamine hypotaurine epinephrine (PHE) is also sometimes added with the heparin and has been shown to assist in maintaining sperm viability and motility, and it increases the number of sperm which undergo the acrosome reaction. Time to fertilization and the concentration of heparin needed for capacitation vary, depending on the presence or absence of PHE and its concentration.

Alternative sperm separation techniques prior to initiation of *in vitro* capacitation and IVF have also included the use of Percoll gradients and glass-wool filtration. Percoll consists of small silica particles, which are used to create density gradients for the separation of cells. Percoll is used as a migration medium, whereby the sperm are layered on an isotonic discontinuous Percoll gradient, centrifuged, and collected from the pellet. In this way, cell debris, bacteria, and malformed sperm are removed and the normal motile sperm selected according to their specific gravity. Percoll gradients for bovine sperm purification have used layering of a 45% Percoll over a 90% Percoll, followed by centrifugation at 700 × g for 15 minutes (Figure 19–1). After centrifugation, the sperm pellet is collected from the bottom of the tube and is washed and re-centrifuged to remove the Percoll. The removal of Percoll is accomplished since long-term incubation in Percoll has in some cases been reported to be toxic to spermatozoa, although Percoll is reported to be chemically inert and does not adhere to cell membranes. Another method of sperm purification has used glass-wool fibers, across which sperm are passed to remove (filter) dead sperm and other material from bull, boar, and turkey sperm. While this technique can yield nearly 100% viable sperm, there is

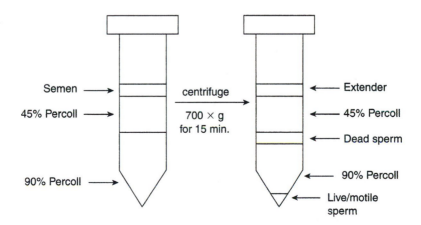

Figure 19–1 A schematic drawing showing the use of Percoll gradients for the separation of live motile sperm for *in vitro* fertilization (IVF).

some concern that glass-wool filtration of sperm may have a deleterious effect on the ultra-structure of sperm. Use of the sperm swim-up and use of Percoll gradients are the most common approaches used today for viable sperm separation prior to IVF procedures.

19–1.2 *Oocyte Collection and* in Vitro *Maturation (IVM)*

While some studies have demonstrated success using IVF of ovulated oocytes, some research indicates that oocytes from preovulatory follicles may, in fact, be more suitable for IVF than ovulated oocytes. With the use of laparoscopic or ultrasound-guided follicular aspiration techniques, oocytes can be taken from preovulatory follicles of superovulated, untreated or even pregnant females. When several oocytes are collected from the same female, each can be fertilized by sperm from different males. This can enhance the progeny testing of females, as is done with males through the use of AI. As applied specifically to the bull and semen output, the use of IVF could further extend the use of sperm from genetically superior sires by 60 to 100 times. Moreover, females with reproductive tract pathologies (e.g., oviductal occlusions) could still be used as donors of oocytes for IVF using these oocyte retrieval techniques. For primarily research purposes, ovaries from cows sent to the abattoir are routinely collected for oocyte retrieval and IVF.

Even though the early IVF and embryo culture was done with ovulated oocytes, development of the embryo seemed to be blocked at the two-cell stage for most species. Consequently, surgical transfer to the ampulla of the oviduct was necessary. More recently, research has been expanded to include aspirated oocytes from preovulatory follicles. Originally, the source of these oocytes was from ovaries of slaughtered females, which were aspirated using an 18-gauge needle connected to a 4.0 kPa (30 mmHg) vacuum or through extraction with a tuberculin syringe. Follicles from 2 mm to 6 mm in diameter are collected, usually yielding 6 to 8 oocytes per ovary in the cow. Techniques have now been developed for the aspirations of oocytes from live cows, referred to as ultrasound-guided follicular aspiration or transvaginal ovum pick-up (OPU; Figure 19–2). The aspiration needle is inserted through a guide within a transvaginal ultrasound probe and then inserted through the vaginal wall and into each follicle while applying vacuum. Six to 8 oocytes can usually be obtained per ovary using this method and has also been used in conjunction with superovulation protocols to assure the presence of multiple follicles for aspiration. Theoretically, even without superovulation, genetically superior cows can provide a harvest of 10 to 20 oocytes every 10 to 14 days without stimulation, which might yield 2.5 to 5 transferable embryos in cattle. Scarring and adhesions from frequent collections can damage the ovary; therefore, the use of an experienced technician is requisite to assure an efficient collection with little trauma to the ovary. One problem recognized with aspirated oocytes versus ovulated oocytes is that some of the follicles aspirated will have begun the atresia process, and early studies suggest that some of these oocytes may not develop or mature normally. This may account for some of the differences in the percentage of normal embryos obtained for ovulated versus aspirated oocytes. Nevertheless, IVF technicians today routinely aspirate 4 mm to 6 mm follicles that result in viable oocytes, most likely due to improved media formulations for *in vitro* maturation (IVM) and IVF. Oocytes are also selected from the collected pool based on the presence of a compact aggregation of cumulus cells around the oocyte. Cumulus expansion observed at oocyte collection may be an indication of follicular atresia or premature meiotic resumption of the oocyte, which would indicate the oocyte may not be suitable for IVF.

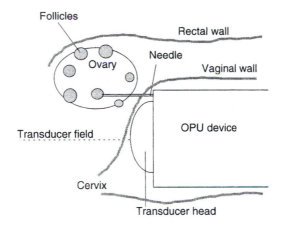

Figure 19–2 Schematic representation of ovum pick-up (OPU). The technician maintains the ovary in close contact from the transducer probe. The ovarian follicles are visible on an echo-graph screen, as well as a line fitting the course of the aspiration needle. The needle is pushed through the vaginal wall to reach a follicle through ovarian stroma. The aspiration system is turned on at that time and follicular fluid, as well as cumulus oocyte complexes, is collected in a tube connected to the needle. *Source:* Reprinted from *Encyclopedia of Dairy Sciences*, 2, Mermillod, P., In Vitro Fertilization, p. 1180, 2002, with permission from Elsevier Science.

In vitro fertilization results with aspirated oocytes were poor to nil when they were subjected to the same techniques used for ovulated ova. Success was not achieved until it was discovered that the aspirated oocytes had to be matured *in vitro* before attempting to fertilize them. This is accomplished by culturing the oocytes in a balanced salt solution (e.g., TCM 199 medium with Earle's salts supplemented with estradiol-17β, FSHp, sodium pyruvate, Gentamicin, and 10% heat-treated fetal calf serum) for 24 hours at 39°C in a CO_2 incubator with 5% humidified CO_2 in air. During the maturation process, the first meiotic division takes place and the first polar body is extruded. Following maturation of the aspirated oocytes, IVF procedures are the same for ovulated and aspirated oocytes.

19–1.3 In Vitro *Fertilization (IVF)*

Researchers have recognized the value of IVF to reproduction for many decades. The first offspring born as a result of IVF was reported in 1959, with the rabbit. Since that time, IVF has been accomplished in a number of animal species, domestic and wild. The first IVF in humans culminated in the birth of the first "test-tube baby" in 1978, and others since then have received considerable publicity for two reasons: first, they involve humans; second, these techniques assist couples dealing with infertility problems—an advantage of IVF and ART procedures in general.

In cattle, *in vitro* fertilization success has been higher in recently ovulated oocytes when compared with follicular oocytes. In research which resulted in the birth of a normal calf, the oocytes were incubated in 4 ml of DM containing 1×10^6 capacitated sperm. *In vitro* inseminations and all incubations of oocytes were carried out in small glass, sealable tissue culture dishes under paraffin oil. After the fertilization period (usually 18 to 24 hours), oocytes were transferred to a 10% serum solution for an additional 22 to 24 hours. They were then examined for cleavage, and a decision was made regarding further incubation or transfer to recipient for *in vivo* development. Transfers were done surgically with embryos placed about 2.5 cm into the oviductal ampulla.

In vitro fertilization is accomplished by diluting the matured oocytes, or ovulated oocytes, in several changes of TALP-HEPES without glucose and placing them in fertilization medium composed of glucose-free TALP. Aliquots of capacitated sperm containing 1×10^4 to 1×10^5 sperm per oocyte are then added to the fertilization medium containing the oocytes, and the mixture is incubated as described in the preceding paragraph for 18 to 24 hours.

Following incubation of the oocytes and sperm, the presumed zygotes are stripped of their cumulus cells by vortexing in 200 µl of TALP-HEPES for 90 seconds, diluted in TALP-HEPES, and placed in groups of six or more in 50 µl droplets of CR1 + aa defined embryo culture medium with 3 mg/ml Bovine Serum Albumin (BSA) and 15 µl/ml Gentamicin (antibiotics) under Parrafin oil and cultured at 39°C in 5% CO_2 in air. CR1 is a commercially available embryo culture medium, and the "aa" designates the supplementation with amino acid cocktail mixtures. HEPES is a buffer commonly used in cell and embryo culture systems and provides better stability of pH during freezing and thawing. On day 2 of culture, with the day of fertilization being day 1, initial cleavage is evaluated by noting the number of zygotes greater than the two-cell stage. The following steps were developed to overcome the early problem of not being able to get *in vitro* embryonic development to progress beyond the two-cell stage. Zygotes showing evidence of cleavage are packaged in sterile vials containing sterilized CR1 + aa embryo culture medium, with culturing continuing as previously described. If the culture medium being used does not contain serum, 10% fetal calf serum (FCS) is added on day 5 and culture continued until day 7. The embryos that develop to the blastocyst stage by that time are ready for nonsurgical embryo transfer. They can be packaged (one or two per straw) in 0.5-ml plastic straws for transfer with a standard embryo transfer straw gun, which has a discharge opening on the side rather than at the end. Progress has also been made with the freezing of embryos (Section 18–2.4). The steps involved in the production of embryos *in vitro* are shown in Figure 19–3, and the timing of *in vitro* embryo development in a system using CR1 culture medium is shown in Table 19–2.

It should be noted that some abnormalities have been reported in cattle as a result of *in vitro* embryo production (IVM/IVF) and transfer. Specifically, calves tend to be larger (large-calf-syndrome), which can translate into slightly longer gestations, dystocia, and higher perinatal mortality. This has been a greater problem for *in vitro*–produced cloned embryos (Section 19–3). In sheep, this syndrome has been clearly linked to the presence and quantity of serum in the embryo culture medium. The factor or combination of factors specifically responsible for these effects on embryonic/fetal development is not fully understood.

19–1.4 In Vitro *Culture of Embryos*

The *in vitro* culture of embryos during initial stages of development to the blastocyst stage has been difficult. In early studies of swine, only 4.3% to 7.3% of one-cell porcine embryos developed to the blastocyst stage in various modified culture media. This inefficency with

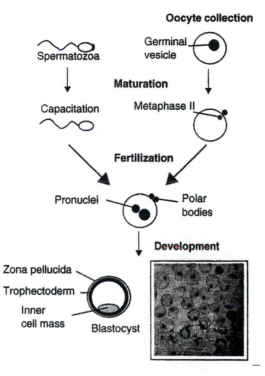

Figure 19–3 Schematic representation of *in vitro* production of embryos in domestic mammals. Four major steps are represented. Oocytes are collected at the germinal vesicle stage of meiosis and reach the metaphase II stage after maturation. They are fertilized by capacitated sperms and cultured for 7 to 9 days to reach the expanded blastocyst stage. A batch of *in vitro*–produced bovine blastocysts is represented. *Source:* Reprinted from *Encyclopedia of Dairy Sciences,* 2, Mermillod, P., In Vitro Fertilization, p. 1176, 2002, with permission from Elsevier Science.

the culture of early developing embryos has posed a problem for the application of gene transfer and other biotechnologies in livestock. Initially, early cleavage embryos from cattle were embedded in agar and surgically transferred into the oviducts of sheep or rabbits for 5 to 6 days. They were then surgically recovered, evaluated for stage of development, and transferred into recipient cows or frozen.

As an alternative to this more invasive approach, the co-culture of embryos with oviductal epithelial cells, oviductal fluid, or granulosa cells has also been used for development of early cleavage embryos in rabbits, cattle, sheep, and swine. The oviductal cells or secretions provide a favorable environment for the embryo with sources of energy and nutritive and growth factors, as might be provided *in vivo*. Use of an *in vitro* mouse oviduct culture system in one study permitted 78.1% of one-cell porcine embryos to develop to the morula and blastocyst stages. Therefore, cross-species co-culture of livestock embryos with excised tissues or flushings obtained from laboratory animals (rats, mice, rabbits) has permitted the *in vitro*

Table 19–2   *Time of* in vitro *fertilization events and embryo development*

Time postsperm addition		
Hour	Day	Event
	−1	Oocyte aspirated and placed in culture medium
0	0	Sperm washed, added to oocytes and capacitated (if not prior capacitated)
24	1	Moved to development medium, two-cell
48	2	Two- to four-cell
72	3	Four- to eight-cell
96	4	Compacting morula
120	5	Serum added to culture medium, compact Morula
144	6	Morula—early blastocyst
168	7	Early—expanded blastocyst

From Parrish. *Proc. 15th Tech. Conf. Artif. Insem. Reprod.* NAAB, 1994.

development of livestock embryos to be more efficient than previous surgical implantation and recovery procedures. More recently, synthetic oviductal fluid (SOF) medium or potassium simplex optimized medium (KSOM) supplemented with sheep or cow serum collected at estrus or BSA has also been used with success for embryo culture.

19–1.5 *Intracytoplasmic Sperm Injection (ICSI)*

Intracytoplasmic sperm injection (ICSI) was developed in the early 1990s as an ART procedure to assist infertile couples, with a particular emphasis on overcoming problems related to male infertility. This procedure involves the placement of a single spermatozoon directly into the cytoplasm of an oocyte. This bypasses normal barriers to sperm penetration, including the cumulus cell matrix, zona pellucida, and plasma membrane. This reduces the requirement for millions of sperm to achieve fertilization when using AI or IVF to just a single sperm cell. Even nonmotile sperm can be used for fertilization with ICSI if necessary; however, determinations of live cells that are immotile versus dead cells has been a problem. To achieve injection of sperm into the oocyte, a glass holding pipette of 40 to 50 microns in diameter is used to hold the embryo using gentle vacuum. Active sperm are placed in a droplet of polyvinyl pyrrolidone solution (PVP), which is placed in mineral oil or some other viscous medium. This slows the motility of the sperm and serves as a cleanser. While active sperm are chosen for placement in the PVP, a spermatozoon with the least amount of activity once in PVP-oil solution is often chosen for use in ICSI procedures. This prevents damage to the oocyte following injection from the whipping action of the tail, and the tail of the sperm is sometimes pinched-off or crushed to immobilize it for injection. The sperm is injected into the oocyte using a glass microinjection needle with an outer diameter of only 5 to 6 microns (Figure 19–4). Care is taken when injecting the sperm into the oocyte to ensure against excess media being injected into the oocyte with the sperm and to ensure that the sperm in not drawn back into the injection pipette on withdrawal of the needle from the oocyte.

One problem encountered with using ICSI in some species, including farm livestock, has been the fact that sperm injection bypasses steps required for activation of the oocyte for continued development. Fusion of the sperm with the oocyte results in activation, which causes resumption of meiosis, pronuclear formation, and the first cleavage division. The use of chemical reagents to activate oocytes during the ICSI procedure has provided a means

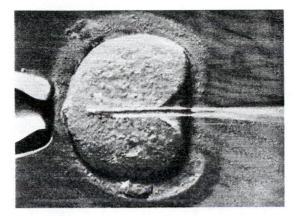

Figure 19–4 Intracytoplasmic sperm injection (ICSI) (Courtesy of S. Jindal, Hackensack Medical Center, Hackensack, NJ.)

of bypassing the requirement for the spermatozoa to perform this function (i.e., bind to the zona pellucida and plasma membrane). Equine oocytes have been activated with a variety of chemical stimulants, including ionomycin, ethanol, thimersol, and inosital 1,4,5-triphosphate. These chemical stimulants can alter the pattern of intracellular Ca^{2+} changes within the oocyte facilitating activation and normal fertilization postsperm injection. In both sheep and cattle, 50% to 80% of oocytes subjected to ICSI will cleave to the two-cell stage when stimulated chemically to induce activation, yet further development of these embryos is much less than those produced by conventional IVF techniques. In one study in the bovine, the rate of development from the two-cell stage to the eight-cell stage following ICSI was 38%, which is about half of what can be achieved with conventional IVF. This higher activation rate of oocytes versus those that cleave to the eight-cell or greater stage is due to the chemical induction of parthenogenesis, which is continued initial development (cleavage) in the absence of spermatozoa (chemical induction only) or without sperm head decondensation. As many as 40% to 70% of bovine oocytes after artificial activation chemically may exhibit parthenogenic cleavage and eventually cease further development.

Fertilization rates in humans using ICSI are good, at approximately 65%, although actual pregnancy rates following transfer are much lower (7% to 18%). Fertilization rates across four studies conducted in the equine using oocytes matured *in vitro* and injected with sperm ranged from 12% to 30%. In a recent study, an initial pregnancy rate of 38% from microinjected equine oocytes at 30 days posttransfer was achieved; however, following several incidences of pregnancy loss, the overall pregnancy rate at 150 days of gestation fell to 13%. While this technique has promise as a clinical treatment for infertility by reducing the requirement for large numbers of spermatozoa, its widespread use in the reproductive management of production livestock may be limited.

19–2 SEX DETERMINATION AND CONTROL

19–2.1 *Determining the Sex of Embryos*

Predetermination of the sex of embryos has been high on livestock producers' and embryo transfer practitioners' "wish list" for a long time. Sexing of offspring using ultrasonography in cattle has been conducted at around day 60 of gestation with good accuracy (> 90%) from a trained technician or clinician. A drawback of fetal sexing with ultrasonography is that the cow is already pregnant. If the sex of the offspring is not desired, a decision of whether or not to terminate the pregnancy needs to be made by the producer. Preselection of offspring sex prior to embryo transfer would be much more desirable, provided the technique was relatively accurate in its predictive ability and did not compromise embryo viability.

The first success in the development of an embryo sexing technique involved the use of karyotyping, in which a picture of the chromosomes from embryonic cells are obtained, showing the entire chromosome complement of the cells during mitotic metaphase. In 1976, Hare and coworker demonstrated that elongated 14- to 15-day-old bovine embryos could be biopsied and sexed by karyotyping within approximately 3.5 hours. However, only about 60% of embryos provide usable karyotypes and the need for removal of a relatively large number of cells to provide a usable metaphase spread often compromised embryo viability. The fact that this procedure required hatched, elongated blastocysts also made this technique impractical for use in embryo transfer programs.

Two other techniques for embryo sexing were developed in the early to mid-1980s, the X-linked enzyme method and H-Y antigen procedure. However neither procedure has developed into a commercially viable technique for use in livestock. The X-linked enzyme method was based on the hypothesis that the ratio of X-linked enzyme activity to total cellular enzyme activity will be higher in female (XX) than male (XY) embryos. In a study attempting to sex preimplantation mouse embryos with this technique, correct identification of male and female embryos was 72% and 57%, respectively, using the X-linked enzyme glucose-6-phosphate dehydrogenase. In a second study of embryos examining X-linked hypoxanthine phosphoribosyl transferase enzyme activity, accuracy of sexing was 91% for females and 100% for males. This technique was very accurate (for mice) in determing the sex of embryos and could be accomplished using only one blastomere. However, mortality rates were high in both studies, presumably due to the dyes used and/or biopsy procedures. Our current lack of knowledge concerning the timing of X-inactivation in domestic livestock and the variability in cellular enzymatic activity has prevented further development of this technique for use in livestock. The H-Y antigen procedure (histocompatability Y antigen) has an advantage as an immunological approach in that a biopsy is not required, and the technique is rapid (2 hours) and relatively simple. In this procedure, embryos are exposed to primary (H-Y) antibody for 30 minutes, followed by reaction with a secondary antibody to which fluorescein isothiocyanate (FITC) has been conjugated. Embryos are then evaluated for the presence or absence of the FITC tag under a fluorescent microscope. Despite the use of newer (monoclonal) antibodies, the accuracy of predicting the sex of embryos with H-Y antigen immunoassays has not exceeded 87%. Research continues in the development of antibodies against embryo outer surface sex-specific proteins (SSPs), yet to date no additional diagnostic procedures of note have been developed.

The method of embryo sexing that seems to have the greatest potential is through the amplification and detection of repetitive, male-specific DNA sequences that are present on the Y chromosome. The presence of these sequences from a biopsied embryo would indicate a male, whereas their absence would indicate a female. The method has been refined to the point that only one to four cells are required. This method uses the polymerase chain reaction (PCR) to amplify minute quantities of DNA and has increased the efficiency with which embryos can be sexed. PCR was first developed in the early 1980s, and its developer, Kary Mullis, received the Nobel Prize in Chemistry for his discovery in 1993.

The purpose of PCR is to make a huge number of copies of a specific gene—in this case, a gene sequence specific to the Y chromosome (e.g., the btDYZ-1 region of the bovine Y chromosome). It allows one to have a small starting quantity of DNA (i.e., one to four cells from an embryo), with the end result producing enough quantity of DNA to permit biochemical detection of a specific sequence or to provide a DNA template to determine an unknown sequence of DNA. There are three major steps in a PCR reaction, which are repeated for 30 to 50 cycles on an automated cycler, which can heat and cool the tubes with the reaction mixtures in a very short period of time. The DNA is first denatured (92°C to 94°C), at which time the double-stranded DNA melts open to single-stranded DNA. Primers that are specific to the gene sequence of interest are then annealed or hybridized to the single-stranded DNA (45°C to 63°C), from which DNA polymerase can attach and start copying the DNA template. Finally, extension (72°C) of the primers with polymerase then occurs (i.e., DNA synthesis), filling in complementary bases to create multiple copies (several million) of the sequence targeted. The absence of a target sequence would result in no amplification of Y-specific sequences and thus indicate a female embryo (Figure 19–5). This technique was first reported for embryo sexing in the bovine using radioactive probes for the detection of the amplified Y-specific DNA sequences by Bondioli and coworkers in 1989. A total of 1,331 embryonic samples were assayed with this initial procedure, of which a determination as to whether the embryo was male or female was made in 1,252 (94%) of the samples (Table 19–3). From these samples, 197 pregnancies were monitored, and sexing by ultrasound indicated a 94% to 100% accuracy of determination for those embryos classified prior to transfer as female or male, respectively. Of these 197 pregnancies, 111 resulted in the birth of live calves, from which those that were classified as male or female had an accuracy of determination of 95% and 93%, respectively (Table 19–4).

Since the time of this first embryo sexing study by PCR, the sexing of bovine embryos has been greatly simplified. The original procedure required 8 days to complete and used radioactivity to quantify results. Today, more simplified PCR-based approaches

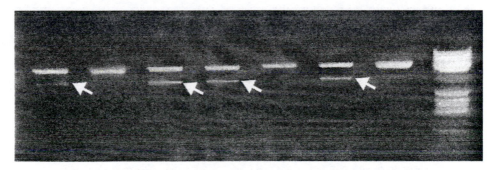

Figure 19–5 Electrophoretic characterization of polymerase chain reaction products separated through an agarose gel. The resulting bands of amplified DNA were stained with ethidium bromide for fluorescence visualization. Y-chromosome-specific bands from male embryos are indicated (arrows). *Source:* Reprinted from *Encyclopedia of Dairy Sciences*, 2, Hasler, J. F. & Garner, D. L., Sexed Offspring, p. 1195, 2002, with permission from Elsevier Science.

Table 19–3   *The effect of sample size on sex determination rate by amplification of a bovine Y chromosome–specific sequence*

Number cells in sample	Number samples	Number determinations
2	476	438 (92%)
3	213	202 (95%)
4	343	329 (96%)
5	299	283 (95%)
Total	1,331	1,252 (94%)

From Bondioli. 1992. *J. Anim. Sci.* 70(Suppl. 2): 19.

Table 19–4   *Confirmation of sex prediction of embryos by amplification of Y chromosome–specific sequences by birth of live calves or ultrasound pregnancy diagnosis*

Sex determination	Number embryos	Live calf results		Accuracy of determination
		Male	Female	
Female	40	3	37	93%
Male	64	61	3	95%
Female?	0	———	———	———
Male?	3	2	1	66%
Undetermined	4	3	1	———
		Ultrasound results		
Female	84	5	79	94%
Male	100	100	0	100%
Female?	1	1	0	0%
Male?	4	3	1	75%
Undetermined	9	7	2	

From Bondioli. 1992. *J. Anim. Sci.* 70(Suppl. 2):19.

Female? and Male? determinations resulted from a sample having fewer than two cells of DNA as determined by hybridization with the nonsex-specific probe but a tentative determination was possible. Undetermined samples did not contain any DNA as determined by hybridization with the nonsex-specific probe.

have been developed that use nonradioactive probes (fluorescence; Figure 19–6) and require only 2.5 to 3 hours to complete. On-the-farm embryo biopsy and sex determination kits are commercially available and, while not as widely available in the United States as in other countries, sexed embryos can be purchased. In France, the transfer of this technology has been rapid, and many farmers in that country will no longer transfer embryos without having them sexed. The costs of buying and transferring sexed embryos are justified relative to the savings of the cost of maintenance of pregnant recipients carrying the undesired sex, with particular reference to the need for replacement heifers in dairy op-

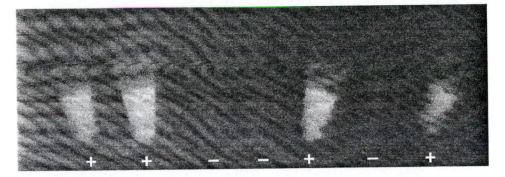

Figure 19–6   Polymerase chain reaction (PCR) determination of the presence of the Y chromosome in biopsied tissues from seven embryos using ethidium bromide-labeled Y-specific PCR primers. Fluorescent illumination is used to identify the male embryos by the pinkish-red stain (+), while female embryos do not fluoresce (2). *Source:* Reprinted from *Encyclopedia of Dairy Science*, 2, Haster, J. F. & Garner, D. L., Sexed Offspring, p. 1196, 2002, with permission from Elsevier Science.

erations. When coupled with IVF efforts and cloning, embryo sexing may play a significant role in future reproductive biotechnology applications.

19–2.2 *Sexing of Spermatozoa*

One of the first scientific studies to be conducted in sex preselection in mammals was reported by J. L. Lush in 1925. His research was based on a possible differential density between X- and Y-bearing sperm in the rabbit. However, this initial attempt did not yield a viable method with which to sex sperm, and researchers have pondered this problem for more than 75 years. Centrifugation, sedimentation, electrophoresis, selective killing, pressure changes, pH changes, viscosity, filtration, and other techniques have been used in attempts to separate X and Y chromosome–bearing sperm into separate fractions, only to frustrate researchers.

Scientists at the Beltsville National Research Laboratory have worked for several years with high-density flow cytometric measurement (FCM) of DNA of sperm nuclei that are stained with a DNA-specific dye, Hoechst 33342. They determined that X and Y chromosome–bearing sperm differ in DNA content by 3% to 4%. This difference, though small, allows a sorting system coupled with the FCM to divert the X chromosome–bearing sperm into one collection tube and the Y chromosome–bearing sperm into another. Both nucleated sperm cells and viable, intact sperm can be analyzed and sorted. The sperm pass through a laser beam, where the DNA analysis determines which ones contain X chromosomes and which contain Y chromosomes. The stained X chromosome–bearing sperm emit proportionately brighter fluorescence due to their higher DNA content than the Y_2 chromosome–bearing sperm. The flow stream leaving the laser is vibrated, causing the stream to break into small, uniform droplets. These droplets carrying no more than a single sperm pass through an electric field, where those containing an X chromosome are given a positive charge, while those containing a Y chromosome are given a negative charge. Droplets containing no sperm are left uncharged. The positive droplets are pulled to one collection tube while the negative droplets are pulled to another. The collection tubes contain a small amount of semen diluter for holding the sorted sperm. The uncharged droplets and dead sperm which are differentiated from live sperm by uptake of a membrane-impermeable second dye are allowed to drop into a central discard tube (Figures 19–7 and 19–8). Flow cytometric analysis to determine sperm sex ratios of semen with this method has been used effectively in a number of species, excluding humans. Human sperm are characterized by a more angular or bullet-shaped head, which makes orientation difficult. Also, the DNA difference between the Y and X chromosome–bearing sperm is less than 3%, which necessitates increased precision in the analysis.

The current sorting process permits up to 40% of the sperm that pass through the sorter to be sexed, at a rate of 20,000 total sperm per second. This represents up to 4,000 live sperm per second for each sex sorted simultaneously, sorting 10 to 13 million live sperm per hour of each sex. Accuracy of the sort is 85% to 95% live sperm for each sex. Table 19–5 illustrates the accuracy for separating all sexed sperm (sperm nuclei) and viable, intact sperm by reanalysis of FCM-sorted sperm with FCM again for the bull, boar, and rabbit. Note that 76.2% to 80.8% of intact sperm previously sorted as Y sperm were again identified as Y sperm, and 85.9% to 90.0% of X sperm were again identified as X sperm.

Trials with low-dose inseminations of 1,000 heifers with sexed semen (1 to 3×10^6 frozen-thawed sperm/dose) from 22 bulls selected for semen quality produced pregnancy rates at 2 months of 47%, compared with 60% for control, unsexed semen at normal semen doses (20×10^6 frozen-thawed sperm/dose). Accuracy of producing the desired sex approaches 90% overall (73% to 95%). The staining dye does not seem to adversely affect the viability, including motility and fertilizing ability of sperm, but does seem to adversely affect the viability of the embryo *in vitro*. One report in which X- and Y-bearing chromosomes were used for IVF of aspirated IVM oocytes showed cleavage rates of about 80% for both X and Y sperm, but a greatly reduced percentage of those cleaved oocytes developed into normal blastocysts (17% for sexed sperm, compared with 35% for controls that were fertilized with frozen-thawed unsexed sperm). This work supports earlier research with rabbits and pigs, in which lower implantation rates of embryos produced using sexed sperm were obtained following surgical transplantation. Researchers have theorized that the Hoechst 33342 dye probably contributed to the lower pregnancy rates with sexed sperm. Nevertheless, in field trials with cattle, pregnancy losses prior to 2 months of gestation have not been different between sexed pregnancies (8.8%) and control pregnancies (6.2%). Data from more than 2,000 calves born from sexed semen also indicate no gross abnormalities.

Samples of semen that were prepared by numerous "physical separation" methods have been analyzed for DNA content, and it is generally accepted that a 50:50 ratio of Y to X chromosomes is observed. However, some research was reported for both bulls and boars, showing that the ratio of Y and X sperm can vary between ejaculates from the same sire and for ejaculates between sires of the same species. The percentage of sperm bearing the Y chromosome ranged from 24% to 84%. One-fifth of the ejaculates differed significantly from the overall mean. Semen from the bulls and boars in this study was subsequently used to breed cows and sows. The percentage of males per ejaculate and the percentage of males per litter and DNA analysis by the PCR method showed that every ejaculate did not contain an equal number of sperm bearing the X and Y chromosomes. This natural skewing of the sex ratio may account for a number of reported methods for separating X- and Y-bearing sperm that failed to hold up under repeated research through the years.

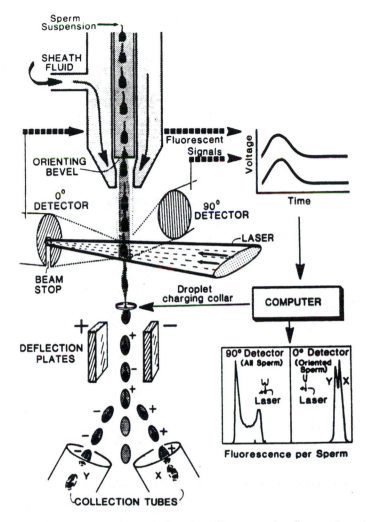

Figure 19–7 This schematic drawing illustrates the flow cytometric analysis and sorting system as modified for measurement of DNA in sperm. The sample of suspended sperm is drawn into the flow cell through a stainless steel tube, where it is injected into sheath fluid from the beveled end of the insertion tube; both streams exit the orifice of the flow cell nozzle. The properly oriented sperm flow in a single file and interesect the laser beam, which excites the fluorescent dye. The light given off is collected by the two optical detectors. Analysis of the sample is now complete. If sorting is done to the sample, circuits are activated so that a charging pulse (+ or −) is given the respective X- or Y-bearing sperm, which are encased in the liquid droplets resulting from the high-speed vibration of the flow cell. As the droplets fall, they pass through an electrostatic field that pulls the charged droplets containing the sperm into different tubes. The collection tubes contain a small amount of Test-Yolk semen diluter to receive the sorted sperm. An aliquot of the sorted sperm is taken for reanalysis to determine the degree of purity of the sort. *Source*: From Johnson. 1992. *J. Anim. Sci.* 70([Suppl. 2]:8.

Preparation of Sperm for Flow Sorting and Reanalysis	
Sorting intact sperm	Reanalysis of sorted sperm for DNA
10×10^6 sperm ⇓ Dilute ⇓ Hoechst 33342 (5 µg/10^6 sperm) ⇓ Incubate 1 hr 35°C ⇓ Sort into Test-Yol ⇓ Surgical insemination *In vitro* fertilization	2×10^5 sperm ⇓ Sonicate (for 15 sec) ⇓ Add 2.5 µg of Hoechst 33342 ⇓ Flow cytometric DNA analysis ⇓ For proportions of X and Y sperm ⇓ % X and Y sperm

Figure 19–8   This chart illustrates the means by which viable sperm are prepared for flow sorting based on DNA and for reanalysis of the sorted sperm for DNA content. (From Johnson. 1992. *J. Anim. Sci.* 70[Suppl. 2]:8.)

Table 19–5   *Comparative flow cytometric reanalysis for DNA of sorted nuclei and sorted, intact sperm from three different species*

Species	Mean X-Y DNA difference, %	% of Y sperm in Y sort, +/− SEM	% of X sperm in X sort, +/− SEM	n
		Sperm nuclei		
Boar	3.7	91.2 +/− 2.6	92.7 +/− 1.6	4
Bull	3.9	92.8 +/− 0.9	90.4 +/− 1.4	9
Rabbit	3.0	84.3 +/− 5.7	88.0 +/− 2.2	3
		Intact sperm		
Boar	—	76.2 +/− 4.3	90.0 +/− 0.7	5
Bull	—	80.5 +/− 1.9	88.9 +/− 1.9	6
Rabbit	—	80.8 +/− 1.9	85.9 +/− 0.8	10

From Johnson, 1992. *J. Anim. Sci.* 70(Suppl. 2):8.

19–3 CLONING

19–3.1 *Embryo Splitting*

In 1900, Driesh separated daughter cells of a fertilized egg and showed that they could each develop into an embryo, disproving preformation theory (Chapter 1). Today, this separation of blastomeres uses microsurgery in which a fine knife or glass needle is used to achieve the embryo split. Separated blastomeres, often referred to as demiembryos, are often placed into an empty zona pellucida or embedded in gelatin or agar. However, demiembryos not placed in a zona pellucida or other protective media seem to survive equally as well. The best success rates using embryo splitting are achieved from bisecting the embryo into two halves, whereas further segmentation decreases embryo developmental viability. The split embryos that develop produce clones (identical twins) since each transferred blastomere originated from the same, single embryo. Using this method, identical twins have been achieved from splitting two- and four-cell-stage embryos in goats, two-cell-stage embryos in sheep, and up to morula-stage embryos in cows.

19–3.2 *Nuclear Transfer*

Nuclear transfer offers another means of obtaining identical individuals. In 1952, developmental biologists Briggs and King developed a cloning method referred to as nuclear transplantation, or nuclear transfer, which was first proposed in 1938 by German scientist Hans Spemann. In this method, the nucleus of an unfertilized oocyte is removed, a procedure known as enucleation, and cells from a trophoblast (from which as many as 200 cells can be obtained) are placed into the enucleated oocyte. These nuclear transfer embryos can then be cultured *in vitro* to the morula or blastocyst stage (Section 19–1.4) and transferred to recipients. This process is often referred to as cloning and, in fact, is the cloning of an embryo. It is necessary to differentiate this process from true cloning, which involves taking cells (somatic or body cells) from an individual at some point after its birth (or at least using differentiated tissue as a cell source) in order to produce another individual. Some invertebrates, including various types of earthworms and starfish, can be cloned by dividing them into segments, and each segment can regrow into a complete organism. The cloning of vertebrates, however, has been much more difficult. Nevertheless, the original nuclear transfer experiments by Briggs and King were, in fact, this type of true cloning, in which body cells from frogs were used to produce several cloned tadpoles. These, and later experiments, seemed to suggest that, even though cells differentiate and specialize, they may, in fact, remain *totipotent*. That is, under certain circumstances, already specialized cell types can direct the development of a complete organism. Totipotency implies that, since all of a fully developed organism's cells contain a complete set of genes (a blueprint for development), differentiated cells might be able to be reprogrammed.

It wasn't until 1996 that this hypothesis became a reality following the birth of the first true mammalian clone, a sheep named Dolly, in an experiment by Ian Wilmut and coworkers of the Roslin Institute near Edinburgh, Scotland. They produced a viable lamb from cell populations established from the mammary cells of a 6-year old ewe, as well as other lambs derived from differentiated fetal tissue and stem cells from a 9-day old embryo. Tissue from all cell sources was grown in tissue culture before being exposed to enzymes to disperse the individual cells. The cells were grown through three to eight changes until the modal chromosome number was 54. At that point, the serum in the culture medium was reduced from 10% to 0.5% and the diploid cells were incubated for 5 days, causing them to exit the growth cycle and become quiescent. In essence, this process made it possible for the differentiated cells to be reprogrammed by oocyte cytoplasm to produce a whole animal when deposited into an enucleated oocyte rather than continuing to produce only the tissue from which it had been derived.

In the meantime, recipient oocytes were recovered from other ewes. They were recovered in calcium- and magnesium-free PBS containing 1% fetal calf serum (FCS), enucleated as soon as possible, and transferred to calcium-free M2 medium containing 10% FCS at 39°C.

The quiescent donor diploid cells were transplanted into the enucleated oocytes, which were then activated with electrical pulses. Some of the reconstructed embryos were incubated in ligated oviducts of live ewes, and some were cultured in a chemically defined medium with similar results. There was a lower percentage of the nuclei from mammary cells that developed into morula and blastocyst than nuclei from embryo stem cells of fetal fibroblast. However, when the ones that did develop were transplanted into recipient ewes the percentage producing live lambs was very similar. Four, three, and one (Dolly) lambs were born, respectively, from embryo-derived, fetal fibroblast-derived, and mammary-derived cells. Almost 300 attempts to produce a viable clone using mammary cells were conducted. Embryos either rejected the mammary cell and did not begin to develop, or they died early in development. Lambs that were born were abnormal and died, yet one (Dolly) developed normally and survived. All of the lambs born, regardless of the originating cell type, had the morphological characteristics of the nucleus donors and not that of the oocyte donors or that of the recipient ewes. Additionally, DNA microsatellite analysis confirmed that each lamb was derived from the cell population used as the nuclear donor.

Six genetically identical calves were produced in the United States. Those calves were developed from fully developed fibroblast cells from a 50-day-old bovine fetus. They were cultured and induced to quiescence before being transferred to enucleated bovine oocytes, by much the same process as that used for the Scottish sheep. Another calf was also born using cells from a 30-day-old bull fetus. This was accomplished using two successive nuclear transfer procedures, with the initial cloned embryos from the first nuclear transfer used as the material for the second nuclear transfer. It is believed this "double" nuclear transfer technique may enhance the reprogramming of cells and increase the success rate of the cloning procedures. However, these successes in cattle, while important, did not replicate what was accomplished by the Scottish scientists who used adult body (somatic) cells instead of cells from an embryo or a fetus. It was not until a separate research team produced more than 50 cloned mice using adult cumulus cells that this feat was replicated and verified. This was followed shortly thereafter by the cloning of pigs, an endangered wild ox (a gaur), and a cat. An overview of cloning by nuclear transfer in the bovine with cells of embryo, fetal, or adult (somatic) cells is represented in Figure 19–9.

19–4 GENETIC ENGINEERING (TRANSGENICS)

The possibility of introducing genes into livestock that may enhance production performance has been discussed for many years. This was popularized when scientists in the 1980s created transgenic mice that produced human growth hormone and grew to be 25% to 30% larger than normal mice. Since then, creation of transgenic laboratory animals has produced a wealth of animal models for elucidating the functions of genes and as models of growth, development, and disease. Similarly, transgenic livestock have been used to produce pharmaceutical compounds in their milk, and a few transgenic animals and genetic lines have been developed which show promise in production-based settings.

The primary method used to introduce foreign genes into a given species is by microinjection of the DNA into the pronucleus of a fertilized oocyte (Figure 19–10). Generally, 200 to 300 copies of the transgene are injected, yet how the transgene gets integrated into the fertilized oocyte is often impossible to direct. In cattle, the use of slaughterhouse

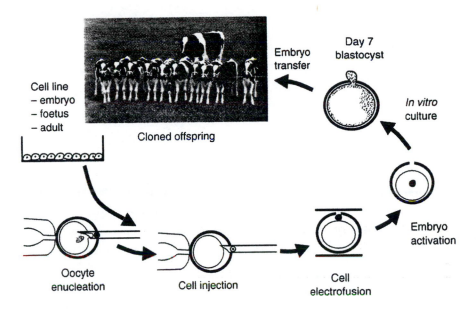

Figure 19–9   Production of cloned calves following nuclear transfer.
Source: Reprinted from *Encyclopedia of Dairy Sciences*, 3, Jordan, B. R., Molecular Genetics and the Dairy Industry, p. 2068, 2002, with permission from Elsevier Science.

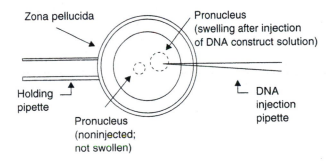

Figure 19–10   Microinjection of DNA into the pronucleus of a zygote.
Source: Reprinted from *Encyclopedia of Dairy Sciences*, 2, Gwazdauskas, F. C., Transgonic Animals, p. 1189, 2002, with permission from Elsevier Science.

ovaries for the collection of oocytes has been integral to the production of transgenic offspring due to the need for large numbers of oocytes that can be collected and the low efficiency of success with pronuclear injection. In one study, 11,500 IVF-derived oocytes were microinjected with DNA. Only 9% developed to the morula or blastocyst stage. Of these, 478 embryos were transferred to recipients, 90 of which produced calves and only 10% were found to be transgenic, with only one heifer expressing the gene appropriately in her milk. This equates to a

0.08% rate of transgenesis in cattle. The use of pronuclear injection as a means of transgenesis has recently been successful in swine for the production of a genetic line of pigs geared toward solving a specific production-based problem associated with waste management. In Canada, scientists have genetically modified pigs that produce manure containing up to 75% less phosphorus, called "enviropigs." Their bodies can absorb a normally indigestible form of phosphorus, thus reducing their fecal phosphorus levels to between 50% and 75% of that of normal pigs. To accomplish this, the scientists took an *E. coli* gene that makes the enzyme phytase and a mouse gene that controls the secretion of protein from the salivary glands, fused them together into a DNA construct, microinjected the DNA into the pronucleus of a pig embryo, and transferred the embryos into recipients. The gene allows the pig to make phytase in the salivary gland and then secrete it into its saliva, where it is swallowed with food. The phytase releases phosphate in the animal's gut that can be absorbed by the bloodstream. This was the first genetically modified farm animal engineered to solve an environmental production problem.

Retroviruses have also been used to incorporate a transgene. To do so, the retrovirus with its RNA-based genome is transcribed by the virus's reverse transcriptase into DNA in the infected cells, which then becomes integrated into the host cell's genome. Zona-free embryos have been incubated with retroviruses containing the gene of interest for 16 to 24 hours, and incorporation of the gene has been documented. However, the rate of transgenesis with retroviruses is not much better than that with the use of pronuclear microinjection (< 1%). The use of retroviruses also has limitations in the size of the gene construct that can be transferred (< 9.4 kilobases in length) and in the degree to which integration within the genome of the host can be controlled.

Use of embryonic stem cells, undifferentiated cells derived from early embryos, has also been considered as a means to achieve transgenesis. As these cells can be propagated in culture, the ability to make not only additions but also deletions to the genome holds great promise for transgenics and gene-specific manipulations. Genes can also be targeted in this manner to try to create germ-line integrations that would assure transfer of the gene later on to offspring. These are often referred to as germ-line chimeras. The modified embryonic stem cell is injected into the cavity of a blastocyst and through subsequent divisions produces a chimera, a living organism that contains two or more genetically distinct tissues. In mice, up to 30% of the chimeras produced are germ-line chimeras containing the genotype of the cell line. While this has worked well in mice, isolation of embryonic stem cells to achieve cell lines for widespread use in livestock is only now being achieved. Thus, the practical applications and efficiency of this technique for use in livestock remain to be seen yet could enhance the efficiency with which germ-line transgenic livestock are produced to achieve greater integration of the gene in offspring.

Nuclear transfer (Section 19–3.2) for cloning using transgenic donor cells that have the gene of interest incorporated into them is an alternative way to produce transgenic livestock. Use of bovine fetal fibroblasts with transgenes incorporated into them by electroporation have been fused with oocytes, with 10% developing to the blastocyst stage. Other techniques have used DNA microinjection into donor cells or liposome-mediated transfer to achieve transfer of the gene of interest into the cell line to be used in the nuclear transfer procedure. The liposome-mediated gene transfer technique was used recently by the Roslin Institute in Scotland to produce two lambs that contained a mammary gland–specific expression vector that produces human Factor IX, a human blood clotting protein useful for treating hemophilia. These two lambs (Molly and Polly) were the first two cloned transgenic animals to contain a human gene of pharmaceutical importance, with human Factor IX secreted into their milk for

Table 19–6   *Selected listing of milk gene promoters and expressed proteins*

Promoter-expressed protein	Animal	Expression per ml milk
Bovine α-lactalbumin	Rat	2.4 mg
Bovine α-lactalbumin	Mouse	1.5 mg
Goat α-lactalbumin	Mouse	1 μg
Human α-lactalbumin	Cow	2.4 mg
Bovine α$_{s1}$-casein		
hEPO[a]	Mouse	0.2 mg
hIGF-I[b]	Rabbit	1 mg
hLactoferrin	Cow	Not reported
Goat β-casein	Mouse	22 mg
hLA tPA[c]	Goat	1.5 mg
hAnti-thrombin III	Goat	3.2 mg
Bovine β-lactoglobulin	Mouse	1.5 mg
Sheep β-lactoglobulin		
hAAT[d]	Mouse	5 μg–21 mg
hAAT	Sheep	5 μg–35 mg
hFactor IX	Sheep	25 ng
hInterferon-γ	Mouse	20 ng
hFibrinogen	Sheep	5 mg
Mouse whey acidic protein		
hGH[e]	Mouse	3.5 mg
Protein C	Mouse	3 μg
Protein C	Pig	1 mg
hFactor VIII	Pig	2.7 mg

Adapted from Ayares 2000.

[a]hEPO, recombinant human erythropoeitin.

[b]hIGF-I, recombinant human insulin-like growth factor-I.

[c]hLA tPA, recombinant human long-acting tissue plasminogen activator.

[d]hAAT, recombinant human α-1-antitrypain.

[e]hGH, recombinant human growth hormone.

Source: Reprinted from *Encyclopedia of Dairy Sciences,* 2, Gwazdauskas, F. C., Transgenic Animals, p. 1191, 2002, with permission from Elsevier Science.

collection and purification. This type of nuclear transfer–transgene cloning has since been used to produce transgenic goats and cattle for the production of foreign proteins in milk (Table 19–6). Use of the mammary gland as a bioreactor in this fashion to produce foreign pharmaceutical proteins has been termed "pharming." Application of these techniques for targeting of transgene expression in other tissues to produce similar results will surely follow, with direct application to livestock production problems. The use of nuclear transfer alone or in combination with cloning is still relatively inefficient, with a low number of embryos transferred that actually survive and develop to term. However, the production of offspring assured to carry the transgene targeted to a specific site of expression represents a significant gain over the chance incorporation and testing required with other transgenic procedures.

Sperm-mediated gene transfer is another approach investigated for creating transgenic livestock. It was first reported in 1989, yet the initial failure of other laboratories to replicate the procedure cast doubt on the use of this method. It involved incubating naked DNA with sperm so that the DNA could bind to the sperm cells, and then IVF was performed to create transgenic embryos. To enhance the efficiency of the binding, liposome-DNA complexes were formed or electroporation conducted to increase sperm cell uptake of the DNA constructs. Another approach to sperm-mediated gene transfer was the development of procedures for spermatogonial cell transplantation or transfection of male stem cells with DNA. Liposomes are incubated with DNA to form complexes, which are injected into the seminiferous tubules. In mice, about 10% of sperm contain the transgene, while in swine about 20% of sperm contain the transgene. This procedure is only a transient transfection and does not create a lasting effect, as this "seeding" lasts only a short period of time. An alternative to these previous attempts at sperm-mediated gene transfer is the development of novel linkers (mAb C), which, like those using electroporation or liposomes, use sperm as the vector for the delivery of DNA. Sperm are first incubated with the mAb C linker and then combined with the linearized DNA fragment containing the gene of interest. The importance of this new approach is that, after forming the linked DNA-sperm associations, the scientists who developed the technology used standard artificial insemination to deliver the sperm rather than *in vitro* techniques. With this technique, a high germ-line transmission of 30% to 40% has been achieved in mice, pigs, and chickens. In one study of cattle and goats, four of five calves born and four of nine kids born with this technique contained the transgene. In pigs, using linker-based sperm-mediated gene transfer, 60% of pigs produced contained the transgene with 37.5% confirmed as germ-line transgenic pigs. Subsequent breeding of the F1 generation of transgenic pigs also demonstrated that the transgene was stably transmitted to the next generation (F2). If these results are confirmed with respect to the efficiency of creating transgenic livestock using this new linker-based method of gene transfer coupled with traditional artificial insemination, the feasibility of widespread use of transgenic technologies may become a reality.

Having described the current status of technologies for the development of transgenic livestock, it should be noted that there are animal welfare and public health and safety concerns with respect to the development of genetically modified organisms (GMO) for mass consumption. In Europe, there are labeling restrictions with respect to whether animals are transgenic or have consumed transgenic feedstuffs. If markets are not amenable to the use of transgenics in livestock, the further development of such technologies for enhancing production performance or carcass traits may be irrelevant. Nevertheless, the use of transgenic animals for the production of milk gene promoter-mediated protein expression will likely continue and provide great benefits to human medicine through the efficient production of therapeutic proteins (Table 19–6). Another disadvantage of transgenics as directed toward conferring disease resistance or the overexpression of a specific genetic trait is the potential for the loss of genetic variation. A single new disease could decimate whole herds of transgenic livestock unable to confer some resistance to the new disease because of reduced genetic variability. Whether this or similar scenarios might occur is mere speculation but cannot be discounted as we move into a new era of genetic control in livestock.

19–5   GENE DISCOVERY—MARKERS FOR REPRODUCTION

Genetic (DNA) information is routinely used in livestock for determination of parentage (DNA fingerprinting) and for a variety of other tests from the determination of traits for coat color (e.g., MCR1 coat color test—red versus black) to the identification of genetic diseases (severe combined immunodeficiency [SCID] in Arabian horses). Due to the low heritability of reproductive traits, genetic selection through breeding for high fertility or other parameters to improve reproductive efficiency have been greatly hampered. However, the use of new technologies that permit marker-assisted selection through the identification of specific genes, or combinations of genes, that may contribute to a given trait may assist these efforts. DNA tests could be used to sort livestock and properly match a genetic profile with management decisions.

Within the chromosomes of most mammals, it is estimated that the entire DNA sequence is 3 billion base pairs in length, coding for 30,000 to 60,000 different genes. An animal inherits two copies of every gene (except those on the sex chromosomes) from each parent, and these two copies differ from each other in their exact DNA sequence. There may be several million locations within the genome where individuals may differ. Where these differences cause different proteins to be produced or control alternative expression patterns of various genes, they may cause a variation among animals in their performance. Detection of these variations and their functional significance to the growth and reproductive performance to livestock is the basis for marker-assisted selection efforts. The mapping of farm animal genomes will greatly expand the use of marker-assisted selection (Section 19–6). The following are examples of how selection based on variations in specific DNA sequences among individuals or populations may be used to enhance reproductive performance in livestock.

Selection at the estrogen receptor (ESR) locus in pigs has been associated with litter size and can be selected for. There are two common alleles (any of two or more alternative forms of a gene occupying the same chromosomal locus), A and B. The B allele when increased within a population appears to increase litter size in pigs. Thus, using selection to increase specifically the frequency of the B allele within a population and using selection to incorporate the B allele into a population that does not carry it are both predicted to increase litter size. Selection for ESR genotypes is currently being conducted commercially, with a reported 30% increase in the rate of genetic progress by incorporating the ESR genotype in selection indices for various dam lines. Moreover, the increase in average litter size is also observed in cross-bred animals derived from these selected lines.

Markers for genes controlling sperm freezability in the boar have also been identified, demonstrating a genetic basis for variations among individual boars in postthaw semen quality. Sixteen candidate molecular markers have been linked to genes controlling semen freezability. This has been accomplished through genomic analysis of boars with "good" or "poor" semen freezability using a molecular technique called amplified restriction fragment length polymorphism (AFLP). AFLP is based on the principle of selectively amplifying a subset of gene fragments after digestion of the genomic DNA with restriction enzymes (Figure 19–11). The presence or absence of specific nucleotide sequences, or DNA fragments, of different lengths (polymorphisms) provides information as to the individual's genetic profile as related to the trait in question (i.e., semen freezability; Figure 19–12). These markers are shown in Table 19–7, in which the correlations between each marker and the identification of good and bad freezers (G/B) or specific sperm quality traits (progressive motility, intact plasma membranes, etc.) are identified. The use of AFLP markers to define genetic differences between boars with "good" and "poor" semen freezability may ultimately permit identification of the biophysical components of spermatozoa that are essential for successful cryopreservation. Through a greater understanding of the relationship

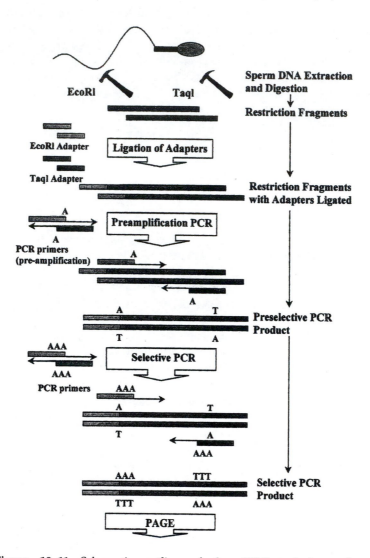

Figure 19–11 Schematic outline of the AFLP technique. *Source:* Thurston, L. et al. 2002. *Biol. of Reprod.*, 66:545. [© 2002, http://www. biolreprod. org/].

between freezability-related genes and sperm function, such findings may lead to better protocols for freezing semen to minimize the detrimental effects of the freezing process.

Other quantitative trait loci (QTL), which are polymorphic loci that contain alleles that differentially affect the expression of a phenotypic trait, have also been identified for other reproductive traits in swine. These markers describe a statistical association with the quantitative variation of a particular phenotypic trait that is controlled by the combined actions of alleles that may be found at multiple locations on the chromosomes. Evidence of QTL affecting ovulation rate, number of CLs, number of stillborn pigs, and age at puberty

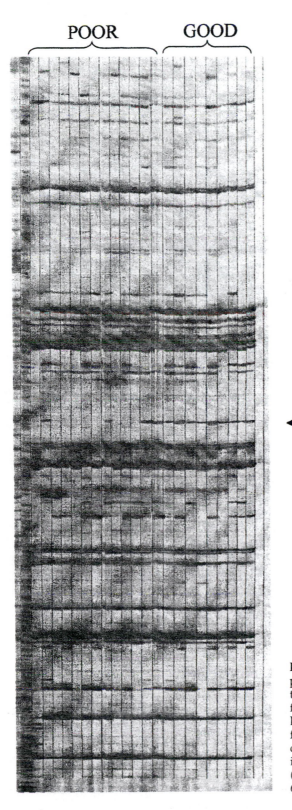

POOR   GOOD

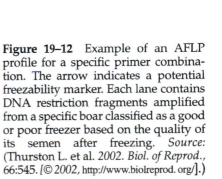

Figure 19–12 Example of an AFLP profile for a specific primer combination. The arrow indicates a potential freezability marker. Each lane contains DNA restriction fragments amplified from a specific boar classified as a good or poor freezer based on the quality of its semen after freezing. *Source:* (Thurston L. et al. *2002. Biol. of Reprod.,* 66:545. [© 2002, http://www.biolreprod. org/].)

Table 19–7   *Logistic regression analysis of the presence or absence of AFLP markers with classifications of good or bad freezability and semen quality assessments*

Marker	Variable[*]	Regression coefficient	SEM	Significance of variables (P)	Significance of logistic model (P)
1	G/B	0.599	1	0.005	0.005
2	G/B	0.643	1	0.005	0.003
3	G/B	0.650	1	0.005	0.004
4	G/B	0.740	1	0.001	0.0007
5	G/B	0.589	1	0.005	0.005
6	G/B	0.759	1	0.001	0.0001
7	G/B	0.639	1	0.005	0.005
7	SYBR14 (%)	0.775	0.1	0.0009	
8	G/B	0.639	1	0.005	0.005
8	SYBR14 (%)	0.436	0.1	0.04	
9	G/B	0.641	1	0.005	0.005
9	SYBR14 (%)	0.752	0.07	0.001	
10	G/B	0.663	1	0.005	0.003
11	G/B	0.662	1	0.004	0.004
11	Motile (%)	0.503	0.12	0.02	
11	Progressive motility (%)	0.436	0.41	0.04	
11	SYBR14 (%)	0.639	0.06	0.005	
12	G/B	0.600	1	0.003	0.005
13	G/B	0.662	1	0.006	0.005
14	G/B	0.797	1	0.0008	0.005
15	G/B	0.727	1	0.001	0.004
16	G/B	0.752	1	0.001	0.0008

Source: Thurston et al. 2002. *Biol of Reprod.*, 66:545 (© 2002, http://www.biolreprod.org/)

[*]G/B are classifications of good and bad freezers, SYBR14 (%) refers to the percentage of spermatozoa with intact plasma membranes in the thawed ejaculate.

in swine have been observed. Therefore, accuracy of selection for ovulation rate, age at puberty, and litter size may be enhanced by the use of marker-assisted selection using QTLs in breeding programs. Similar QTLs and marker-assisted selection criteria are also being investigated and applied to cattle and sheep for a variety of production parameters.

19–6   TECHNOLOGIES FOR THE FUTURE—DEFINITIONS

A new vocabulary has emerged (genomics, proteomics, microarrays, bioinformatics) that links the use of molecular tools to applied problems, together with procedures for interpreting and integrating these data into usable forms of information. While reproductive biologists and animal scientists are just now learning how to tap into these new disciplines, a renewed understanding of how the reproductive system is integrated and how traits controlling reproductive efficiency might be selected for may come from these advancements. A brief description of each technology is provided in this section as an introduction to the current status and potential of these areas of expertise.

19–6.1 *Genomics*

The mapping, sequencing, and analyzing of genomes, which is the complete gene complement of an organism contained in a set of chromosomes, is referred to as genomics. Genome analysis can be divided into two disciplines, structural genomics and functional genomics. Structural genomics involves the construction of genetic and physical maps of an organism, with the ultimate goal of a complete DNA sequence. "Functional genomics" refers to the development and application through experimental approaches of gene function, which uses the information provided by structural gene maps. The sequencing of animal and plant genomes began in the late 1970s and continues today with collaborative efforts among universities and government-sponsored research organizations. These will provide the genetic "blueprint" for various organisms, including livestock. In February 2001, a 90% complete draft of the human genome was published, with completion anticipated in 2003. The National Center for Biotechnology Information (NCBI) lists completion of 97 microbial genomes and current sequencing projects complete or nearing completion for a number of plant species, the fruit fly, the mouse, the rat, the zebrafish, and several viruses. Cattle, swine, sheep, and horse genome projects are also currently underway as directed by the National Animal Genome Research Program (NAGRP) and are reported in a web-based format in ArkDB (i.e., Ark database). These projects will initially use bacterial artificial chromosomes (BAC) as a vector to clone DNA fragments for sequencing in *E. coli* cells. BAC libraries have been made from Holstein bull DNA and Hereford bull DNA that will then be DNA fingerprinted to produce a sequence. The 280,000 BAC clones that have been produced from the two libraries constructed contain about 170,000 bases of cattle DNA each. The sequencing of these fragments will then be aligned to identify overlapping sequences, from which a continuous sequence can be developed once all the gaps between the sequences have been filled in and joined. By having these complete gene maps for the different livestock species, the selection of livestock for specific traits may be more accurate and DNA fingerprinting, marker-assisted selection, and transgenic technologies improved.

19–6.2 *DNA Microarrays*

There are thousands of genes present and expressed in livestock that we know nothing about. To gain insight into the function of genes, changes in gene expression are being studied throughout embryonic development, as an organism matures, through the aging process, and during disease progression and treatment. To obtain this information faster, DNA microarrays, or "DNA chips," are being developed to screen changes in gene expression that may occur for thousands of genes at a single time. DNA probes are arrayed in known positions on a solid support ("chips") and the sample DNA to be tested labeled with a fluorescent tag and hybridized with the array. Positive fluorescence at a given location on the array indicates hybridization and that the sample DNA contains the DNA complementary to the probe attached to the solid surface. Microarray technology allows tens of thousands of nucleic acid sequences to be investigated at one time and is sensitive enough to detect a single base pair difference between two DNA samples. This technology can be used to determine which mRNAs are present in different cell types under different conditions. This is referred to as gene expression profiling and can be used for identifying gene expression changes or specific sequences associated with diseases or other genetic traits. This allows one to determine under what conditions genes may be turned on or off and, more specifically, what other genes are turned on or off at the same time. The ability to screen thousands of genes at one time with these methodologies will greatly advance our understanding of how genes are linked, as well as how modifications to the organism's environment may influence the expression of these genes.

19–6.3 *Proteomics*

The study of qualitative and quantitative comparisons of proteins produced under different conditions as part of complex biological processes is referred to as proteomics. While the genome may have 3 billion base pairs encoding 30,000 to 60,000 genes, a given cell may actively express only a small proportion of these genes. From these expressed genes, mRNA transcripts are produced that code for the production of proteins critical to cell survival and the biochemical integration of the organism. These mRNA transcripts may be spliced in different ways, allowing a single gene to give rise to several different protein products. While only specific or a limited complement of genes may be expressed in a given cell, several-fold magnitudes of protein products may be produced through posttranscriptional and posttranslational modifications (enzymatic cleavage, glycosylation, phosphorylation). Like genomics and the use of DNA microarrays, how modifications to the organism's environment may influence changes in the proteome of a cell or an organism is a natural extension from the expression of genes. As protein products are the ultimate effectors of gene expression events in biological processes, whether directly as a hormone or indirectly as an enzyme, proteomics may facilitate the selection of livestock based on protein expression patterns of specific tissues in conjunction with their overall gene map.

19–6.4 *Bioinformatics*

Also referred to as computational biology, bioinformatics is the application of computer technology to the management of the vast quantities of biological information produced by genomics and proteomics. Computers are used specifically to gather, store, analyze, integrate, and distill this information for further applications. Bioinformatics incorporates molecular biology into information technology (computer science) and enables the practical use of genomic and proteomic information for understanding complex biological processes. Genome sequencing and proteome profiling produce enormous amounts of information about gene positions on chromosomes and their linkages to other genes, as well as the vast complement of proteins that can be produced within and across species for specific cells or tissues under specific environmental conditions. Computational algorithms are used in bioinformatics to process genomic sequences to identify genes and predict their structure, identify mRNA and protein products, and pinpoint changes in gene and protein expression patterns spatially over time. This information, together with genetic experimentation on the role of genes in the development and physiology of livestock, could create a clearer picture, gene by gene, of cell and tissue functions (i.e., protein expression patterns). More important for livestock production, this information may indicate how these genes and their functions might be manipulated to enhance reproductive and production performance. Most bioinformatic databases are being produced in common domains for everyone to have access to worldwide and can be updated indefinitely as more information is compiled.

SUGGESTED READING

AMOAH, E. A. and S. GELAYE. 1997. Biotechnological advances in goat reproduction. *J. Anim. Sci.,* 75:578.

BONDIOLI, K. R. 1992. Embryo sexing: A review of current techniques and their potential for commercial application in livestock. *J. Anim. Sci.,* 70(Suppl. 2):19.

BONDIOLI, K. R., S. B. ELLIS, J. H. PRYOR, M. W. WILLIAMS, and M. M. HARPOLD. 1989. The use of male-specific chromosomal DNA fragments to determine the sex of bovine preimplantation embryos. *Theriogenology,* 31:95.

BRACKETT, B. G., D. BOUSQUET, M. L. BOICE, W. J. DONAWICK, J. F. EVANS, and M. A. DRESSEL. 1982. Normal development following *in vitro* fertilization in the cow. *Biol. Reprod.,* 27:147.

BREDBACHER, P., A. KANKAANPAA, and J. PEIPPO. 1995. PCR-sexing of bovine embryos: A simplified protocol. *Theriogenology,* 44:167.

CASSADY, J. P., R. K. JOHNSON, D. POMP, G. A. ROHRER, L. D. VAN VLECK, E. K. SPIEGEL, and K. M. GILSON. 2001. Identification of quantitative trait loci affecting reproduction in pigs. *J. Anim. Sci.,* 79:623.

CHANDLER, J. E., H. C. STEINHOLT-CHINEVERT, R. W. ADKINSON, and E. B. MOSER. 1998. Sex ratio variation between ejaculates within sire evaluated by polymerase chain reaction, calving, and farrowing records. *J. Dairy Sci.,* 81:1855.

CRAN, D. G., L. A. JOHNSON, and C. POLGE. 1995. Sex preselection in cattle: A field trial. *Vet. Rec.,* 136:495.

CUNNINGHAM, E. P. 1999. The application of biotechnologies to enhance animal production in different farming systems. *Livestock Production Science,* 58:1.

GANDOLFI, F. and R. M. MOOR. 1987. Stimulation of early embryonic development in the sheep by co-culture with oviduct epithelial cells. *J. Reprod. Fert.,* 81:23.

GWAZDAUSKAS, F. C. 2002. Gamete and embryo technology-transgenic animals. *Encyclopedia of Dairy Science.* eds. H. Roginski, J. W. Fuquay, and P. F. Fox. Academic Press, an Imprint of Elsevier Science.

HARE, W. C. D. and K. J. BETTERIDGE. 1978. Relationship of embryo sexing to other methods of prenatal sex determination in farm animals: A review. *Theriogenology,* 9:27.

HASLER, J. F. and D. L. GARNER. 2002. Gamete and embryo technology-sexed offspring. *Encyclopedia of Dairy Science.* eds. H. Roginski, J. W. Fuquay, and P. F. Fox. Academic Press, an imprint of Elsevier Science.

HOHENBOKEN, W. D. 1999. Applications of sexed semen in cattle production. *Theriogenology,* 52:1421.

JOHNSON, L. A. 1992. Gender preselection in domestic animals using flow cytometrically sorted sperm. *J. Anim. Sci.,* 70(Suppl. 2):8.

JORDAN, B. R. 2002. Molecular genetics and the dairy industry. *Encyclopedia of Dairy Science.* eds. H. Roginski, J. W. Fuquay, and P. F. Fox. Academic Press, an imprint of Elsevier Science.

KATO, Y. and Y. TSUNODA. 2002. Gamete and embryo technology-cloning. *Encyclopedia of Dairy Science.* eds. H. Roginski, J. W. Fuquay, and P. F. Fox. Academic Press, an imprint of Elsevier Science.

KRISHNER, R. L., R. M. PETERS, and B. H. JOHNSON. 1989. Effect of oviductal condition on the development of one-cell porcine embryos in mouse or rat oviducts maintained in organ culture. *Theriogenology,* 32:885.

LIU, A. and R. H. FOOTE. 1995. Development of bovine embryos in KSOM and added superoxide dismutase and taurine and with five and twenty percent O_2. *Biol. Reprod.,* 53:786.

MERMILLOD, P. 2002. Gamete and embryo technology-*In Vitro* fertilization. *Encyclopedia of Dairy Science.* eds. H. Roginski, J. W. Fuquay, and P. F. Fox. Academic Press, an imprint of Elsevier Science.

MONK, M. and A. H. HANDYSIDE. 1988. Sexing of preimplantation mouse embryos by measurement of X-linked gene dosage in a single blastomere. *J. Reprod. Fert.,* 82:365.

PARRISH, J. J., J. L. SUSKO-PARRISH, M. L. LEIBFRIED-RUTLEDGE, E. S. CRITSER, W. H. EYESTONE, and N. L. FIRST. 1986. Bovine *in vitro* fertilization with frozen-thawed semen. *Theriogenology,* 25:91.

POLGE, C. 1996. Historical perspectives of AI: Commercial methods of producing sex specific semen, IVF procedures. *Proc. 16th Tech. Conf. Artif. Insem. Reprod.,* p. 7. NAAB, Columbia, Mo.

ROTHSCHILD, M. F., C. JACOBSON, D. VASKE, C. TUGGLE, L. WANG, T. SHORT, G. ECKARDT, S. SASAKI, A. VINCENT, D. MCLAREN, O. SOUTHWOOD, H. VAN DER STEEN, A. MILEHAM, and G. PLASTOW. 1996. The estrogen receptor locus is associated with a major gene influencing litter size in pigs. *Proc. The National Academy of Science,* 93:201.

SEIDEL, G. E. JR., J. L. SCHENK, L. A. HERICKHOFF, S. P. DOYLE, Z. BRINK, R. D. GREEN, and D. G. CRAN. 1999. Insemination of heifers with sexed sperm. *Theriogenology,* 52:1407.

THIBIER, M. and M. NIBART. 1995. The sexing of bovine embryos in the field. *Theriogenology,* 43:71.

THURSTON, L. M., K. SIGGINS, A. J. MILEHAM, P. F. WATSON, and W. V. HOLT. 2002. Identification of amplified restriction fragment length polymorphism markers linked to genes controlling boar sperm viability following cryopreservation. *Biol. of Reprod.,* 66:545.

VAN VLIET, R. A., A. M. VERRINDER-GIBBINS, and J. S. WALTON. 1989. Livestock embryo sexing: A review of current methods, with emphasis on Y-specific DNA probes. *Theriogenology,* 32:421.

WACHTEL, S. S. 1984. H-Y antigen in the study of sex determination and control of sex ratio. *Theriogenology,* 21:18.

Reproductive Management

Management plays an important role in the reproductive efficiency obtained from both females and males. Unfortunately, reproductive efficiency approaching 100% is not possible even with the very best management; however, poor management can result in drastic decreases in reproductive efficiency.

20–1 Measurements of Reproductive Efficiency

Some guidelines for measuring reproductive efficiency are necessary in order to determine the effects of management practices.

20–1.1 *Services per Conception*

The measurement of services per conception is determined on a herd or flock basis by dividing total services by the number of pregnancies. Services per conception has little value for a large population of animals but is a valid measurement for a single herd or an individual female. On a herd basis, unidentified sterile females will make the calculation less meaningful.

20–1.2 *Parturition Rate*

Calving rate is calculated by dividing the total number of cows bred by the number that calved. It is also expressed as percent calf crop. Lambing, kidding, farrowing, and foaling rates are calculated in the same manner. This measurement of reproductive efficiency is frequently inflated by culling known open females after the breeding season and using the remainder in the calculation. Such inflated values are meaningless in evaluating reproductive efficiency. For multiparous species, the average number of live young produced per pregnancy must also be considered.

20–1.3 *Nonreturn Rates*

With the advent of AI, a means of evaluating the fertility level of semen in the shortest possible time was recognized as a serious need. Pregnancy examination information was too scattered and not readily available. Actual calving rates were too expensive to obtain and came too late to be of greatest value. Artificial insemination organizations began calculating nonreturn (NR) rates at intervals following inseminations. The NR is the percentage of females that do not return to estrus or receive a second service within a designated time interval. The time intervals most commonly used are 28- to 35-days, 60- to 90-days, and 150- to 180-days. Obviously, the shorter intervals provide earlier information, but the longer intervals provide more accurate information. The difference between 28- to 35-day NR rate and 60- to 90-day NR rate ranges from 10 to 15 percentage units. The 150- to 180-day NR rate is only 1 to 2 percentage units lower than the 60- to 90-day NR rate. For this reason, it is not often used.

Nonreturn rates are always higher than actual pregnancy rates because some nonpregnant cows are not reinseminated. Some are bred naturally and some are culled or die without being reinseminated. Even though NRs are relative, they do provide valuable information on males used in AI.

20–2 MANAGEMENT RELATED TO THE FEMALE

20–2.1 *Size and Age at First Insemination*

The main concern relative to when young females should be inseminated or bred for the first time is size. The size at the time of breeding is important because it influences the size of the animal at first parturition. The significance of size at parturition relates to both uncomplicated parturitions and productivity of the female. Dystocia is a serious problem with undersized females (Table 23–2). Larger females within a breed are more profitable producers. The effect of plane of nutrition on puberty and desired size at breeding is discussed in Chapter 23. The level of nutrition greatly affects the age at which puberty occurs, but once the female reaches puberty, neither size nor age affects conception rate within acceptable ranges of management. There are data indicating that cows bred for the first time between 4 and 5 years of age experience a significant increase in reproductive problems. It is extremely important that females grow at a rate that will allow them to reach desired size compatible with the desired age at first breeding. The data in Table 20–1 show the desired

Table 20–1   *Recommended body weight and size of heifers at puberty, first breeding, and first calving for the dairy breeds and selected beef breeds*

| Breed | Puberty (kg) | 1st breeding | | 1st calving (kg) |
		Weight (kg)	Heart girth (cm)	
Ayrshire	232	284	152	432
Brown Swiss	272	340	160	500
Guernsey	215	272	150	410
Holstein	272	340	160	500
Jersey	170	250	147	385
Angus	260	280	151	400
Hereford	260	280	151	400
Brahma	300	320	148	420

weight at puberty, first breeding, and first parturition for the dairy breeds and some selected beef breeds. Heifers of the dairy breeds should reach the desired first breeding weight at an average of 15 months so that they can calve at approximately 24 months of age. Heifers calving at older ages through 36 months will produce slightly more milk during first and possibly second lactations than heifers calving earlier. Heifers that calve at 24 months on the average will have a higher lifetime production than those calving later.

Managers of some commercial beef cattle operations have followed a practice of having their heifers calve for the first time at 3 years of age. The major and perhaps only reason for this practice is to have the heifers large enough to avoid calving difficulties at first parturition. More managers have taken a look at the total cost of carrying the heifer to 3 years of age for first calving versus the cost of growing them fast enough so that they will be large enough to calve at 2 years of age. In addition to an earlier economic return, there is the added advantage of a shorter generation interval. The reader is referred to Section 5–1 for recommended size at first breeding for the other species.

20–2.2 *Detection of Estrus*

In herds or flocks where artificial insemination is to be practiced, one of the most important management practices is detecting estrus so that insemination can be performed at the proper time. Synchronization of estrus as described in Chapter 18 may relieve the problem somewhat, especially with dairy cows, beef cows, sheep, goats, and swine.

20–2.2a Detection of Estrus in the Cow

The problem related to detection of estrus in cows is more critical than it is with other species because of their shorter and more variable length periods of estrus (Chapter 5). Research from Missouri indicates that herd managers need to improve their detection efficiency for estrus because on average they are detecting estrus in only about half of the estrus cycles in their herds. A surprising number of cows are being inseminated when not in estrus. The data in Table 20–2 illustrate the need for frequent observation for detecting estrus. Using twice daily checks at 6:00 A.M. and 6:00 P.M. as a basis for comparison, an additional check at 12:00 noon increased efficiency by 10%. A fourth observation at 12:00 midnight gave an increase in efficiency of 19.9% over the twice daily checks. Estrus expectancy lists were used as an aid in the detection of estrus. Not only does checking cows for estrus four times a day detect a higher percentage of cows in estrus so that they can be inseminated, but the beginning of estrus is

Table 20–2 *Cows detected in estrus when checked three or four times daily, compared with twice daily*

	Time checked				
Number of checks	A.M.	Noon	P.M.	Midnight	Increase (%)
2	6:00		6:00		Base
3	6:00	12:00	6:00		+10
4	6:00	12:00	6:00	12:00	+19.9

From Hall et al. *J. Dairy Sci.,* 42:1086, 1959.

Table 20–3   *Cows detected in estrus during A.M. versus P.M.*

	Number	Percent
A.M.	32,405	72.5
P.M.	12,302	27.5
Total cows	44,707	100.0

Adapted from Foote. *Search,* 8:1. Cornell University Agricultural Experiment Station, 1978.

more nearly determined so that insemination can be timed more accurately. The early morning check for estrus (as soon after daylight as possible) is the most important. More cows come into estrus between 2:00 A.M. and 5:00 A.M. than any other similar period of time during the day (Table 20–3).

   Checking cows for estrus should not be combined with other chores. It needs the full attention of the individual doing the checking. If feeding is done in connection with checking for estrus, the cows will have their minds on eating rather than demonstrating symptoms of estrus. The individual observing cows for estrus should be thoroughly familiar with all of the physiological and psychological symptoms of estrus (Chapter 5). He or she should move among the animals to be checked, causing as little distraction as possible. During the early morning check, if the cows are still lying down, they should be gotten up and moved around briefly and then carefully observed (Figure 20–1 and Color Plate 22).

   A number of aids are available that will reduce the likelihood of missing cows when in estrus. Of these, mount detectors are used the most extensively. A simple form of mount detector is to mark the tailhead with grease-type cattle marker or spray with paint. This method works well for lactating dairy cows because they go through the milking parlor regularly and can be remarked as needed. Frequently, rain will make remarking necessary. A number of mount detectors that can be glued on the tailhead are available on the market. All have a built-in signaling device to indicate if a cow has been mounted. This signal might be a capsule that turns red from the pressure of mounting (Figure 20–2 and Color Plate 23), a

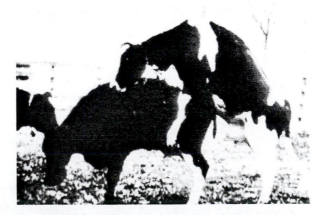

Figure 20–1   When checking cows for estrus, the one that stands when mounted is in estrus.

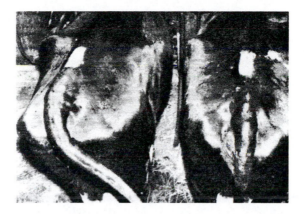

Figure 20–2 KAMAR® mount heat detectors aid detection of estrus. The detector on the right has turned red due to pressure from mounting cow.

blinking light, a flag that stands up, or an electronic signal transmitted to a microcomputer via a fixed radio antenna. The advantage of an electronic system is that it can indicate when the cow was first mounted and how many mounts were received. Some questions remain unanswered concerning cost: benefit ratio and the reliability and durability of the equipment. A disadvantage of mount detectors that are glued to the tailhead is that they are sometimes lost. Some give false-positives due to a false mount or pressure from rubbing on a tree or other structures. Other aids include pedometers to monitor level of walking activity and probes that measure the resistance of the vaginal mucus. Herd managers should choose an aid that will be accurate and cost-effective in their management system. The cost of failing to detect estrus is too high not to use one of the available aids.

For a mount detector to be effective, the cow or heifer must be mounted. Synchronization of estrus (Section 18–1.1) and managed breeding programs (Section 18–1.1e) are of benefit in detecting estrus because groups of animals will be in estrus at the same time, creating more mounting activity. Altering a male, such as a redirected prepuce (Section 20–4.4 and Color Plate 24), will provide an aggressive mounting animal. Such males are often fitted with a chin-ball marking harness, which eliminates the need for other types of mount detectors. Some livestock managers prefer to use cull heifers that have been treated with androgens as estrus checkers rather than using altered bulls. Androgenized heifers are safer, especially where dairy animals are concerned. Continued treatment provides an effective animal for long periods and androgen injections are easier and less expensive than some of the surgical procedures. In addition, the androgenized female poses no disease threat.

One procedure for treating cull heifers that has been used successfully is as follows: dissolve testosterone propionate in corn oil and inject 200 mg of the hormone intramuscularly every other day for a total of 10 injections. Thereafter, inject 1 gram of testosterone enanthate dissolved in corn oil intramuscularly at 14-day intervals for maintenance. Use of androgen-based, growth-promoting implants has worked well, also.

The androgenized heifers can be fitted with chin-ball marking devices. However, frequent observation so that cows in estrus can be observed standing while being mounted will help timing of inseminations.

Enzyme immunoassay methods for milk progesterone are available in kits that can be used at the farm. Results can be available in about 1 hour at a nominal cost. The procedure employs enzyme labeled progesterone which competes with the progesterone in the milk sample for binding sites on an antiprogesterone antibody bonded to a test paper (Section 4–10). The kits have their greatest economic value when used with genetically superior problem cows. Milk from these cows can be assayed for progesterone 21 to 24 days postbreeding to detect cows that have failed to conceive (Section 21–1.2). A second approach is to assay milk samples twice weekly beginning on day 18 postbreeding and continue until the progesterone level drops or until the cow can be confirmed pregnant by rectal palpation. Another application of the kits is in herds where management has to rely on a marginal labor force for detection of estrus. If the estrus status is uncertain, a high progesterone concentration would indicate that the cow is not in estrus, and a low concentration would indicate that the cow may be in estrus. When combined with other signs of estrus, it can help confirm a diagnosis. A veterinarian may use the kits as a training tool in client herds when detecting estrus is a problem but not perceived as a problem by the manager.

20–2.2b Detection of Estrus in the Ewe

Ewes do not demonstrate any signs of estrus when separated from the ram. Therefore, it is necessary to use an altered ram to detect ewes in estrus if AI is to be used. The vasectomized ram has been used most frequently, but rams with redirected prepuce are preferred because of reduced possibility of disease transmission. A dye material painted on the brisket or harness of the ram is usually used to identify the estrus ewe (Figure 20–3 and Color Plate 21). The ewe flock should be checked for estrus at least twice daily.

20–2.2c Detection of Estrus in the Doe

Does seldom show strong symptoms of estrus in the absence of the buck. Does occasionally mount each other, but not often. Pheromones from the buck's scent glands (Section 5–5) attract does and intensify their expression of estrual symptoms. Altered bucks can be used to check does for estrus as

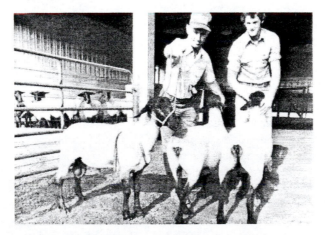

Figure 20–3 The ewe on the left has green chalk on the rump from the ram's harness. This technique can be used to record natural breeding dates or to detect ewes in estrus for AI.

with ewes. Bucks have also been placed in cages in the doe paddock. Estrus does will congregate around the cage, and other symptoms can be used to verify estrus. These include tail wagging, bleating, frequent urination, swelling of the vulva, and discharge of mucus.

20–2.2d Detection of Estrus in the Sow

Sows usually demonstrate sufficient symptoms of estrus to be detected. The vulva of the estrus gilt swells noticeably and the increased vascularity causes a reddish color, particularly in the white breeds. There will be no visible discharge of mucus from the vulva. Sows demonstrate the symptoms of estrus more plainly when boars are kept within hearing and smelling range. Both sows and boars produce pheromones that can be detected by the sense of smell. Sows respond to pheromone odor and the visual presence of, as well as noise made by, the boar. Sows can be checked to determine whether they are in standing estrus by applying pressure to the lumbar region. If she is in standing estrus, she will assume the mating stance (Figure 20–4 and Color Plate 20). The final sign of standing estrus is the "ear popping response," where the sow's ears will repeatedly jump to an erect position as she assumes the mating stance (Figure 20–4).

20–2.2e Detection of Estrus in the Mare

Usual symptoms of estrus in mares are frequent urination, followed by a series of contractions of the vulva which expose an erected clitoris—a process referred to as "winking" (Figure 20–5). The winking may continue for 2 to 3 minutes. Because of the variability in the behavior of mares, the most

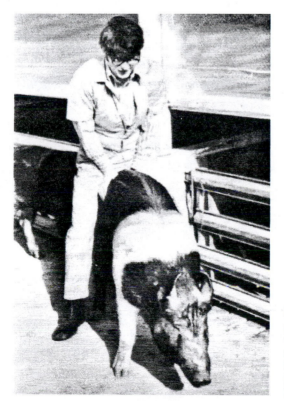

Figure 20–4 Method for detecting estrus in the sow. Note erect ears, wrinkles between eyes, and rigid stance with pressure applied to back in presence of boar. (From Pork Industry Handbook No. 64, Purdue University.)

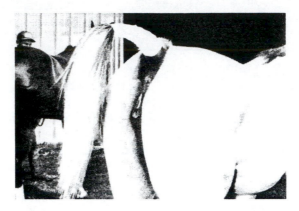

Figure 20–5   Estrus mare demonstrating the "winking" phenomenon following urination.

accurate means of detecting estrus involves teasing the mare with the stallion. In order to protect the stallion and the handler from being kicked by the mare, the teasing should be done over a teasing rail or half wall (brisket high). If the mare is in estrus, she will permit the stallion to bite her and will lower her rump and lift her tail to one side, in addition to frequent urination and winking. If she switches her tail and attempts to fight the stallion, she probably is not in estrus. Frequent urination and winking may occur during winter anestrus or during proestrus. Horse breeders should know the behavior of their mares, especially during estrus. Some mares show strong signs of estrus, while a few never accept the stallion. In the latter case, the breeder should palpate the ovaries to follow follicle growth so that the mare can be bred artificially when a follicle reaches 35 mm.

20–2.3   *Timing of Insemination*

Proper timing of artificial insemination or hand mating is essential for optimum conception rate. The length of sperm life in the female reproductive tract, sperm capacitation, and viable life of the ovum have been discussed in previous chapters, but all relate to the optimum timing of insemination. For most species, sperm life in the female tract is considered to be about 24 hours. It is reported to be longer in horses. Sperm capacitation in the rabbit takes about 4 hours but may require a longer time in other species. The ovum remains viable up to 8 to 12 hours, with a better chance of survival when a capacitated sperm comes in contact with it soon after ovulation. The length of the estrus cycle and the time of ovulation in relation to the beginning of estrus also play an important role in the timing of insemination. Within these confines, recommendations will be given for each of the five species (further discussion in Chapter 8).

20–2.3a Cows   Figure 20–6 shows the conception rate from inseminations performed at intervals from the beginning of estrus until after ovulation. It should be noted that the best conception rate is obtained from approximately the middle of estrus until about the end of estrus. The conception rate for those inseminations performed near the beginning of estrus is considerably lower indicating that, in many cases, sperm have lost their viability

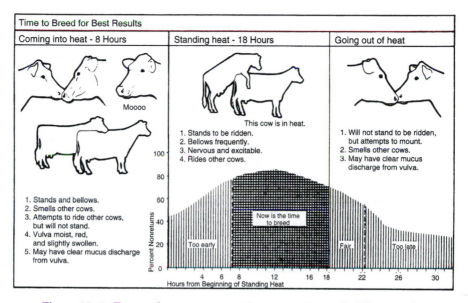

Figure 20–6 Expected average conception rates at intervals following the beginning of estrus. (From Asdell and Bearden. *Cornell Ext. Bull.*, 737, 1959.)

prior to the time of ovulation. It also appears that inseminations occurring less than 6 hours prior to ovulation also result in lowered conception. Ova may have aged before sperm capacitation is completed in such cases. Some conceptions may result from inseminations performed after presumed ovulation has occurred. Part or all of these may result from cows ovulating considerably later than expected.

A good rule of thumb to follow in a practical management situation is for cows first observed in estrus in the morning to be bred late the same day. Those cows first observed in the afternoon should be bred early the next morning. When cows are observed for estrus at midday, those detected in estrus for the first time should be inseminated as late as possible the same day (Tables 20–4 and 20–5). Accurate diagnosis of estrus is essential for proper timing of breeding. The data in Table 20–6 show the difference in nonreturn rate for cows in four management systems related to estrus detection. Cows turned out once and twice daily for estrus detection showed 5 and 6 percentage units higher nonreturn rate, respectively, when compared with those that remained in stanchions 24 hours a day. These data did not measure the difference in undetected estrus, but on the basis of the data in Table 20–2, one can assume a significant increase in percentage of detected estrus for those cows turned out twice daily.

20–2.3b Ewes Scientists still disagree as to when ewes should be inseminated for best conception. There seems to be more support for inseminating 12 to 18 hours after the onset of estrus than at other times. Most research has shown that two inseminations 24 hours apart will increase both conception rate and twinning rate. However, many do not feel that this increase is worth the extra time and effort required.

Table 20–4　*Time of insemination and 150- to 180-day percentage of nonreturns*

Time observed in estrus	Time inseminated	Number of cows	Nonreturns
Morning (A.M.)	Before noon, same day	1,308	67.1%
	Noon to 6 P.M., same day	27,320	69.9%
	After 6 P.M., same day	3,509	68.9%
	Before noon, next day	268	62.7%
Evening (P.M.)	Before noon, next day	6,893	69.9%
	Noon to 2 P.M., next day	4,948	67.4%
	After 2 P.M., next day	461	63.8%

From Foote. *Search*, 8:1. Cornell University Agricultural Experiment Station, 1978.

Table 20–5　*Recommended time for breeding cows and sows in relation to onset of estrus*

	Time to breed		Too late to breed	
Onset of estrus	Cow	Sow	Cow	Sow
A.M.	Same day	Next A.M.	Next day	Next P.M.
Noon	Late same day	Late next day	Noon next day	Late next day
P.M.	Early next day	Next P.M.	Late next day	Second P.M.

Table 20–6　*Effect of winter turn-out management on nonreturn rate in cows*

Practice	1st services	Number of herds	Nonreturns
No turn out	9,412	494	64.1%
Out once daily	47,365	3,237	69.5%
Out twice daily	4,070	348	70.4%
Pen stable	1,084	58	68.3%

From Bearden. *N.Y. Artificial Breeder's Cooperator,* 132, 1956.

20–2.3c Does　The length of the estrus cycle in the doe appears to be highly variable; however, some of this may be due to interpretation, since estrus in the doe is not well defined. The most commonly reported estrus period length is about 36 hours. Ovulation is generally reported as occurring a few hours after the end of estrus. A single insemination should be performed toward the end or soon after the end of standing estrus. There may be some advantage to two inseminations—the first 8 to 12 hours after the onset of estrus and the second 12 to 18 hours later.

20–2.3d Sows　The preferred time for breeding the sow when a single breeding, either natural service or AI is used, is approximately 24 hours after the onset of estrus (Table 20–5). The period of estrus in the sow lasts for 2 or 3 days (estrus in gilts is usually 24 hours shorter), with ovulation occurring at approximately midestrus or a little later. Multiple inseminations starting 12 hours after onset of estrus seems to be standard practice because double inseminations increase farrowing rate by 8% to 12% and litter size by 0.2 pigs. However, gilts that remain in estrus less than 2 days fail to show increased reproductive performance with multiple inseminations. Based on the latest research, a better approach is to inseminate all sows and gilts on day 1 and, only if they are still in estrus on the second day, inseminate a second time.

In swine, a large volume of semen is deposited directly into the uterus and induces an inflammation response in the form of an influx of neutrophilic granulocytes beginning 2 hours after insemination. Excess semen and inflammatory products need to be eliminated from the uterus to ensure a favorable environment for the embryos before they descend. Inseminations made during late estrus and during metestrus may result in the embryos reaching the uterus during the peak of the inflammatory period. Such inseminations have resulted in a decrease of 20% in farrowing rate and 1.1 pigs per litter.

20–2.3e Mares   The optimum time for inseminating or hand breeding the mare is more difficult to determine than for the other species. Ovulation occurs near the end of estrus whether the mare has a 3-day or an 8-day estrus period. Best results without palpation are obtained by multiple breedings starting on the third day and repeating at 48-hour intervals until the mare is no longer in estrus. When only one breeding is desired because of a heavy breeding schedule for the stallion, it is recommended that the mare be palpated and bred when she has a 35-mm follicle. She should be palpated 2 days later to see if ovulation occurred and, if not, she should be rebred. When two follicles are present, ovulation will occur when the follicles are about 25 mm in diameter. An ultrasound transducer is available for intrarectal use. It is held against the ovary with the palpating hand to accurately measure the diameter of the follicle. The practice of whether or not to breed a mare when two large follicles are present has changed. Breeding these mares increases conception from 50% to 75%. Doing so requires the use of ultrasound at 15 days postbreeding. When twins are diagnosed and both are in the same horn, nothing needs to be done. In almost all cases, one will be reabsorbed; however, these mares should be reexamined 25 days later. If both twins are still living, the mare should be aborted. When the fetuses are in different horns, one should be manually destroyed. Twins allowed to continue are usually aborted and, when they are carried to term, they are so small and weak that they do not survive. Some breeders inject LH at the time of breeding to ensure ovulation while sperm are viable.

20–2.4 *Rest After Parturition*

Sexual rest following parturition is more of a problem with dairy cows than with other species because they resume cycling before uterine recovery is completed. As described in Chapter 9, uterine involution in the cow includes the return of the uterus to the pelvic area, return to its nonpregnant size, and a recovery of normal uterine tone. The average time required for this is 45 days (Figure 10–4). However, histological studies have shown that another 15 days may be required before the endometrium is histologically normal. Dairy herd managers should palpate the involuting uterus at 35 days postpartum to determine whether normal progress is being made. Treatment should be provided for those cows not making normal progress.

On the basis of this information, researchers have for many years recommended that cows not be bred until the first estrus occurring after 60 days postpartum. The conception rate at this time will be 10 to 15 percentage units higher than those cows bred one estrus

Table 20–7   *Relationship of postpartum breeding interval to percent nonreturns and interval to conception*

Interval, calving to 1st breeding (days)	Number of cows	150- to 180-day nonreturns	Interval, calving to conception (days)	Projected calving interval (days)
0–19	47	40%	64	342
20–29	208	46%	58	336
30–39	459	45%	64	342
40–49	1,170	51%	70	348
50–59	2,203	59%	76	354
60–69	3,192	65%	85	363
70–79	3,412	66%	93	371
80–89	2,899	69%	103	381
90–99	2,059	69%	113	391
100	3,984	71%	156	434
All	19,633	66%	102	380

Adapted from Foote. *Search,* 8:1. Cornell University Agricultural Experiment Station, 1978.

period earlier (Table 20–7). Following this recommendation, about 90% of the cows in a well-managed herd will maintain an average calving interval of approximately 12 months. The remaining 10% are classified as problem cows and, even with veterinary assistance, up to 50% of these cows may never conceive.

During recent years, a few individuals have recommended that cows be bred at the first estrus after 40 days postpartum. This recommendation has been made for herds with average calving intervals of 14 to 15 months as a means of shortening the calving interval as near to 12 months as possible. To the authors, this is an attempt at finding a solution while avoiding the real problem, which in most cases is poor management. We do not think that the introduction of a questionable management practice to camouflage other poor management is acceptable. Perhaps 45% to 50% of the cows bred between 40 and 60 days postpartum will conceive to first service, and these cows will have an average calving interval of only 330 days (50 plus 280). In high-producing herds, all calving intervals as short as 330 days should be avoided for optimum milk production, and certainly there is no justification for having 40% of a herd with calving intervals that short. Furthermore, the same cows that become pregnant to the service between 40 and 60 days would also conceive to first service between 60 and 80 days and, in the latter case, would have acceptable calving intervals.

Short postpartum intervals usually are not a problem with beef cattle. The beef cattle manager usually is more concerned with getting the cows started cycling so that they can be serviced early enough to maintain 12-month calving intervals. Refer to Section 25–3 for treatment for anestrus.

Mares will come into estrus from 7 to 12 days after parturition (foaling heat) and can usually be rebred with good results. However, mares should be bred at this time only if they have been given a careful examination to determine if there has been adequate recovery since parturition. Mares considered ready for rebreeding will have as good a chance of conceiving at the foal heat as at later estrus periods. A good rule of thumb is to check the mare on day 7 and, if there is any question about her recovery, wait until the next estrus, which will occur about 30 days postpartum. Reasons not to breed at foaling heat include (1) bruised cervix; (2) lacerations of the cervix or vagina; (3) vaginal discharge; (4) lack of uterine tone; or (5) placenta retained more than 2 hours.

Sows have a farrowing heat a few days after parturition. Fertilization is low at this time because of failure to ovulate. The next estrus will occur about 7 days following weaning, and, if sows are well nourished, uterine recovery will be complete. Ovulation and conception should be normal. Following late fall and winter weanings, some sows enter a period of anestrus. An injection of PG 600 (PMSG 400 IU and hCG 200 IU) should initiate cycling. Some managers prefer to breed sows at the second estrus following weaning of pigs.

20–2.5 *Reproductive Records*

A complete set of records is absolutely essential for good reproductive management. Records which should be kept on each female are (1) permanent identification; (2) parturition date; (3) date of first estrus after parturition and all subsequent estrus dates; (4) breeding dates with identification of service sire; (5) results of preliminary pregnancy checks between 35 and 40 days postbreeding; (6) results of final pregnancy check at 60 days or as soon thereafter as possible; (7) calculated due date; (8) date to turn dry (dairy); (9) actual parturition date; and finally (10) identification, sex, and disposition of offspring. In addition, notation should be made at parturition of abnormal occurrences such as dystocia and retained placenta. Any abnormal discharge, including cloudiness or flakes in estrual mucus, should be noted. Record all treatments, whether performed by the livestock manager or by a veterinarian, along with a diagnosis and the date. A general herd health record is desirable and can be maintained along with the reproductive records. Include such items as diagnosis and treatment for mastitis, all vaccinations, and the diagnosis and treatments performed for any other health problem.

We recommend that a daily barn sheet be filled out (Figure 20–7). A record station should be established at a convenient location so that daily events may be recorded as they occur. A pocket notebook and pencil should be carried so that notes may be made while going about daily routines. These notes will help make the daily barn sheet record more accurate and complete. The manager should check the daily barn sheet at the end of the day to ensure that all information has been recorded. The daily records are temporary and should be transferred to a permanent record system.

The livestock manager needs to organize records so that the reproductive status of the animal can be monitored daily, simply, and easily. For dairy herds, a good management tool, the *Dairy Herd Monitor,* is available (Figure 20–8). It is designed as a revolving circle, divided into the 12 months with the respective number of days for each month. Color-coded, self-adhesive, removable stickers are used to identify each cow's breeding status. Blue represents cows that have not been bred since calving. Red represents bred cows and cows programmed for breeding. Previous estrus dates remind the manager when to expect cows in estrus. First and repeat breedings are registered by recording the service sire's name or number on the sticker. Green represents confirmed pregnancy. Yellow represents dry cows. The manager is reminded to dry treat for mastitis and it gives a countdown of days to parturition. The revolving circle is rotated one space daily to correct calendar date. With this tool, no cow is lost with respect to reproductive status. The herd manager is constantly reminded of what needs to be done, when it needs to be done, and what to expect and when.

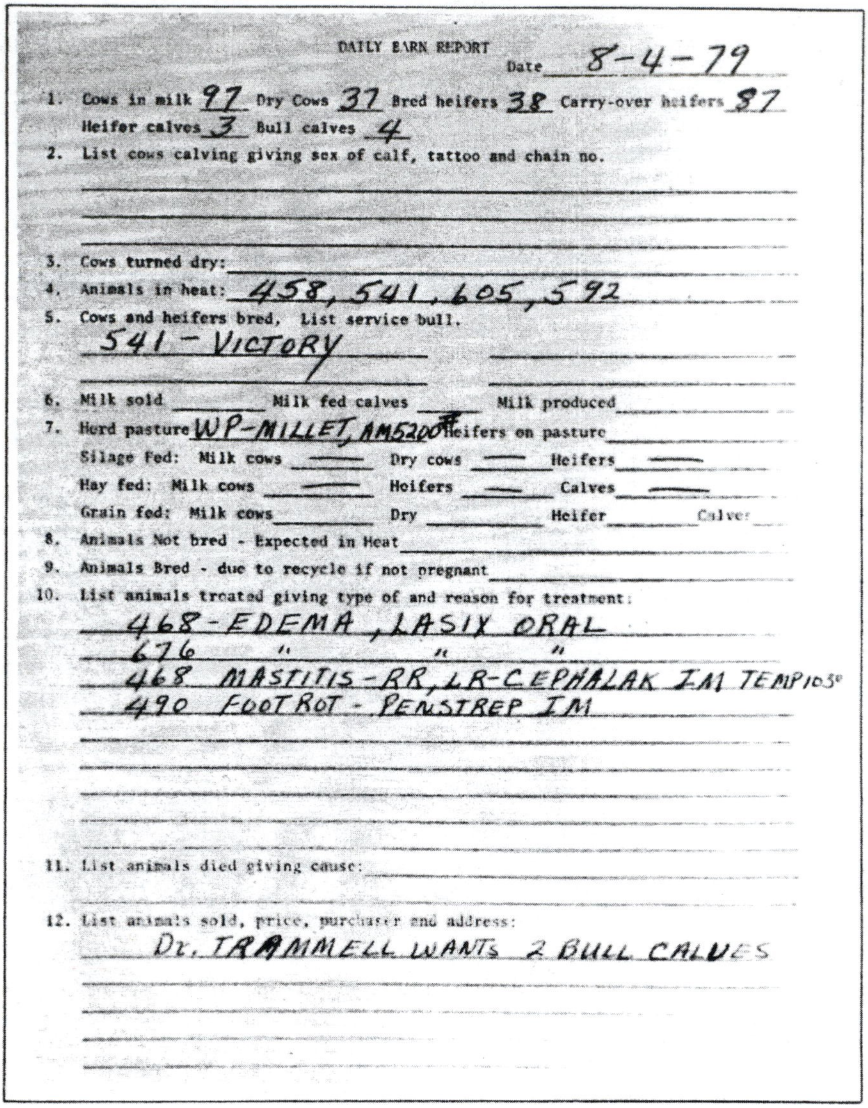
DAILY BARN REPORT

Date 8-4-79

1. Cows in milk 97 Dry Cows 37 Bred heifers 38 Carry-over heifers 87
Heifer calves 3 Bull calves 4
2. List cows calving giving sex of calf, tattoo and chain no.
3. Cows turned dry:
4. Animals in heat: 458, 541, 605, 592
5. Cows and heifers bred, List service bull.
541 – VICTORY
6. Milk sold ______ Milk fed calves ______ Milk produced ______
7. Herd pasture WP-MILLET, AM5200 Heifers on pasture ______
Silage Fed: Milk cows —— Dry cows —— Heifers ——
Hay fed: Milk cows —— Heifers —— Calves ——
Grain fed: Milk cows ______ Dry ______ Heifer ______ Calves ______
8. Animals Not bred - Expected in Heat ______
9. Animals Bred - due to recycle if not pregnant ______
10. List animals treated giving type of and reason for treatment:
468-EDEMA, LASIX ORAL
676 " " "
468 MASTITIS-RR, LR-CEPHALAK IM TEMP 105°
490 FOOTROT - PENSTREP IM
11. List animals died giving cause:
12. List animals sold, price, purchaser and address:
Dr. TRAMMELL WANTS 2 BULL CALVES

Figure 20–7 A daily barn sheet used in a dairy herd.

Data from the daily barn sheet should be transferred to permanent records on a regular basis. Permanent records include

1. *Individual female card.* The information pertinent to each female should be transferred from the daily barn sheet to the individual female card. This card provides a lifetime breeding and health history (Figure 20–9).
2. *Breeding book.* This should be a hardback ledger book. Each breeding should be recorded in chronological order. The date, female identification number, service number, and service sire identification should be recorded for each breeding. Not only is

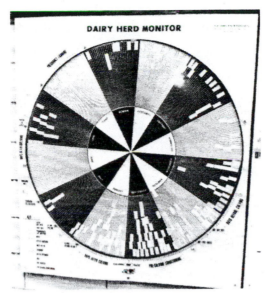

Figure 20–8 The Dairy Herd Monitor gives a graphic picture of the reproductive status of a herd.

HERD NO. 631
GP 83 (5-13-74)
MAGNOLIA ARCHIES GEM 7515888
EMPEROR DUKE ARCHIE 1320310
MAGNOLIA ALERT GEM 6292470
DATE OF BIRTH 8-2-69
TATTOO OR EAR TAG RIGHT E589 LEFT E589
MASTITIS & UDDER HEALTH
BREEDING RECORD
CALF RECORD
20cc Forte II in Udder 12/2/71 12/15/71
10cc Forte II & 10cc 1/25/72 3/1/71
4/14/74 2/12/73 Elevation
11/6/71 Dead
12/12/72 F
DIAGNOSIS AND TREATMENT BY VETERINARIAN
REPRODUCTIVE DISEASES
OTHER DISEASES
12/1/71 Uterine Infection 150cc Furacin, Penstrep, & Estrodiol
12/14/72 Fresh Neomycin Bols in uterus
1/25/73 Estrus 40cc Furacin in uterus for Experiment
Post Breeding 40cc Penstrep, 120cc. Furacin. I.U.
11/2/74 Penstrep & Furacin Intra V.
8/22/75 Uterine Inj.
8/5/74 Severe Mastitis Sulfa Boluses orally, Penstrep IM
8/6/74
8/9/74
8/10,11,
8/21/74

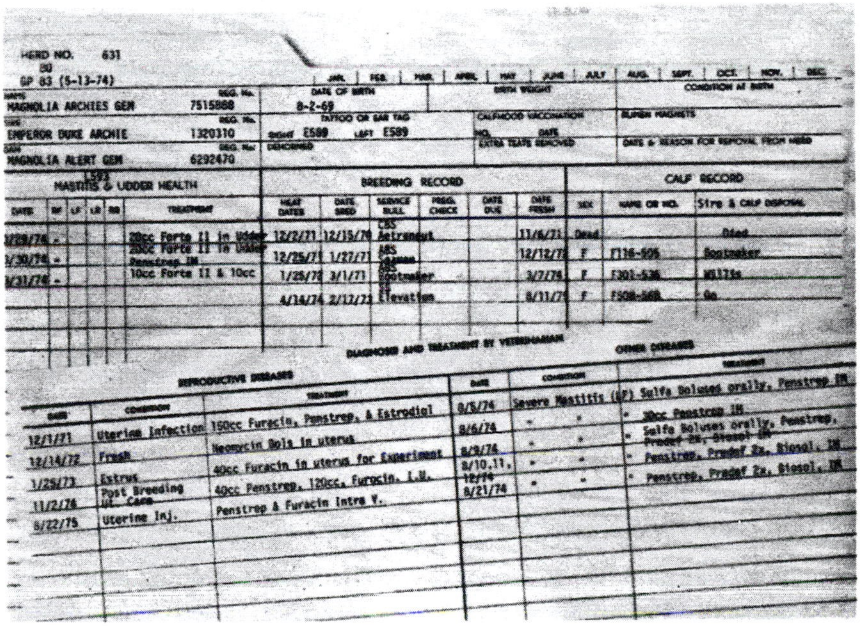

Figure 20–9 Lifetime record card used for individual animals.

this information valuable from a reproductive point of view, but it is also essential in providing the necessary information for registering offspring in a purebred herd (Figure 20–10).

3. *Offspring book.* This should also be a hardback ledger book. A sample page from an offspring book is shown in Figure 20–11. On the left-hand sheet, tattoo number, date

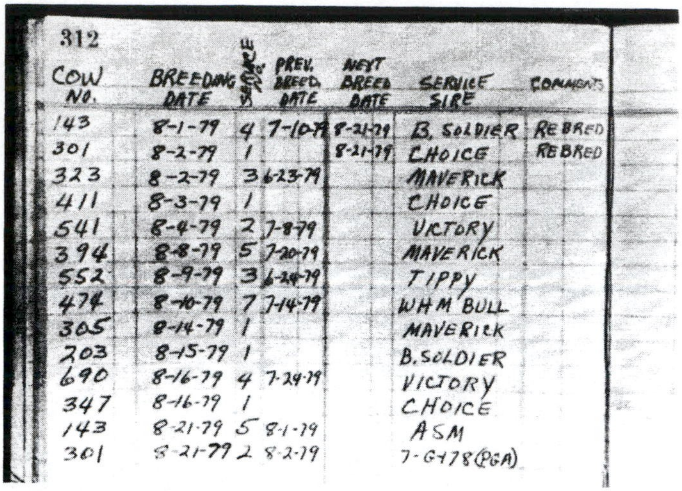

312

COW NO.	BREEDING DATE	SERVICE	PREV. BREED. DATE	NEXT BREED DATE	SERVICE SIRE	COMMENTS
143	8-1-79	4	7-10-79	8-21-79	B. SOLDIER	REBRED
301	8-2-79	1		8-21-79	CHOICE	REBRED
323	8-2-79	3	6-23-79		MAVERICK	
411	8-3-79	1			CHOICE	
541	8-4-79	2	7-8-79		VICTORY	
394	8-8-79	5	7-20-79		MAVERICK	
552	8-9-79	3	6-24-79		TIPPY	
474	8-10-79	7	7-14-79		WHM BULL	
305	8-14-79	1			MAVERICK	
203	8-15-79	1			B. SOLDIER	
690	8-16-79	4	7-29-79		VICTORY	
347	8-16-79	1			CHOICE	
143	8-21-79	5	8-1-79		ASM	
301	8-21-79	2	8-2-79		7-G178 (PGA)	

Figure 20–10 Sample page from a breeding ledger book.

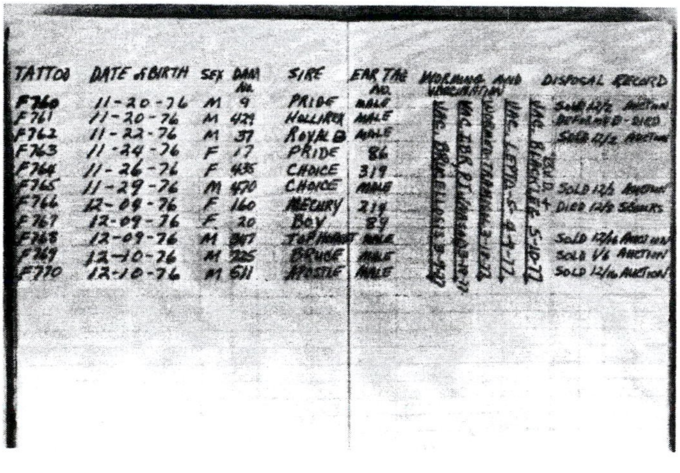

TATTOO	DATE of BIRTH	SEX	DAM No.	SIRE	EAR TAG No.	DISPOSAL RECORD
F760	11-20-76	M	9	PRIDE	MALE	SOLD 12/2 AUCTION
F761	11-20-76	M	429	HALLIREX	MALE	DEFORMED-DIED
F762	11-22-76	M	37	ROYAL B	MALE	SOLD 12/2 AUCTION
F763	11-24-76	F	17	PRIDE	86	
F764	11-26-76	F	435	CHOICE	319	
F765	11-29-76	M	470	CHOICE	MALE	SOLD 12/2 AUCTION
F766	12-09-76	F	160	MECURY	219	DIED 12/3 SCOURS
F767	12-09-76	F	20	BOY	89	
F768	12-09-76	M	347	TOP HONOR	MALE	SOLD 12/16 AUCTION
F769	12-10-76	M	325	BRUCE	MALE	SOLD 1/6 AUCTION
F770	12-10-76	M	611	APOSTLE	MALE	SOLD 12/16 AUCTION

Figure 20–11 Sample pages from an offspring ledger book. Note the vaccination and worming record on the right.

of birth of offspring, sex, and dam and sire identification are recorded. The right-hand page is used for ear tag number, immunization and worming records, and disposal records.

The record system outlined here is highly recommended in its entirety for dairy herds. Since dairy herds are more intensely managed than most beef herds and the other species, managers may want to use the portions best suited to their needs or make modifications. Regardless of the record system used, all of the information listed will be useful in managing any species.

The Dairy Herd Improvement Association (DHIA) record program is available to dairy herd managers. This is an official computerized record-keeping program sponsored by the state agricultural colleges. In addition to production records, certain information pertaining to the reproductive status of the individual cow and the entire herd is provided. Information is recorded on a monthly barn sheet, which is mailed to a regional dairy record processing center. A computer printout is mailed back to the dairy manager in about 10 days. The record on reproductive status of the individual cow is updated monthly and shows the number of days open (not pregnant) or number of days pregnant along with the last breeding date. A reproductive efficiency summary is provided for the herd. The number of cows open less than 60 days, the number open for 60 to 100 days, and the number open more than 100 days are shown. Total number of pregnant cows, average days open, projected minimum calving interval, number of breedings during the past 12 months, conception rate, and percentage of problem cows are also provided.

There are some other computerized record systems. Some are sponsored by the Cooperative Extension Service and some are commercial. These systems usually provide production and management information and a complete set of financial records.

20–2.6 *Detecting Reproductive Problems*

Records mentioned in the preceding section are absolutely essential for early detection of reproductive problems. Early detection is necessary for two reasons: (1) problems are much easier to correct when detected early, and (2) problems corrected early result in less loss of reproductive time and money.

Before one can detect problems, it is necessary to have standards for comparison. The following criteria can be used for this purpose in dairy herds and can serve as guidelines for beef cattle and other species.

1. At least 90% of the cycling cows (after 40 days postpartum) should be detected each estrus period. This will require at least two and preferably three checks for estrus per day.
2. From 60% to 65% of the cows will calve to first service. Pregnancy diagnosis at 60 days postbreeding will also reflect these percentages.
3. There should be no more than 10% of the cows classified as problem cows at any one time. Problem cows are those that (1) fail to conceive to three services, (2) continue to have abnormal discharges and/or uninvoluted uteri beyond 60 days postpartum, or (3) open more than 100 days.
4. The number of cows leaving the herd because of failure to breed should not exceed 5% in any 12-month period.
5. The average number of services per pregnancy should be 2 or fewer. In a 100-cow herd, this allows for 100 first services to which 60 cows become pregnant, 40 second services with 20 becoming pregnant, and 20 third services with 10 becoming pregnant. This accounts for 90 cows with 160 total services and leaves up to 40 services for the remaining 10 problem cows. The actual number of services utilized will depend on the extent of the problems and how soon the nonbreeders are eliminated from the herd.

Managers should be especially alert for

1. Abnormal discharge (blood or pus) at any time. A small amount of blood without pus about 24 to 36 hours after estrus is probably normal metestrus bleeding and should cause no alarm.

2. A nonpregnant cow not observed in estrus by 50 days postpartum. The cow may be in anestrus, but, if palpation reveals a corpus luteum on an ovary, she is cycling but not being detected in estrus.

3. An estrus cycle of irregular length (less than 18 days or more than 24 days). Short cycles are an indication of ovarian dysfunction, and long cycles are an indication of embryonic or fetal loss or undetected estrus.

4. Continuous or prolonged estrus (more than 24 hours). This condition is an indication of follicular cysts.

5. Retained placenta. From 5% to 15% retained placentae can be expected in healthy herds. There seems to be a breed difference between dairy breeds, as well as a lower incidence in beef cattle than with dairy cattle (Table 20–8).

6. Observable abortions. Every cow that aborts should be suspected of having a contagious disease. A veterinarian should be called in to make a diagnosis in each case.

7. Cows that have not settled to three services. These cows are classified as problem cows and veterinary assistance may be desirable.

In most herds, problem situations are usually related to individual cows. Any one of the mentioned symptoms is serious for that particular cow, and she should be handled as an individual case. These symptoms do not necessarily indicate an infectious disease. However, disease should not be ruled out, as many of the listed symptoms can be caused by one or more infectious diseases. If more than 10% of the herd is affected by a combination of these symptoms, a herd problem probably exists. Whether the problems relate to individual cows or the entire herd, it is essential to act quickly to correct the problems. Early treatment increases the likelihood of successful correction of the problem and reduces losses from delayed breeding and sterility.

Prevention is far superior to cure. A good herd health program carried out in conjunction with a veterinarian is by far the most economical approach to maintaining a healthy herd. In such a program, the veterinarian should visit the herd at least once a month to provide the following services: (1) examine all cows between 30 and 60 days postpartum to determine if the uteri are involuting properly; (2) administer calfhood vaccination for brucellosis and perhaps other vaccinations, depending on the expertise of the livestock manager; (3) examine and/or treat cows with mastitis problems; (4) examine and/or treat

Table 20–8   *Incidence of retained placenta in the Mississippi State University dairy herd by breed (Jan. 1971–Dec. 1977)*

Breed	Mean percentage
Ayrshire	25.5
Jersey	2.3*
Guernsey	28.2
Holstein	22.1
Brown Swiss	27.3

Watts et al. *Proceedings So. Div. ADSA,* 1979.

*Means differ ($P < .05$).

cows with reproductive problems; and (5) perform pregnancy diagnosis if the livestock manager is not proficient in this practice. A herd health program of this nature should reduce the number of emergency visits by the veterinarian to treat acute problems.

20–3 MANAGEMENT RELATED TO THE MALE

20–3.1 *Age and Size Factors in Semen Production*

The age at puberty was discussed in Chapter 6 and will not be covered here, except to reemphasize that level of feeding can hasten or delay the onset of puberty. Size is also affected by level of feeding and, from the time of puberty until the mature age is reached, it is difficult to separate age and size, particularly in well-managed herds. The data in Table 20–9 show semen characteristics of a Holstein bull during the 4 years following puberty. The ejaculate volume and total sperm produced per year more than doubled between the first and fourth years. Sperm concentration increased between the first and second year but remained essentially constant for the remaining years. The size of the bull is not given, but it is reasonable to assume that the bull continued to grow even through the fourth year.

A number of studies have shown a highly significant correlation of 0.90 between testes size and body weight. Even though the relationship between testes size and body weight diminishes after puberty, larger males of the same species will usually have larger testes than smaller males.

The relationship between testes size and sperm output has a significant correlation of 0.80. It is apparent, then, that, the larger the male, the larger the testes will be and the greater the output of sperm. Most work of this nature has been done with bulls but it also relates to the other species.

20–3.2 *Bull Handling Techniques*

Bulls in general, and dairy bulls in particular, can be dangerous and should be handled accordingly. Dairy bulls should never be allowed to run in a pasture or paddock where humans need to enter. The student is referred to Section 13–1 for facilities needed for handling bulls.

Table 20–9 *Semen characteristics of a Holstein bull ejaculated three times per week, 4 consecutive years following puberty*

Characteristic	Year			
	1st	2nd	3rd	4th
No. ejaculates	153	151	143	135
Av. volume/ejaculate ml	2.8	3.8	5.0	6.0
Sperm concentration (10^6/ml)	1,089	1,530	1,513	1,451
Total sperm produced (10^9)	523	898	1,093	1,197

From VanDemark et al. *J. Dairy Sci.*, 39:1071, 1956.

The frequency of collection of semen for artificial insemination will depend a great deal on the need for semen from a particular bull. If the goal is maximum spermatozoa harvest, the bull may be collected as often as his libido will allow. Bulls have been collected daily for an extended period (300 days) with no decrease in semen quality or conception rate. The volume and total sperm collected per day decreased in some bulls to the point of not being practical for commercial processing. In such situations, two ejaculates may be collected every other day to achieve similar sperm harvest with a greater number of sperm available each processing day. The major U.S. bull studs are routinely collecting individual bulls twice or three times a week. Three ejaculates are collected per day for the twice weekly group and two ejaculates per day for the three times a week group. There are some bulls that cannot maintain acceptable volume or sperm numbers when collected that often. Those with superior genetic value are collected less frequently, but lesser-quality bulls are soon culled.

In natural mating, it is desirable to match each bull with the number of cows that he can handle without exhaustion during the specified breeding season. These bulls may be ejaculating several times per day for several consecutive days, and, if there are too many cows in estrus at one time, some may not be bred or the bull's sperm supply may become depleted before all the cows have come into estrus.

Proper nutrition is extremely important for both the young, growing bull and the mature bull. Overfeeding and underfeeding adversely affect health and libido of males. Further discussion can be found in Chapter 23.

Exercise was once thought to be essential for maintaining semen quality and fertility levels. More closely controlled experiments have disproven this idea by showing that bulls maintained for 6 months or more in tie stalls or box stalls maintain conception rates equal to those that were forced to exercise for 30 minutes per day. This is not to imply that exercise is unnecessary, however. It is reasonable to expect that bulls that have an opportunity to exercise regularly will experience less lameness and will require less hoof trimming. There may be other beneficial effects from exercise related to maintaining a healthy animal.

Transporting bulls from one location to another need not be a factor in maintaining fertility. Care should be taken to maintain comfortable conditions for the bull that is being transported and to prevent injury. Moving the bull from familiar quarters to unfamiliar quarters does not seem to have any affect on fertility. Care should be taken to prevent stress when moving and handling bulls.

20–3.3 *Reproductive Management of the Stallion*

Young stallions should be separated from fillies when they are weaned. They will not have reached puberty by weaning, and separation at this time is easy to incorporate into the management routine. As 2-year-olds, they should be limited to four or five mares. The goal of the breeder is to give the 2-year-olds training and experience. Three-year-olds can be used three or four times weekly, permitting 20 to 30 mares to be scheduled to them during the breeding season. Older stallions can be used once per day for 5 or 6 days a week or twice a day three times per week. This will permit the scheduling of about 40 mares to an older stallion during a breeding season. Frequency of use will usually be limited by libido rather than by semen quality.

If demand for a stallion is high, his total services can be increased by a factor of about 10 during a breeding season through use of AI. Approximately 5 billion sperm can be collected from a stallion in a day. Using the recommended 500 million sperm per insemination, 10 inseminations per day is possible. To gain maximum utilization of semen from an AI program, synchronization of mares should be scheduled to ensure that enough mares are in estrus when the semen is collected. Twice as many mares can be bred if they are palpated and inseminated when the follicle is 35 mm, as compared with breeding every other day without palpation. The palpation technique applies to both AI and natural mating. Ultrasonography can be used to supplement palpation to determine when the follicle is approaching maturity.

When a stallion is evaluated for purchase or use in a breeding program, several items should be on the evaluation checklist. The first three items are best evaluated during the breeding season. (1) Semen quality tests should include concentration (no less than 50×10^6 sperm per ml), motility (no less than 40% progressive), volume (preferably 40 ml or more), and morphology (no more than 25% total abnormal sperm). See Chapter 15 for procedures for conducting these tests. (2) Reaction time or libido of the stallion should be checked with an estrus mare. During the breeding season, expected reaction time is about 2 minutes. During the winter, his reaction time may be about 10 minutes. (3) The temperament of the stallion is important, as to both ease in handling and whether he chews excessively on the mares during teasing. Other items to evaluate include (4) his past breeding record, (5) his health record, and (6) his conformation. See Chapter 26 for diseases that cause reproductive problems in equine.

20–3.4 *Breeding Fitness Tests for Males*

A high percentage crop of offspring in herds and flocks being mated naturally is dependent to a large degree on using males capable of producing semen that has a high fertility level. Unfortunately, there is no laboratory test that will determine the fertility level of semen (Chapter 15). The best that can be done is to collect semen from the male and subject it to certain quality tests. The quality tests normally performed are gross examination and motility. In some cases, concentration and morphology of the sperm are also determined. The student is referred to Chapter 15 for procedures for conducting these quality tests. Other factors to consider are genetics-related traits, whether the individual is free of transmissible diseases (especially those affecting the reproductive processes), and the results of a physical examination.

A satisfactory sample of semen will have a good concentration as indicated by an opaque, milky-white color. The sample should have 40% or greater progressive motility, and if morphology is performed, the sample should have less than 25% abnormal sperm. Semen that falls below the satisfactory standards on one or more of the three criteria would be classified as questionable. Samples that are clear or watery, indicating few or no sperm, would be classified as cull. Samples with good concentration but with an extremely high level of abnormal sperm or very low motility should also be classified as cull.

Bulls producing questionable or cull-quality semen may be rechecked 1 month later if the owner desires. Experience shows that only about 1 out of every 30 bulls classified as questionable or cull will improve enough that the semen can be classified as satisfactory. Rechecks can be justified only on genetically superior bulls.

The semen from young bulls should be checked, but one should remember that beef bulls usually reach puberty later than dairy bulls. Most bulls of the European breeds can be checked for semen quality at about 14 months of age, but other breeds should not be checked until they are about 18 months old. Ejaculates from young bulls will have a lower volume and usually a lower concentration than ejaculates from older bulls.

Semen quality checks should be made on bulls 2 months before the breeding season. This will allow time for retest, should such be desirable, and it will also allow time to find replacement bulls for those that need to be culled.

Transmissible diseases should always be of concern in a natural mating program. The easiest way to maintain a disease-free herd once this status is attained is to maintain a closed herd. This means introducing no breeding animals, either male or female, from outside the herd. This frequently is not possible, so it is necessary to use safeguards. When buying bulls for breeding, it is safer to buy prepuberal bulls and keep them isolated until health checks can be performed. If breeding age bulls must be purchased, it is absolutely essential that they be tested for certain communicable diseases. They must be tested for brucellosis, vibriosis, leptospirosis, and trichomoniasis (Chapter 26). In addition, it is desirable to test for the three more common viruses, infectious bovine rhinotracheitis, bovine virus diarrhea (BVD), and parainfluenza-3. The bull should be tested prior to purchase and kept isolated from the rest of the herd for 30 to 60 days until a second test can be performed.

One genetic trait that can be quantified is scrotal circumference. Thresholds by age groups are as follows:

15 months or less	30 cm
15 to 18 months	31 cm
18 to 21 months	32 cm
21 to 24 months	33 cm

Scrotal circumference directly reflects testes diameter, which in turn determines amount of sperm-producing tissue. Bulls not meeting these thresholds would likely be poor sperm producers.

Mating behavior should be evaluated because a male that scores well on other fitness criteria may not have high libido. The male should be observed in the presence of females that are in estrus. The evaluation could include time until the first copulation, time to repeated copulation, number of copulations until sexual exhastion is reached, and time needed to recover from sexual exhaustion.

Based on these breeding fitness tests, bulls can be classified into three categories:

1. *Satisfactory*—equal or surpass the minimum thresholds for scrotal circumference and sperm quality tests and do not show genetic, infectious disease, or other faults that could compromise breeding ability or fertility.

2. *Unsatisfactory*—below one or more of the thresholds and highly unlikely to ever improve their status; also, bulls that show genetic faults or irrevocable physical problems (including infectious disease) that would compromise breeding ability or fertility.

3. *Classification deferred*—do not fit into either of the preceding categories and could benefit from a retest. As stated previously, a bull would have to be of superior genetic value to justify a retest.

Much of the information presented for the bull and the stallion can be adapted to the boar, ram, and buck. The proper semen characteristics and appropriate diseases can be found in other chapters.

20–4 ALTERING MALE REPRODUCTION

There are two practical reasons for altering male reproduction. The most common, castration, is performed for the purpose of producing a higher-quality carcass in meat animals. Other alterations have been performed to produce males that can be used to assist in detecting estrus.

20–4.1 *Castration*

Castration involves surgical removal of the testes and epididymides or a treatment which causes degeneration of the testes. The castrated, immature male, in addition to being sterile, fails to develop the secondary sex characteristics of the intact male. The accessory sex glands, aggressiveness, and sex drive typical for the intact male do not develop. Castration of the mature male results in sterility, loss of sex drive in a short period of time, and regression of the secondary sex glands. However, the secondary sex characteristics remain at the stage of development they had attained at the time of castration. For this reason, castration in horses is deliberately delayed until the secondary sex characteristics are developed.

Equipment commonly used for castration is shown in Figure 20–12. Surgical castration of lambs, young bucks, and calves is best accomplished by cutting away 1 cm of the

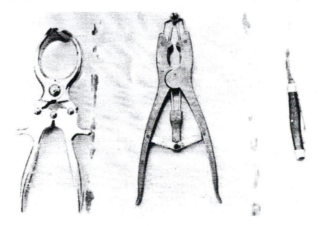

Figure 20–12 Equipment commonly used for castration. Left to right: emasculator, rubber band applicator, and knife.

bottom of the scrotum (Figure 20–13). This cuts through the tunica vaginalis, exposing the testes. Each testis is then pushed through the opening, gripped with the thumb and forefinger, and removed with a quick jerk, making sure that the spermatic cord breaks inside the scrotum. When the blood vessels of the spermatic cord are broken in this manner, the stretching involved results in the lumen's closing to prevent bleeding. The Newberry castrator, an instrument that grips the bottom of the scrotum and makes a vertical incision into both scrotal pouches, is available. The testicles are removed in the manner just described. When pigs are castrated, an incision is made near the bottom of each scrotal pouch to expose the testes and the epididymides. The testis is separated from the tunica vaginalis and the spermatic cord is macerated rather than cut to prevent bleeding.

Nonsurgical procedures may be used for castrating lambs, young bucks, and calves. Emasculation is a procedure in which a special instrument called an emasculator is used to sever the spermatic cord without breaking the skin (Figure 20–13). This process disrupts blood and nerve supply to the testes, resulting in degeneration. Rubber bands of a special design with an instrument for application are also available. The instrument (Figure 20–13) stretches the rubber band so that it can be slipped over the testes and released on the scrotum above the testes, stopping the blood supply to the testes, again resulting in degeneration.

Castration of stallions requires an individual with experience, since the stallion is not castrated until after puberty. One of the short-acting general anesthetic regimens should be used instead of a casting harness.

The surgical procedure is much the same as that used for the pig.

20–4.2 *Vasectomy*

Vasectomy is a surgical procedure in which the vasa deferentia are severed (usually a section is removed), which results in sterility. Since the blood and nerve supply to the testes are not interrupted, the male remains normal in all other respects. The vasectomized male has been used to aid the detection of estrus in the female when AI is being used in the herd or flock. The animal is effective in identifying the estrual female, but there is a distinct disadvantage in that he can spread venereal diseases, since he is able to copulate. For this reason, penilectomy is sometimes done.

20–4.3 *Penile Block*

The penile block is a simple procedure in which a plastic tube is inserted into the sheath. A trocar and cannula are used to punch a hole through the sheath in line with an opening through the plastic tube (Figure 20–14). The stainless steel cannula serves as a pin to hold the tube in place. The tube and pin prevent the protrusion of the penis and thus inhibit copulation. The procedure is effective for a relatively short time, but, since the male is unable to copulate and ejaculate, most tend to lose sex drive rather rapidly. Pain may be a factor in loss of libido. There is also some problem related to infection of the sheath where the puncture was made.

Penilectomy has been used to alter bulls and rams for use in checking females for estrus. It has an advantage over the penile block of not being as subject to infections. However, these males lose their sex drive in about the same length of time.

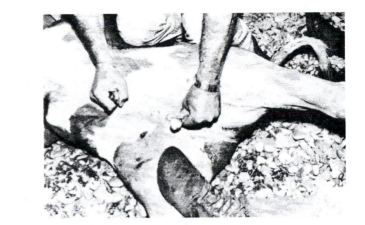

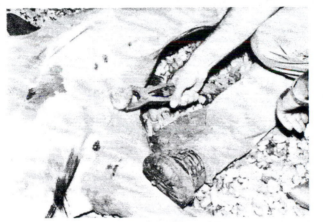

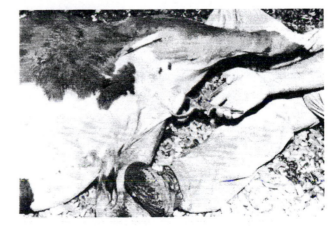

Figure 20–13 Three castration procedures: (*a*) knife is used to open scrotum so testes can be removed; (*b*) rubber band is placed around scrotum above testes; (*c*) emasculator is used to pinch spermatic cord.

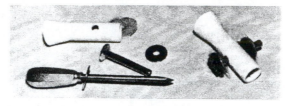

Figure 20–14   Left: unassembled penile block. Trocar is used to punch hole through sheath for application. Right: assembled.

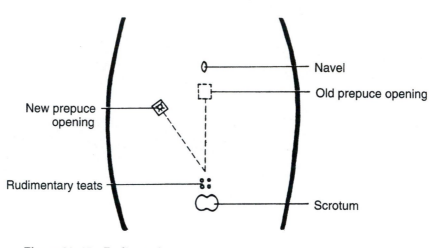

Figure 20–15   Redirected prepuce procedure.

20–4.4 *Redirecting the Prepuce*

Redirection of the prepuce has been performed on bulls but can also be done for rams and bucks. The purpose is to move the opening of the prepuce to one side so that the penis fails to line up with the vulva of the female, thus preventing copulation. It is accomplished by excising a small section of skin around the prepucial opening. An identical section of skin is removed 10 cm to 20 cm to one side. From this second opening, a probe is used to loosen the skin from the abdominal wall so the sheath with the penis and the section of skin can be brought through to the new location and the skin sutured into place. The section of skin removed from the new location is used to cover the opening left at the old location (Figure 20–15 and Color Plate 24). Males with redirected prepuce are much more satisfactory for detecting estrus females than either the vasectomized males or males with penile blocks. Copulation is prevented, thus reducing the chance of spreading diseases. An additional advantage is that pressure of the male resting on the rump of the female allows the male to make an ejaculatory thrust and ejaculate. This prevents the male from losing sex drive, thus providing a useful tool over a much longer period of time.

SUGGESTED READING

BEARDEN, H. J. 1956. Improving your herd's conception rate. *N.Y. Artificial Breeder's Cooperator,* 13:2.

DRANSFIELD, M. B. G., R. L. NEBEL, R. E. PEARSON, and L. D. WARNICK. 1998. Timing of insemination for dairy cows identified in estrus by a radiotelemetric estrus detection system. *J. Dairy Sci.,* 81:1874.

FOOTE, R. H. 1978. Reproductive performance and problems in New York dairy herds. *Search,* 8:1. Cornell University Agr. Exp. Sta.

GINTHER, O. J. 1988. Using a twinning tree for designing equine twin-prevention programs. *Equine Vet. Sci.,* 8:101.

GINTHER, O. J. 1989. Twin embryos in mares II: Post fixation embryo reduction. *Equine Vet. J.,* 21:171.

HALL, J. G., C. BRANTON, and E. J. STONE. 1959. Estrus, estrus cycles, ovulation time, time of service and fertility of dairy cattle in Louisiana. *J. Dairy Sci.,* 42:1086.

KIDDY, C. A. 1979. Estrus detection in dairy cattle. *Beltsville Symposia in Agricultural Research. 3. Animal Reproduction,* p. 77. ed. H. W. Hawk. Allanheld, Osmun and Co., Publisher; Halsted Press, a division of Wiley and Sons.

MADDOX, L. A., A. M. SORENSEN, JR., and U. D. THOMPSON. 1961. Testing bulls for fertility. *Texas Agr. Exp. Sta.—Texas Agr. Ext. Service Bull.* 924.

MCKINNON, A. O. and J. L. VOSS. 1993. *Equine Reproduction.* Lea and Febiger.

MORROW, D. A., S. J. ROBERTS, and K. MCENTEE. 1969. A review of postpartum ovarian activity and involution of the uterus and cervix in cattle. *Cornell Vet.,* 59:134.

PICKETT, B. W. and J. L. VOSS. 1973. Reproductive management of the stallion. *Proc. 18th An. Conv. Am. Assoc. Equine Pract.,* p. 501. ed. F. J. Milne.

ROSEBOOM, J. D., M. H. T. TROEDSSON, G. C. SHURSON, J. D. HAWTON, and B. G. CRABO. 1997. Late estrus and metestrus insemination after estrual inseminations decreases farrowing rate and litter size in swine. *J. Anim. Sci.,* 75:2323.

SALISBURY, G. W., N. L. VANDEMARK, and J. R. LODGE. 1978. *Physiology of Reproduction and Artificial Insemination of Cattle.* (2nd ed.) W. H. Freeman and Co.

TRIMBERGER, G. W. and H. P. DAVIS. 1943. Conception rate in dairy cattle by artificial insemination at various stages of estrus. *Nebraska Agr. Exp. Sta. Res. Bull.* 129.

VANDEMARK, N. L., L. J. BOYD, and F. N. BAKER. 1956. Potential services of a bull frequently ejaculated for four consecutive years. *J. Dairy Sci.,* 39:1071.

WATTS, T. L., J. W. FUQUAY, and C. J. MONLEZUN. 1979. Season and breed effects on placenta retention in a university dairy herd. *Proc. An. Mtg. So. Div. ADSA.*

YOUNGQUIST, R. S. 1992. Breeding soundness evaluation of bulls. *Proc. An. Gen. Meeting, Soc. for Theriogenology.*

21

Pregnancy Diagnosis

21–1 COW

The economic value of an early diagnosis of pregnancy in the cow is quite clear. Whether one is dealing with dairy cattle or beef cattle, the ultimate goal is an average 12-month calving interval for the herd. Every management practice that contributes to attaining this goal is well worth consideration. Pregnancy diagnosis is one of these tools. Most cows that fail to conceive will return to estrus in approximately 21 days postbreeding. Due to a number of different causes, a small percentage do not. The members of this latter group are the ones that need to be discovered by pregnancy diagnosis as early as possible. Regardless of how good a management program might be, not all cows that return to estrus are detected. These cows also need to be discovered early so that additional attention can be given to heat detection so that they can be rebred.

The ideal pregnancy test would be one that is inexpensive and highly accurate, that could be conducted at the farm by farm personnel, utilizing milk, urine, or other easily obtained specimens that would detect pregnancy at 17 to 19 days postbreeding. No such test is available today. The milk progesterone assay test shows that progress is being made. This test is conducted on milk samples taken 21 to 24 days postbreeding. These tests can be conducted in a laboratory with appropriate equipment or on the farm with a commercial enzyme immunoassay progesterone kit. Pregnancy diagnosis by rectal palpation remains one of the more practical means for detecting pregnancy in cattle.

Some authors have recommended that diagnosis of pregnancy by rectal palpation be done by practicing veterinarians. We disagree and feel strongly that pregnancy diagnosis by rectal palpation is a good management tool that all progressive livestock managers should utilize. We would like it clearly understood that all cattle operations should have a good preventive herd health program in which the veterinarian is an integral part. A good relationship between the herd owner and the veterinarian will usually identify the practices that should be carried out by the manager and those that should be relegated to the veterinarian. A wise veterinarian will work with clients to help them become more proficient with their management tools.

21–1.1 Rectal Palpation

In order for pregnancy diagnosis to be of greatest benefit, it is necessary to set up a workable schedule and follow it rigidly. We recommend for dairy herds and beef herds using artificial insemination that some pregnancy palpations be scheduled each week. This is best accomplished when the same time of the same day each week is designated for this purpose. The next decision to be made is when cows should be palpated following breeding. In herds where AI is used, the first palpation should be made between 35 and 42 days after insemination. Even though palpation at this stage requires greater expertise, the main interest should be to identify those cows that are not pregnant so that they can be observed more carefully during the next few days when they should be returning to estrus. Many cows that are open (not pregnant) at this time probably were in estrus 21 days postbreeding but were not detected. All questionable cows at this time should be placed in a group to be observed carefully for estrus. All cows that have not returned to estrus by 60 days postbreeding should be palpated a final time. A few pregnancies (about 5%) at 30 to 35 days will result in embryonic mortality and can be picked up as open at the 60-day check. Very few pregnancies terminate after 60 days except as a result of a disease which causes abortion. Accurate records of each palpation should be maintained for each cow.

The management system used for individual beef cattle operations will dictate to some extent when pregnancy palpations are to be made. If the management tool is to be of value in retaining breeding females in a herd, it must be performed as previously described. Frequently, pregnancy palpation is used simply to determine which cows to cull so that open cows are not carried through the winter. This can be accomplished in connection with other management practices which require running cows through a chute.

21–1.1a Structures to Be Palpated

The *cervix* is chiefly a landmark serving as a guide for locating other structures. It is easily identified by palpation. The position and, to some extent, size give an indication of the stage of pregnancy, but a diagnosis should never be based on the cervix alone.

Most of the diagnosis is based on the *uterus* and its contents. The size of the uterus influences its position in relation to the pelvis and should be noted. The thickness and tone of the uterine wall are important. The uterine wall becomes thinner as pregnancy progresses and is very resilient to touch, compared with the uterus of the open cow. This is particularly important in differentiating between pregnancy and a condition that causes uterine enlargement without pregnancy. A dorsal bulge is detectable from 30 to 50 days in the area of the body of the uterus. The uterine wall is thinnest at this point and the pressure created by the contents of the uterus causes the bulging effect.

The *chorionic membrane* can be detected by gently grasping the uterine wall between the thumb and forefinger and lifting slightly. With some practice, one can feel the membrane slip from between the thumb and finger. Thus, the term "slipping the membrane" has been used to describe this procedure. By 120 days, the placentomes are large enough to palpate through the uterine wall. At first, these will be about the diameter of a dime and become much larger toward the end of pregnancy.

The *contents of the uterus* are the most positive diagnostic structures to be palpated. Between 35 and 50 days, the amnion is quite turgid and can usually be detected by palpating the uterine horns with the thumb and forefinger. This can be done by starting near the tip of the uterine horn and applying gentle pressure as the thumb and forefinger are moved back toward the cervix. After 50 days, the amnion begins to soften, and by 60 days it is no longer detectable. After 60 days, the fetus can be palpated except during a period from 170 to 230 days, when it is too deep in the abdominal cavity to be reached in large cows.

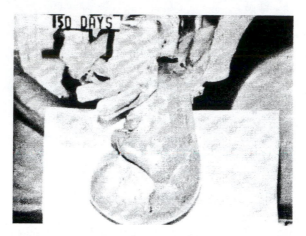

Figure 21–1   Palpation of a simulated middle uterine artery. Note the finger completely surrounding the artery.

The *ovaries* can be palpated up to about 120 days. Structures on the ovary can help confirm either a positive or a negative diagnosis. Pregnancy is always accompanied by a corpus luteum. However, one must remember that a corpus luteum is not always accompanied by a pregnancy. The absence of a corpus luteum would confirm that the cow is not pregnant.

The *pulse of pregnancy* can be helpful in confirming a diagnosis, particularly at certain stages of pregnancy. This pulse is felt in the middle uterine artery which branches from the internal iliac and descends to the uterus via the broad ligament on the right side near the forward edge of the pelvis (Figure 21–1). It is suspended in a fold of this ligament, which permits it to be readily picked up through the walls of the rectum and moved about freely. The middle uterine artery in the nonpregnant cow is 3 mm to 4 mm in diameter and has a clearly defined pulsation. In the pregnant cow, it begins to enlarge when the conceptus is large enough to require an increased blood supply and may reach a diameter of 1 cm to 1.5 cm by the end of gestation. The pulsation in the enlarged artery is much more forceful, indicating a greater volume of blood flow. By 120 days of pregnancy, the middle uterine artery will have enlarged sufficiently to be used as a differential diagnosis in pregnancy determination by rectal palpation.

Palpation at 35 to 40 Days   This stage of pregnancy requires more skill than later stages. However, it can provide valuable management information when used properly. Figure 21–2 shows an open uterus on the floor of the pelvis for reference. The following features should be identified:

1. The uterus is on the floor of pelvis, except in larger cows with elongated reproductive tracts. There is slight enlargement of one horn, with detectable dorsal bulging (Table 21–1). There is thinning of the uterine wall, with a fluid-filled feeling (Figure 21–3).
2. Slippage of the membrane is possible.
3. An amnion about the size of the yolk of a hen egg can be detected.
4. The corpus luteum is present on the ovary adjacent to the horn containing the amnion.

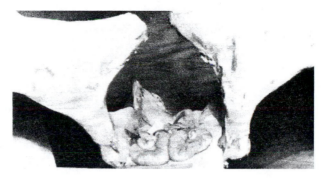

Figure 21–2   Nonpregnant uterus lying on the floor of the pelvic cavity.

Table 21–1   *Diameter of pregnant bovine uterine horn at different stages of pregnancy*

Stage in days	Diameter in cm
30	Slight enlargement and dorsal bulging
60	7
90	8
120	12
150	18

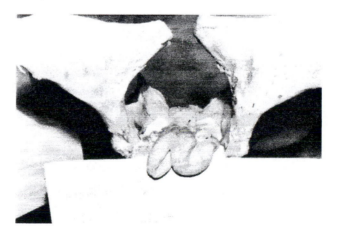

Figure 21–3   Pregnant uterus—35 days. Note bulge in left horn and CL on left ovary.

Palpation at 45 to 50 Days

1. The uterus is still on the pelvic floor. There is a slightly greater difference in the size of the pregnant and nonpregnant horns, with the pregnant horn being 5 cm to 6.5 cm in diameter and the dorsal bulging more pronounced.

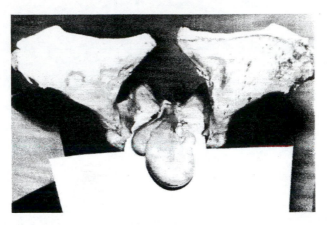

Figure 21–4 Pregnant uterus—60 days. Left horn containing fetus is pulled over brim of pelvis.

2. The amnion is about the size of a small hen egg.
3. The membranes can be slipped in either horn.
4. The corpus luteum is on the ovary adjacent to the pregnant horn.

Palpation at 60 Days

1. The pregnant horn is dropping slightly over the brim of the pelvis and feels like a balloon filled with water (Figure 21–4 and Color Plate 25). The pregnant horn is 6.5 cm to 7.6 cm in diameter and the dorsal bulge is no longer detectable.
2. The membranes can be slipped in both horns, but the amnion is detectable.
3. The fetus (5 cm long) can be bumped by rubbing the hand over the outer curvature of the uterine horn or by pressing against the outer curvature and then moving the hand slightly but quickly posteriorly (Table 21–2).
4. A corpus luteum will be on the ovary adjacent to the pregnant horn.

Table 21–2 *Average size of bovine conceptus at different ages: variation occurs between breeds and within breeds*

Age/days	Crown/rump length in cm
30	1
60	5
90	13
120	30
150	38
180	56
210	71
245	81
280	86

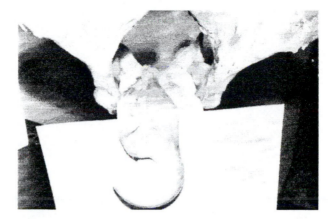

Figure 21–5 Pregnant uterus—90 days. Both horns are pulled over pelvic brim.

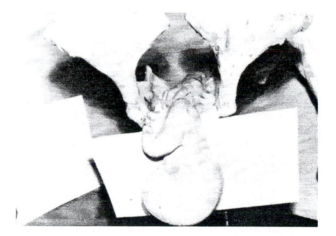

Figure 21–6 Pregnant uterus—120 days. Cervix is pulled to brim of pelvis.

Palpation at 90 Days

1. The uterus is pulled well over the pelvic brim and is 8 cm to 10 cm in diameter (Figure 21–5).
2. The fetus is 10 cm to 15 cm long and is easily palpated.
3. A corpus luteum is on the ovary adjacent to the pregnant horn.

Palpation at 120 Days

1. The uterus is well over the brim of the pelvis, with the cervix pulled almost to the pelvic brim (Figure 21–6 and Color Plate 27).
2. The fetus can be easily palpated and is 25 cm to 30 cm long. Anatomical parts of the fetus can be identified.
3. Small placentomes can be identified.

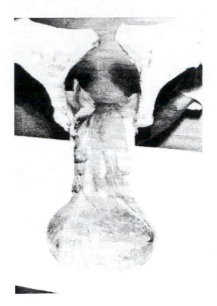

Figure 21–7 Pregnant uterus— 150 days. Cervix may be pulled partially over brim. Uterus is difficult to palpate.

4. The pulse of pregnancy can be detected.
5. The ovaries may be difficult to reach, but a corpus luteum is present on the ovary adjacent to the pregnant horn.

Palpation at 150 Days

1. The uterus is pulled well into the abdominal cavity, and the cervix is located at the brim of the pelvis (Figure 21–7 and Color Plate 28).
2. Distinct placentomes about the size of ovaries can be identified.
3. The fetus is well formed and is 35 cm to 40 cm in length but may be difficult to reach in larger cows.
4. The pulse of pregnancy is quite distinct, with the artery being 6 mm to 1.25 cm in diameter.

Palpation at 170 to 230 Days

1. The cervix is at the brim of the pelvis and may be bent over the edge.
2. The dorsal wall of the uterus is tight and difficult to palpate.
3. The placentomes vary in size and may be difficult to palpate because of the tight uterine wall.
4. The fetus is difficult to palpate, particularly in larger cows due to the depth of the abdominal cavity.
5. There is a strong pulse of pregnancy and the artery is 1.25 cm to 1.4 cm in diameter.

Palpation at 230 to 280 Days

1. The fetus is large enough to extend back within range of the hand. The head and front feet are usually the structures palpated.
2. Movement of the fetus can frequently be detected.

21–1.1b Differential Diagnosis Pregnancy is by far the greatest cause of uterine enlargement, but by no means is it the only cause. At each of the stages, pregnancy must be differentiated from one or more of the other causes of uterine enlargement.

Pyometra Pyometra is a condition characterized by an accumulation of pus in a sealed uterus. The condition occurs when an infectious organism enters the uterus at the time of or prior to the onset of pregnancy. The organism allows pregnancy to be initiated but after a variable period of time causes death of the embryo or early fetus. The conceptus is not expelled and degenerates in the sealed uterus accompanied by the formation of pus. The amount of pus varies from a relatively small amount to several liters. In cases of this sort, the contents of the uterus prevent the release of $PGF_{2\alpha}$, which in turn results in the corpus luteum remaining functional. The condition may remain *status quo* for an extended period of time.

Pyometra differs from pregnancy in that the uterine wall is thicker, spongy, and less resilient. In addition, the pus is more viscous than the fluid of pregnancy and frequently can be moved from one horn to the other. Of course, there is no fetus to palpate. The stages of pregnancy which need to be differentiated from pyometra are 45 days through 120 days.

Metritis Metritis is a nonspecific infection of the uterus characterized by the presence of visible pus. The pus may be seen on the lips of the vulva and on the tail where it rubs across the vulva. The pus may also be seen in estrous mucus as cloudiness or yellow or white flakes. The uterine wall is thickened and spongy to feel. This condition might be confused with the 35- to 40-day stage of pregnancy.

Mummified Fetus Mummified fetus is a condition in which the fetus dies and the fluids and soft tissues are reabsorbed (Figure 21–8). Depending on the stage at which the condition is detected, the mass ranges from a semisolid to a solid ball. It is not difficult to differentiate between a mummified fetus and normal pregnancy at the 90- to 120-day period. However, with a casual palpation one might feel the mummified fetus and misinterpret it for a normal fetus. Additional palpation would reveal the absence of fluid surrounding the mass and provide the differential diagnosis.

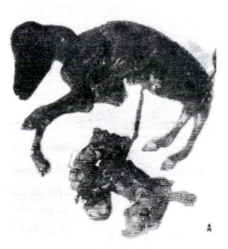

Figure 21–8 A mummified fetus. (From Hafez. 1974. *Reproduction in Farm Animals.* (3rd ed.) Lea and Febiger.)

21–1.1c Restraining Cows   Cows must be properly restrained during rectal palpation. Consideration should be given to protection of the palpator and to the efficiency of the operation. Many dairy producers have work areas with lock-in stanchions, and these serve very well for pregnancy palpation. A work chute narrow enough that cows cannot turn around also works well. The examination area does not have to be a squeeze chute but should have a solid cover so that animals will not try to jump over the sides. A pipe or bar can be used to prevent animals from backing up. A narrow gate (width of the chute) placed immediately behind the examining area is very helpful. When opened, the palpator can step in behind the cow to be palpated and at the same time the gate closes the chute behind him or her protecting the palpator from the cows waiting to be palpated. A squeeze chute, shown in Figure 21–9, may be necessary with some beef cattle.

21–1.2 *Assay of Progesterone in Milk*

Researchers in Great Britain, Germany, and the United States have reported pregnancy testing on the basis of progesterone levels in milk. Milk progesterone levels have been found to parallel blood progesterone levels when samples were taken periodically throughout the estrous cycle. The levels correspond to a pattern set by the corpus luteum. That is, high during midcycle and low just before, during, and just after estrus.

The prediction of pregnancy using this test is based on the progesterone level in a single sample of milk taken at 21 to 24 days postbreeding. For cows producing positive samples (> 11 ng/ml), 80% have been pregnant 40 to 60 days postbreeding as determined by rectal palpation. Essentially, all the cows producing milk negative to the test (< 2 ng/ml) have been open. These progesterone levels are based on whole milk samples. If analyses are made on milkfat or stripping samples, the hormone levels used to designate positive and negative will have to be adjusted accordingly. Since progesterone is a lipid, its levels will be higher in high-fat products than in whole milk samples.

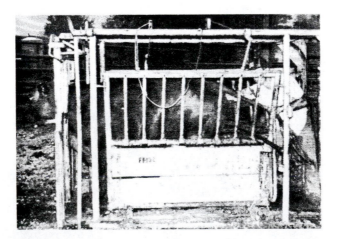

Figure 21–9   A squeeze chute with head gate should be available for palpating beef cows.

Table 21–3 *Fertilization, embryonic survival, and embryonic mortality rates of bulls with histories of either low or high fertility in artificial breeding*

| Histories of bulls in A.B. | 3-day slaughter data | | 33-day slaughter data | | Causes of repeat breedings | | |
	Number of observ.	Percentage of fertilized eggs	Number of observ.	Percentage of normal embryos	Percentage of eggs not fertilized	Estimated percentage of embryonic mortality	Percentage of breeding failure caused by embryonic mortality
High	29	96.6	29	86.1	3.4	10.5	75.5
Low	26	76.9	26	57.7	23.1	19.6	46.3
High-low		19.7		28.4	19.7	9.1	29.2

From Bearden, Ph.D. Dissertation, Cornell University, 1954.

The difference between the predicted pregnancy based on progesterone level at 21 to 24 days compared with actual pregnancy at 40 to 60 days postbreeding has been referred to as a false-positive. In reality, a high percentage of those cows may actually have been pregnant at, or shortly before, the 21- to 24-day sampling period. Embryonic mortality then would be the reason for their not being pregnant when palpated 40 to 60 days postbreeding.

Research has shown that, with virgin heifers free of known reproductive diseases, embryonic mortality accounted for 46% to 75% of the pregnancy failures when the heifers were artificially inseminated during the latter half of estrus (Table 21–3). Many of the embryo deaths occur early enough for the cows to return to estrus at the normal time. However, a significant number of embryos die between 20 and 40 days. When dealing with a cross section of cattle from several herds, one would expect that the difference between predicted and actual pregnancy rate could be caused by embryonic mortality. Some of the positive samples may have been due to nonpregnant cows with long but normal estrous cycles and some may have been due to errors in sampling (wrong cow or wrong time in the cycle). A method that could be used to accurately predict 60-day pregnancies utilizing milk samples taken at 21 to 24 days would be highly desirable. However, due to the problems related to embryonic mortality, the results reported here may be as close as we can come.

The best validated method for measuring progesterone in milk or blood is by radioimmunoassay, which must be done by a trained technician in a laboratory equipped for this procedure (Section 4–10). An efficient laboratory with an adequate volume of samples could deliver results in 3 to 5 days. This would provide earlier detection of open cows than is possible by rectal palpation. However, a central laboratory set up primarily for this purpose is feasible only in areas of high cow population.

Several different enzyme immunoassay progesterone kits are available and are practical for on-the-farm use (Section 20–2.2a). Quantitative kits with accuracy similar to that of radioimmunoassay are best used in large herds where one person can be trained and designated to run all samples. Qualitative kits are more practical for most herds. Easy-to-follow directions are included and results can be obtained within an hour of sampling. While not quantitative, they do distinguish between samples with high progesterone (indicating pregnancy) and samples with low progesterone (nonpregnant).

21–1.3 *Pregnancy-Specific Protein B*

With the discovery, isolation, and partial purification of pregnancy-specific protein B from the placental tissue of cows, an antibody was produced that permitted detection of protein B by radioimmunoassay. Whereas it can be detected in the blood of cows and heifers as early as 24 days postbreeding, it is most accurate when blood samples are drawn after 30 days postbreeding. In one study, when blood samples were drawn 30 to 35 days after insemination, samples that were positive for protein B were 86% accurate in cows and 95% accurate in heifers when pregnancy was confirmed by rectal palpation at about 70 days after insemination. Samples drawn at this time that tested negative for protein B were 100% accurate in identifying nonpregnant cows and heifers.

Much of the lower accuracy for samples that tested positive resulted from embryo mortality that occurred prior to the confirming diagnosis by rectal palpation. This problem was discussed in Section 21–1.2 in relation to use of milk progesterone in diagnosing pregnancy. Embryo mortality may not account for all of the difference between cows and heifers. Immunologically active protein B has been detected in cows for up to 80 days postpartum. This would not be a problem for cows inseminated after 60 days postpartum and sampled after 30 days postinsemination. However, the postpartum activity of protein B could result in false-positives in cows bred before 60 days postpartum. Comparison of this method with the milk progesterone test for pregnancy shows it to be more accurate than milk progesterone in detecting pregnant cows and equally accurate in identifying nonpregnant cows. Protein B must be assayed in a laboratory equipped for radioimmunoassay and therefore is not as practical for most herds as the enzyme immunoassay kits for milk progesterone.

21–1.4 *Ultrasonography*

The use of real-time B-mode diagnostic ultrasound has increased sharply as a diagnostic procedure in animal reproduction. Two factors have contributed to that increase: the cost has become much more favorable, and its imagery is far superior to that provided by the A-mode ultrasound. The real-time ultrasound provides far greater accuracy in diagnosing pregnancy and examining ovarian activity as well as other uses (Figure 21–10).

The choice of frequencies of the transducer is important in obtaining the best scanning results. The lower the frequency of the transducer, the greater the depth at which useful signals can be obtained, but greater depth results in loss of resolution. On the other hand, the higher frequencies greatly improve resolution but result in loss of penetration. A general rule of thumb, when working intrarectally, is to use the 7.5 MHz for early pregnancy detection and for presence/absence of ovarian structures; use the 5 MHz transducer for routine pregnancy diagnosis at 40 days and later; and use the 3.5 MHz transducer for late pregnancy checks and for scanning the uterus immediately after calving. Late pregnancy diagnosis can also be accomplished transcutaneously by applying the 3.5 MHz transducer in the inguinal area, above the udder.

With the real-time ultrasound, one can expect 95% to 100% accuracy when cows are checked for pregnancy between 18 and 24 days postbreeding. A part of the apparent error at this stage is not true error but due to embryonic mortality. At 30 days and beyond, ultrasonic pregnancy detection should be 100%. Comparable accuracy by manual rectal palpation is not achieved until 40 to 45 days. Even though accuracy is less than 100% at 18 to 22 days of pregnancy, an ultrasonic exam during that period will identify some ap-

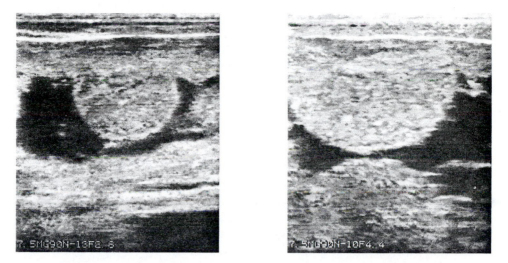

Figure 21–10 Placentomes, which consist of the fetal cotyledon and maternal caruncle, in the pregnant cow as detected by transrectal ultrasonography (7.5-MHz probe).

parently open cows so that they can be watched more closely for estrus and rebred. Ovarian structures will be important in making a diagnosis at this stage. An examination at this time can also be very advantageous in identifying open embryo transplant recipients, which allows them to be recycled sooner, thus reducing the number of recipients needed.

Fetal sex determination can usually be determined between days 55 and 100 of gestation. The key structure in fetal sexing is the genital tubercle (GT). In the male fetus, the GT can be located just posterior to the umbilical cord, and the scrotum can be visualized in male fetuses after day 60 of gestation. The GT is highly echogenic just below the anus of the female fetus.

21–2 EWE AND DOE

21–2.1 *Progesterone Assay*

Research utilizing the progesterone assay method on plasma as a means of diagnosing pregnancy has been reported for the ewe and should work equally well for the doe. Although the assay method on milk has not been reported, the procedure is a viable option for both species. For plasma samples taken from ewes on day 18 postbreeding, the method was 83.5% accurate for pregnant ewes, while the accuracy for nonpregnant ewesapproached 100%. This compares favorably with the data for cows. Progesterone levels were 4.81 ng/ml and 1.41 ng/ml for the pregnant and nonpregnant ewes, respectively. Samples (plasma or milk) should be taken from the doe on days 21 to 23 postbreeding for assay.

21–2.2 *Protein B Assay*

The radioimmunoassay developed to detect protein B in pregnant cows has also detected a similar protein in pregnant ewes and does. Therefore, the placenta of the pregnant ewe and doe produces a pregnancy-specific protein that is immunologically very much like protein B in cows. The practicability of use of this method for diagnosing pregnancy in sheep will need additional study.

21–2.3 *Ultrasonography*

Real-time B-mode ultrasonography equipment and techniques utilized in human obstetrics have been adapted for use on the ewe (Figure 21–11). Wool is shorn from the abdomen from flank to flank 8 cm to 10 cm in front of the udder. The ultrasonic probe is then passed along this line aimed toward the reproductive tract. Positive diagnosis is based on detecting a fetal pulse and swishing of the umbilical cord. Unfortunately, the method is only effective in diagnosing pregnancy in ewes 100 or more days postbreeding.

An intrarectal Doppler ultrasound technique has been developed for the ewe and doe. A small Doppler probe is inserted into the rectum just above the reproductive tract. Diagnosis is based on findings as previously described. In a study involving 1,396 ewes, accuracy on pregnant ewes increased from 80% to 97% as pregnancy advanced from 31 to 120 days. The accuracy of pregnancy diagnosis at 46 days postbreeding was 95% in another study involving 674 ewes. Similar results have been obtained with does (Figure 21–12 and Color Plate 29).

21–2.4 *Vaginal Biopsy*

Vaginal biopsy is a method that has shown up to 97% accuracy in diagnosing pregnancy in the ewe. The method is not one that can be used on the farm. Biopsies must be obtained surgically and processed for histological examination. Vaginal epithelium of the nonpregnant ewe contains 10 to 12 layers of cells. The surface layers are squamous, while the deeper layers are polygonal. The epithelium of the pregnant ewe contains fewer layers, and these are columnar and cuboidal rather than squamous and polygonal. The test can be conducted from 40 days postbreeding to term.

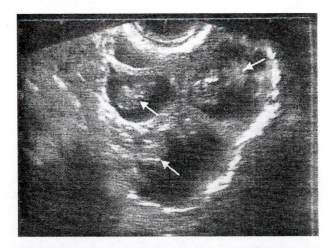

Figure 21–11   Ultrasonographic scan at 40 days of pregnancy of an Afec-Assaf ewe carrying three fetuses (fetuses are indicated by arrows). *Source:* Reprinted from *Encyclopedia of Dairy Sciences*, 4, Gootwine, E., Reproductive Management, 2530, 2002, with permission from Elsevier Science.

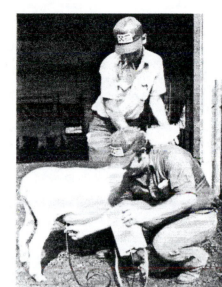

Figure 21–12 A version of the ultrasonic sound equipment used to diagnose pregnancy in the ewe. Note that wool has been clipped from abdomen in front of udder.

21–2.5 *Rectal Abdominal Palpation*

A rectal abdominal palpation technique has been described for diagnosing pregnancy in the ewe. The ewes are fasted overnight. For examination, they are placed on their backs on a laparotomy table, in a tilting squeeze chute or on a flat wood floor. A palpation rod (0.5 cm to 1.5 cm diameter and 50 cm long) is lubricated and inserted through the rectum into the abdominal cavity 30 cm to 35 cm. Insertion is easier when inclined slightly toward the backbone. The rod is manipulated with one hand while the other hand is placed on the posterior abdomen. If the ewe is pregnant, a significant obstruction will be encountered when the rod is moved from side to side or up and down. The obstruction can be palpated between the rod and the hand on the abdomen. In the nonpregnant ewe, no obstruction is found.

This method is only about 50% to 70% accurate at 41 to 45 days but approaches 95% accuracy at 49 to 53 days postbreeding. After 60 days postbreeding, it is essentially 100% accurate.

The rectal abdominal palpation technique of determining pregnancy has one major problem. The palpation rod can cause damage to the rectal wall. In one experiment, the incidence of perforated recta was 18%, 5%, and 1% in three respective trials. The difference could have been due to experience of the operators. The incidence of bruising and abrasions ranged from 8% to 46% in the same experiment. The method is more hazardous with respect to rectal injury and abortion in the doe and is therefore not an acceptable method for practical use.

21–3 MARE

21–3.1 *Rectal Palpation*

The most practical and earliest determination of pregnancy in mares is done by rectal palpation. The most practical time for palpating the mare is 35 days postbreeding. While the procedures are very similar to the rectal palpation method in cows, some differences will be described.

Restraint. Some mares may be palpated without restraint. But being kicked by a mare may be serious if not fatal, so all mares should be properly restrained before palpation. A properly designed breeding stock that protects the examiner may be used (Figure 21–13). A number of commercial as well as improvised breeding hobbles may be used. Any such equipment should provide protection for the examiner, should not cause the mare to become excited, and should be easy and safe to apply and remove. A nose twitch may be effective with some mares but causes additional excitement in others. Very nervous mares may have to be sedated or tranquilized before the application of restraint equipment. The restraint should also prevent the animal from moving from side to side to prevent injury to the elbow.

Lubrication. The rectal mucosa of the mare is much dryer than the mucosa of the cow. Proper lubrication is essential for successful palpation and to prevent damage to the rectum. A tear in the rectum of the mare is very serious and usually causes death.

21–3.1a Structures to Be Palpated

The ovaries, rather than the cervix, serve as a landmark in the mare. A systematic examination is begun with location of one of the ovaries. The right ovary is easier to reach and locate when the left hand is used by the examiner. In nonpregnant and early pregnant mares, the ovaries are located 5 cm to 10 cm anterior to the upper third of the pelvic arch. They can be recognized by their distinct oval and irregular form and rather firm consistency. Detailed examination of the ovaries does not contribute information of significance for pregnancy diagnosis.

Uterus and Its Contents. The diagnostic decision in the mare is based almost entirely on the size of the uterus and its contents. The mare's uterus is bipartite, with the horns joining the body of the uterus almost perpendicularly, resulting in a T-shaped structure. The horns are slightly funnel-shaped and are 10 cm to 16 cm in length. The body of the uterus measures 15 cm to 20 cm in length, with a width of 4 cm to 6 cm. After locating an ovary, the palpator follows the broad ligament down to the top of the uterine horn. A systematic examination of both horns and the body of the uterus is necessary in making the diagnosis. The uterus of the open or early pregnant mare will be located in the pelvic region. As pregnancy progresses, the uterus and its contents will be pulled into the abdominal cavity.

Fetal membranes and placentomes which are positive signs of pregnancy in the cow cannot be used as criteria of pregnancy in the mare because of the diffuse attachment of the

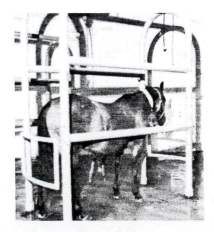

Figure 21–13 Mare being restrained in a stock for palpation.

placenta. Bulging of the uterus caused by the amnionic vesicle is readily detectable between 30 and 50 days postbreeding. Beyond this point, the fetus itself can be palpated.

Pulse of Pregnancy. The demand for an increased blood supply to the uterus causes the same enlargement and increased blood supply in the uterine arteries as observed in the cow. Both the utero-ovarian and middle uterine arteries may be palpated and changes may be detected after 150 days of gestation.

Position of the Ovaries. The change in the position of the uterus involves the broad ligaments and ovaries. As the uterus descends into the abdominal cavity, its weight pulls the broad ligament, which in turn moves the ovaries downward and forward. By the sixth to seventh month of gestation, the ovaries may be level with the pelvic brim.

Palpation at 35 Days   This stage is characterized by the appearance of the amnion, which is about the size of a golf ball, in one of the uterine horns. The remainder of the uterus does not have the fluid-filled feeling as in the cow at this stage. The uterine muscles have good tone.

Palpation at 42 to 45 Days   The amnion at this stage attains a slightly oval form and measures 5 cm to 7 cm in length and approximately 5 cm in diameter. Its position has reached the junction of the horn and body of the uterus (Figure 21–14).

Palpation at 60 Days   Approximately half of the amnionic vesicle is located in the body of the uterus. It has assumed the shape of a football and is 12 cm to 15 cm long and 8 cm to 10 cm in diameter.

Palpation at 90 Days   The entire body of the uterus is involved at this stage. The enlarged area measures approximately 20 cm to 25 cm in length and about 12 cm to 16 cm in diameter. About half of the body of the uterus is pulled over the brim of the pelvis. The fetus is easily palpated at this stage.

Palpation at 3 to 5 Months   The entire uterus is pulled into the abdominal cavity. The ovaries are pulled down and forward. The fetus can still be palpated.

Palpation at 5 to 7 Months   The descent of the uterus continues and is completed toward the end of this period. The ovaries continue to be pulled downward and forward and toward the end of the period are approximately even with the floor of the pelvis. The fetus can be palpated in most mares. The uterine arteries may be palpated as described for the cow.

Palpation at 7 Months to Parturition   The fetus is easily palpated during this period.

21–3.1b Differential Diagnosis   Pathological conditions which might be confused with pregnancy are very rare in the mare. Pyometra, although rare, is relatively easy to distinguish from pregnancy. The uterus can be retracted and the absence of a fetus established. Retention of a dead fetus in the form of mummification has not been encountered in the mare.

21–3.2 *Hormone Assay*

Pregnant mare serum gonadotropin (PMSG) appears in the blood about 40 days postbreeding. Peak levels appear between 50 and 120 days and then begin a gradual decline. A bioassay test using immature female rats (25 to 40 days of age) has been developed for detecting

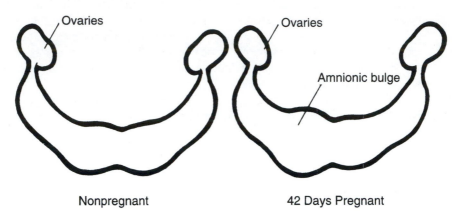

Nonpregnant   42 Days Pregnant

Figure 21–14   Diagram of mare's uterus showing an amnionic bulge typical of a 42-day pregnancy.

the presence of PMSG. These rats are injected with serum from a mare and killed 72 hours later. The ovaries are examined for follicular growth. An immunologic test kit is also available and can be purchased. Both tests give best results when performed between 50 and 100 days postbreeding.

21–3.3 *Progesterone Assay*

Recent research has revealed that mare's milk can be assayed for progesterone to diagnose pregnancy. Since the mare is usually lactating at the time of breeding, milk samples can be obtained. Progesterone assay on blood may also be a possibility. Additional research needs to be performed in this area.

21–3.4 *Ultrasonography*

Pregnancy can be detected in mares as early as 10 to 12 days postovulation with real-time B-mode ultrasound equipment. However, because of natural embryonic loss, it is not practical to check mares that early. The first examination can be done at 18 to 20 days to identify open mares, so they can be checked for estrus for rebreeding. An exception should be made for breeds with a history of high rate of double ovulations. These mares should be checked at 15 to 17 days in order to properly manage embryo reduction (Section 20–2.3e). Additional ultrasound examinations will depend primarily on economics; however, at least one later check between 40 and 60 days should be made to determine whether the mare is still pregnant. This check may be made either ultrasonically (Figure 21–15) or by manual rectal palpation.

21–4 Sow

The ultrasonographic technique will be the only method described for detecting pregnancy in the sow.

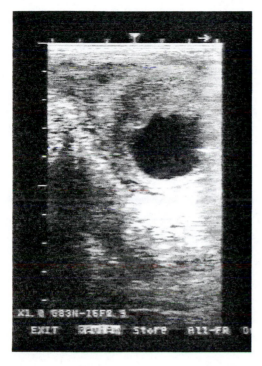

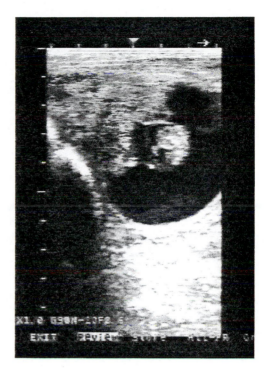

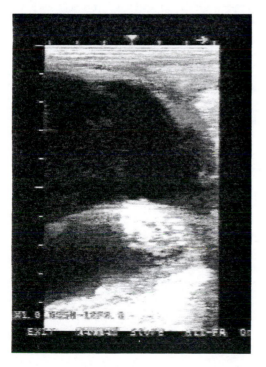

Figure 21–15 Ultrasonography for the detection of pregnancy in the mare at 21 (*top left,*) 35 (*top right*) and 60 (*left*) days of gestation. (Courtesy of P. Ryan, *Animal and Dairy Science,* Miss. State Univ.)

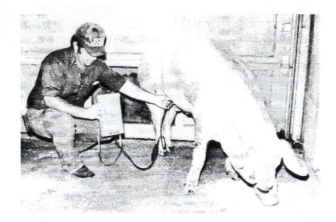

Figure 21–16 Sow being checked for pregnancy with ultrasonic equipment.

The transducer is moved laterally along the abdominal wall just outside the nipple line (Figure 21–16 and Color Plate 30). With the real-time (RTU) unit, you will be looking for walnut-size (at day 30) vesicles that resemble Swiss cheese in the pregnant sow. The two types of ultrasonic equipment, A-mode and real-time (B-mode), were covered in Section 21–1.4, and hereafter the latter will be referred to as RTU. Until very recently, the A-mode equipment was used in most, if not all, swine breeding units that used ultrasound to diagnose pregnancy. The major reason was that initially the RTU units cost $20,000 or more depending on the type and number or transducers purchased. Typically, the A-mode unit cost a few hundred dollars. Now there are two RTU units that sell for $7,000 to $9,000 each. That plus the greater accuracy and a timesaving factor (a contract swine veterinarian states that the RTU easily cuts the time required to check pregnancy in half, compared with the A-mode unit) have caused a rethinking on the economics of checking sows for pregnancy. In a 1,000-sow herd, the same veterinarian checked 45 sows with an RTU unit following an experienced technician using an A-mode unit and found 7 misdiagnosed sows (4 false-positives and 3 false-negatives). This represents an error rate greater than 15%; however, the RTU is not 100% accurate, either. From reported research data, the 5-MHz transducer is from 5% to 10% more accurate at day 21 of the gestation than the 3.5-MHz transducer, with variation between technicians. The following percentages of accuracy were reported for different stages of gestation using an RTU unit with a 5-MHz transducer: days 17 to 20—74.5%, days 21 to 23—97%, days 24 to 30—97.8%, days 38 to 44—98%, and days 52 to 58—98.7%. One consulting veterinarian has calculated that each nonproductive sow day (NDSP) costs $1.50 in feed, labor, and fixed cost. In his opinion, the RTU used properly in a 500-sow herd will reduce NDSP days sufficiently in 1 year to save $7,500, approximately the cost of the unit. On the other hand, if the sows with a false-negative diagnosis are sent to slaughter, they represent lost litters, an additional loss. A staff veterinarian for a 15,000-sow, 12-farm operation reported that they replaced 12 A-mode units with 1 RTU unit. One technician works full-time on RTU duty and checks 1,500 to 1,600 sows per week. He offers the following management lessons:

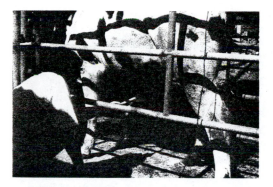

Plate 17 Semen collection in the bull. A Holstein bull being collected by electroejaculation. Note the placement of the collection cone over the glans penis to collect the ejaculate. (Photo courtesy of R. Godfrey, University of the Virgin Islands–St. Croix, USVI).

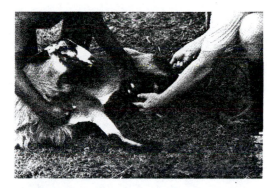

Plate 18 Semen collection in the ram. A Barbados Blackbelly ram being collected by electroejaculation. The ram is restrained manually and the penis, once extended, directed to a funnel attached to a volumetric tube for collection. (Photo courtesy of R. Godfrey, University of the Virgin Islands–St. Croix, USVI).

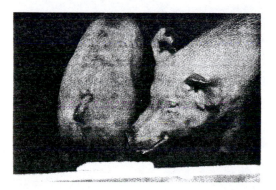

Plate 19 A boar sniffing the vulva of a sow. Note that the vulva may become prominent, reddened and swollen, at estrus as depicted here.

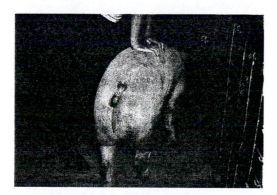

Plate 20 A method for detecting estrus in the sow. When pressure is applied to the back (lumbar region) of the estrus sow, she will assume a rigid mating stance (lordosis).

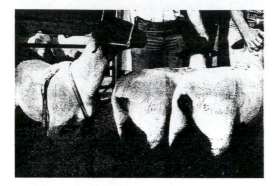

Plate 21 Estrus and mating detection in the ewe. The ram is outfitted with a marking harness containing a green chalk marker located on the brisket portion of the harness. A ewe in estrus that was then mounted by the ram has green chalk on her rump. This facilitates estrus detection and for recording natural breeding dates.

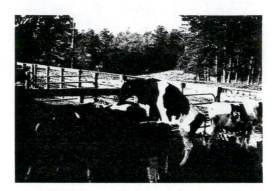

Plate 22 Estrus detection in cattle–I. Homosexual mounting behavior is used frequently in cattle for estrus detection. The heifer in the center depicted here is mounting ("riding") the heifer that is in estrus.

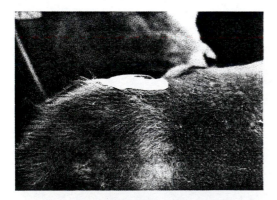

Plate 23 Estrus detection in cattle–II. A K-mar heat detection patch placed on the tail-head of a cow. When mounting occurs (like that depicted in Plate 22) this breaks a seal within the detector causing a color reaction. Use of such devices may prevent animals in estrus from being missed if mounting occurs without observation.

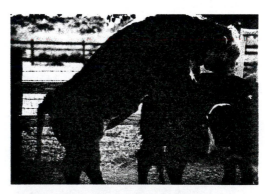

Plate 24 Estrus detection in cattle–III. The penis of the bull can be altered, or redirected, surgically from its normal path to prevent intromission from occurring. Penile deviated heat-check bulls like the one depicted here can be useful for estrus detection. However, they are not infertile without additional surgical measures (e.g., vasectomy or epididymectomy).

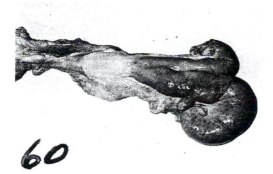

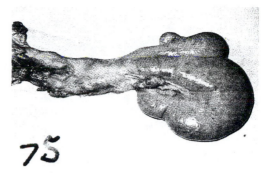

Plate 25 Detection of pregnancy in the cow–I. The pregnant uterus at 60 days of gestation. Note the distended right uterine horn and prominent corpus luteum.

Plate 26 Detection of pregnancy in the cow–II. The pregnant uterus at 75 days of gestation. Note the distended right uterine horn and prominent corpus luteum.

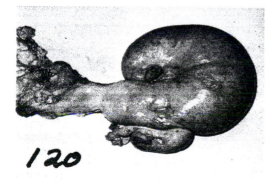

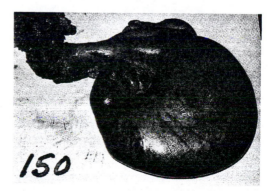

Plate 27 Detection of pregnancy in the cow–III. The pregnant uterus at 120 days of gestation. Note the distended left uterine horn and prominent corpus luteum.

Plate 28 Detection of pregnancy in the cow–IV. The pregnant uterus at 150 days of gestation. Note the distended right uterine horn and prominent corpus luteum.

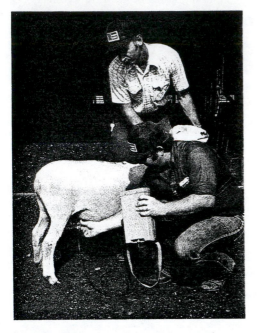

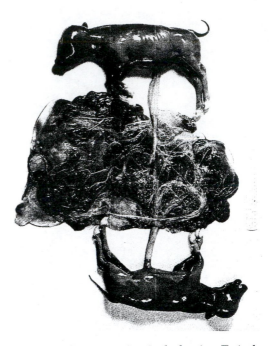

Plate 29 Detection of pregnancy in the ewe. The ultrasonic probe is placed on the shorn abdomen from flank to flank around 8 to 10 cm in front of the udder. Doppler probes detect the fetal and or umbilical pulse, whereas B-mode ultrasonography can provide an image or an indicator light reflecting a pregnancy.

Plate 31 Freemartinism in the bovine. Twin fetuses, one male and one female, which share a common placenta. Had this pregnancy gone to term, the female would have a 90 to 95% chance of being a freemartin with abnormal reproductive tract development. (Photo courtesy of D. Porter, Ontario College of Veterinary Medicine, University of Guelph, and P. Ryan, Department of Animal and Dairy Science, Mississippi State University).

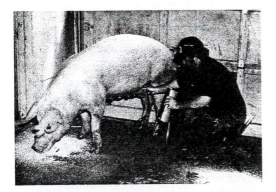

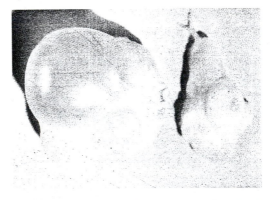

Plate 30 Detection of pregnancy in the sow. The ultrasonic probe is placed on the abdomen in a similar fashion as that described for the ewe in Plate 29. Doppler probes detect the fetal and or umbilical pulse, whereas B-mode ultrasonography can provide an image or an indicator light reflecting a pregnancy.

Plate 32 An ovary with a large thin-walled follicular cyst on left. Normal ovary on the right. (From Asdell and Bearden, 1959, Cornell Ext. Bulletin, 737).

1. The technician must have a positive attitude. Look for open sows rather than pregnant ones because they are the ones costing money; doubtful sows should be temporarily listed as open so vigorous estrus checking will be done, but, if the sow fails to show estrus, she can be checked again in 10 days.

2. Build confidence in the RTU technician; then remove the A-mode unit from the premises.

3. Make one technician responsible for RTU pregnancy checking.

4. Keep aggressively doing 18-day heat checks. Do not let breeding personnel rely too heavily on the RTU results.

5. Apply technology to culling sows. Previously, some pregnant sows were culled, but with RTU, sows are only culled if, indeed, they are open.

6. Prepare for the diagnostic challenges RTU technology will bring. Rather than blaming the "fall out" between day 20 and day 35 on diagnostic error, you can now look for other causes, such as Porcine Reproductive and Respiratory Syndrome.

7. Use what you learn through use of RTU to expand your knowledge of swine reproduction.

SUGGESTED READING

BEARDEN, H. J., W. HANSEL, and R.W. BRATTON. 1956. Fertility and embryonic mortality rates for bulls with histories of either low or high fertility in artificial breeding. *J. Dairy Sci.,* 39:312.

ESTERGREEN, V. L. 1978. A simplified test for milk progesterone and pregnancy testing. *The Advanced Animal Breeder,* 24:10. NAAB, Columbia, Mo.

FOOTE, R. H. 1979. Hormones in milk that may reflect reproductive changes. *Beltsville Symposia in Agricultural Research. 3. Animal Reproduction,* p. 111. ed. H. W. Hawk. Allanheld, Osmun and Co., Publisher; Halsted Press, a division of Wiley and Sons.

HAFEZ, E. S. E. 1974. *Reproduction in Farm Animals.* (3rd ed.) Lea and Febiger.

HULET, C.V. 1972. A rectal-abdominal palpation technique for diagnosing pregnancy in the ewe. *J. Anim. Sci.,* 35:814.

HUMBLOT, P., S. CAMOUS, J. MARTAL, J. CHARLERY, N. JEANGUYOT, M. THIEBIER, and G. SASSER. 1988. Diagnosis of pregnancy by radioimmunoassay of a pregnancy-specific protein in the plasma of dairy cows. *Theriogenology,* 30:257.

KASTELIC, J. P., S. CURRAN, and O. J. GINTHER. 1989. Accuracy of ultrasonography for pregnancy diagnosis on days 10 to 22 in heifers. *Theriogenology,* 31:813.

MCKINNON, A. O. 1993. Diagnosis of pregnancy. *Equine Reproduction.* Lea and Febiger.

RICHARDSON, C. 1972. Pregnancy diagnosis in the ewe: A review. *Vet. Rec.,* 90:264.

SORENSEN, A. M., JR. and J. R. BEVERLY. 1968. Determining pregnancy in cattle. *Texas Agr. Ext. Ser. Bull.,* 1077.

TYRRELL, R. N. and J. W. PLANT. 1979. Rectal damage in ewes following pregnancy diagnosis by rectal-abdominal palpation. *J. Anim. Sci.,* 48:348.

ZEMJANIS, R. 1970. *Diagnostic and Therapeutic Techniques in Animal Reproduction.* (2nd ed.) The Williams and Williams Co.

ZEMJANIS, R. 1974. Pregnancy diagnosis. *Reproduction in Farm Animals.* (3rd ed.) E. S. E. Hafez., ed. Lea and Febiger.

22

Environmental Management

Most animal managers consider adverse stress of any nature to be undesirable in relation to reproductive efficiency. *Stress* can be defined as any environmental change (i.e., alteration in climate or management) that is severe enough to elicit a behavioral or physiological response from the animal. By this definition, the response to stress is not always undesirable. However, this chapter will deal with stressors that lower reproductive efficiency and the management needed to help alleviate undesirable effects of these stressors.

22–1 ENVIRONMENTAL STRESSORS

Of the environmental stressors that affect reproductive efficiency, adverse effects of heat stress are most dramatic and best documented. The response to other types of stressors is more variable with cause-effect relationships not clearly established.

22–1.1 *Heat Stress*

Heat stress will delay puberty in both males and females. Puberty was delayed in Hereford heifers reared at 27°C (80°F) as compared with others reared at 10°C (50°F). Similarly, puberty was delayed in Jersey bulls that were exposed to a 35°C (95°F) environment for 8 hours a day. Gilts born in late spring may have delayed puberty because they undergo their growth before puberty during the summer. Heat stress delays puberty by depressing appetite and slowing growth rate (section 5–1).

Summer conditions in most parts of the world are severe enough to lower semen quality, resulting in lower conception rate. Spermatozoa in semen collected from bulls during the summer show an increase in abnormal morphology (Section 14–1.2) and reduced binding to glycosaminoglycans, such as heparin (Section 6–4). Seasonal effect on fertility in dairy cattle when natural mating was used is illustrated in Figure 22–1. The low point in fertility was late summer, with slow recovery thereafter. Lower semen quality has been reported in bulls exposed to ambient temperatures above 27°C (80°F) for as little as 6 hours per day for several weeks. At 30°C (86°F), semen quality was affected in 5 weeks, whereas at 38°C (100°F) lower quality was observed in 2 weeks. Spermatogenesis will stop when the temperature inside the testes is elevated to as high as that of normal body temperature. When semen quality is reduced by high ambient temperature, several weeks in a thermoneutral environment are needed before semen quality returns to normal.

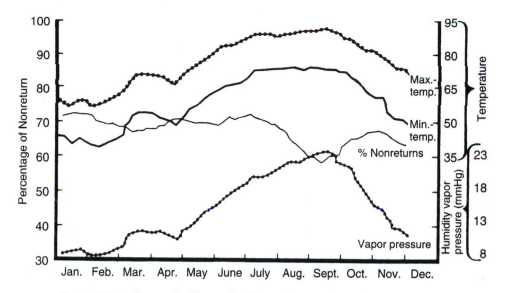

Figure 22–1   Seasonal effect on fertility in dairy cattle in Louisiana using natural mating. (From Johnston and Branton. 1953. *J. Dairy Sci.*, 36:934.)

European-type *(Bos taurus)* cattle exhibit reduced intensity and shorter periods of estrus during heat stress. Recent data suggest that these cows remain cyclic as indicated by patterns of progesterone secretion, but expression of estrus is low (35% to 40% of all cycles) even with intensive observation. This indicates that a high number of quiet ovulations (Section 25–5) occur, although missed detection of estrus may be higher as well. Extended postweaning anestrus occurs more frequently during the summer than in other months in sows.

If cows, ewes, and sows are bred during the summer, lower conception rates will result. While not as pronounced, lower conception rate is seen even if high-quality semen is used during this period. Therefore, heat stress has adverse effects on the female as well as the male. If the ambient temperature is high enough to elevate the rectal temperature of cows or ewes near time of breeding by as little as 1°C, marked reductions in conception rate are seen (Figure 22–2). In superovulated Holsteins, some reduction in fertilization rate is observed in summer as compared with winter. However, most recent research suggests that heat stress has its greatest effect on embryo quality and embryo survival. For cows, ewes, and sows, the time from estrus to a few days thereafter is very critical. An elevated body temperature can affect sperm while capacitating in the female tract or cause damage to cleaving embryos, resulting in lower embryo survival.

Embryos are less sensitive to heat stress by the time they have reached the morula stage. Some recent research supports the concept that this increase in thermal tolerance may be due to the embryo's ability to synthesize specific heat shock proteins or antioxidants such as glutathione. Also, there is evidence that heat stress has other effects on cows that lower conception, with these effects starting the cycle before breeding. This is supported by observations in which short-term cooling around the time of breeding has resulted in less improvement in conception rate than has more extensive cooling before breeding. When heat stress was applied to winter-conditioned heifers 10 days after breeding, embryo survival was not affected.

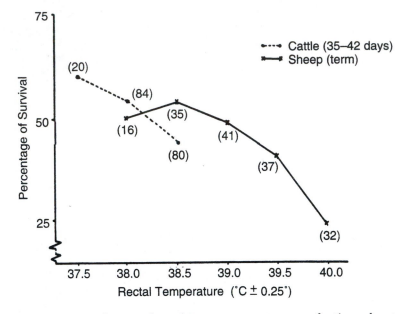

Figure 22–2 Influence of rectal temperatures at or near the time of mating on pregnancy rate in sheep and cattle. Rectal temperatures were taken for sheep at the time of mating and 12 hours after insemination for cattle. The numbers in parentheses represent the number of observations. (From Ulberg and Burfening. 1967. *J. Anim. Sci.*, 26:571.)

Heat stress during late gestation will adversely affect fetal growth in cattle and sheep. Summer-born beef calves in South Africa were smaller than winter-born calves. In Florida, dairy cows that were not shaded had smaller calves than similar cows which were shaded. Ewes that are heat-stressed during late gestation have smaller lambs with higher perinatal mortality, particularly with twin pregnancies. If they survive, weaning weights are similar to lambs not stressed *in utero*. Therefore, compensatory growth occurs postpartum. Heat stress near the end of gestation will increase stillbirths in pigs.

22–1.2 *Other Stressors*

Although heat stress has been identified as the major cause of low reproductive efficiency in the summer, cold stress (low ambient temperature) has not been cited as a cause of the lower reproductive efficiency sometimes reported during the winter except in Zebu cattle. Animals have thermoregulatory mechanisms that maintain internal body temperature at a level compatible with normal reproduction during cold periods. Confinement, affecting both detection of estrus and conception, nutritional deficiencies, or a higher incidence of health disorders may account for winter problems. Photoperiod does not appear to be a factor in polyestrous species such as cattle and domestic pigs.

Animal handling techniques can sometimes adversely affect reproduction. Rearing gilts in individual stalls as compared with group pens has delayed puberty. In one research trial, rearing gilts in confinement reduced the number cycling at 9 months of age by 14 percentage units

(71% vs. 85%). Beef cows isolated and confined in a corral either before or after insemination had lower conception than similar cows left with the herd except for insemination. Transporting animals to a new location has altered estrous cycles and delayed ovulation, as has restraint and mild electrical shock. These examples illustrate that animal handling techniques that are psychologically disturbing to animals will sometimes adversely affect reproductive efficiency.

Both metabolic events and disease states are stressors that may adversely affect reproduction. High milk production in dairy cows has resulted in longer periods of postpartum anestrous (Section 25–3) and more susceptability to ovarian cyst (Section 25–1). This can be exacerbated by metabolic disorders such as fatty liver and ketosis. Acute systemic infections may inhibit reproductive activity. Also, lower conception rate has been associated with mastitis, which is contracted during the first 21 days after breeding.

22–2 PHYSIOLOGICAL RELATIONSHIP OF ENVIRONMENTAL STRESS TO REPRODUCTION

Most researchers believe that general stress exerts its influence through the endocrine system (Figure 22–3). This mechanism is still being debated, but an involvement of the hormones of the adrenal cortex has received considerable attention. It is known that stress will cause the release of ACTH from the anterior pituitary, which, in turn, stimulates release of cortisol and other glucocorticoids from the adrenal cortex. Glucocorticoids inhibit the pulsatile release of

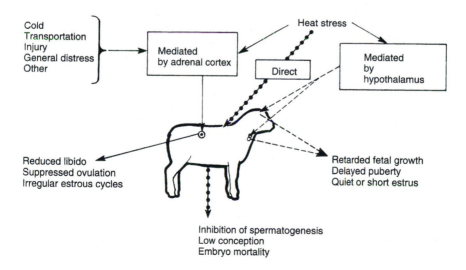

Figure 22–3 Reproductive phenomena impaired by adverse stress and possible physiological mechanisms of action.

LH. Therefore, if an animal is under stress during a critical period of the estrous cycle (late proestrus or estrus), a glucocorticoid-induced suppression of LH is likely to either delay or prevent ovulation and may reduce libido in males. Psychological distress, which may be caused by transportation to new environments, abusive treatment, or isolation, will elicit release of ACTH and glucocorticoids. A similar response may be evoked by a storm or a sudden change in temperature. As the animals adapt to the weather change, glucocorticoids will return to pre-estrus levels.

During negative energy balance, whether caused by underfeeding or high milk production, LH pulsatility is reduced and is the likely cause of the associated extended periods of anestrus after parturition. Acute systemic infections such as those seen with some forms of mastitis cause release of ACTH, which initiates action to inhibit pulsatile release of LH. Acute mastitis may also cause release of $PGF_{2\alpha}$ from the uterus, which could result in termination of pregnancy (particularly early pregnancies) by causing regression of the corpus luteum.

Sudden onset of heat stress may evoke an adrenal response. However, this is a short-term response and is not believed to be a major cause of heat stress–induced infertility. Several other factors may contribute to this problem. One of these is elevated core body temperature. As stated in Section 22–1.1, elevated rectal temperatures are associated with a marked reduction in conception rate. The interference with spermatogenesis appears to be a direct effect of an elevated temperature on the germinal epithelium (Section 3–2). If a female's internal temperature is elevated, there is evidence that damage can occur to (1) the spermatozoa while capacitating in the female tract, (2) the oocyte after ovulation, and/or (3) the embryo during the early cleavages. The damage to the gametes does not interfere with fertilization but results in embryonic mortality before placentation. Research has shown that embryos were more likely to be retarded and/or abnormal when collected from heifers that were subjected to heat stress during estrus as compared with embryos from heifers that were not stressed. Another factor related to the low fertility seen during heat stress is the evidence that the embryo loses its ability to alter prostaglandin synthesis in a manner that favors maintenance of the corpus luteum when under such conditions.

Heat stress causes a depression in progesterone secretion by the corpus luteum. The factors related to this suppression likely start in the previous cycle. Short-term cooling has not resulted in higher luteal progesterone secretion, but cooling for an entire cycle has caused elevation in luteal progesterone in the subsequent cycle. Altered chemistry of the ovulating follicles, which contributes to changes in steroidogenesis, may be involved in this response. In a limited study, injection of GnRH at breeding in lactating Holsteins resulted in an elevation in luteal progesterone during the next cycle as well as increased fertility. Since other factors associated with heat stress–induced infertility were not altered by injection of GnRH, it appears that the suppression of luteal progesterone observed during the summer could be a factor in lower summer fertility.

Heat stress depresses appetite and reduces thyroid activity. This may cause a loss of body condition lasting for 4 to 6 weeks before the animal adapts and may contribute to the lower fertility that occurs during heat stress (Section 23–3). Further, the lower metabolic rate that results from depressed appetite and lower thyroid activity is a major factor in the delayed puberty that occurs during heat stress and may be a factor in the shorter, quieter periods of estrus that are observed. Lower metabolic rate along with reduced blood flow to the uterus are likely causes of the retarded fetal growth that has been observed during heat stress, which results in birth of smaller offspring. The combination of all these factors accounts for the more pronounced effect of heat stress on reproduction than is seen with other stressors.

In understanding the variable reproductive response to stress, one must understand that animals will adapt to specific stressors. Animals maintained in a cold environment will usually reproduce normally. On the other hand, adapting to cold stress may make them more susceptible to other stressors. If, in addition to cold stress, estrous females are subjected to wind and rain or are transported to a new location for insemination, the physiological mechanisms that interfere with reproduction may be triggered. It is important to recognize that stress may interfere with reproduction. Frequently, simple modifications in management will lessen the likelihood of stress occurring around the time of estrus and insemination.

22–3 THERMOREGULATION

Management to alleviate undesirable stress involves recognizing and eliminating the cause of the stress. For most stresses, the most critical period extends from late proestrus through metestrus. Since reduced reproductive efficiency is more dramatic and predictable during heat stress and may include problems in detection of estrus, conception, and fetal growth, a more basic understanding of the animal's response to heat stress is needed. This will help the animal manager adopt practices to increase reproductive efficiency during the summer.

Thermoregulation is defined as the means by which an animal maintains its body temperature (Figure 22–4). It involves a balance between heat gain from metabolism and the environment and heat loss through metabolism and to the environment. Basically, the heat gained from metabolism is that necessary for living, production, and reproduction. Humans have limited control over either heat gain or heat loss from metabolism. This is regulated within the animal, principally through the hypothalamus and related systems. Therefore, the heat gained from the environment must be offset by heat loss to the environment. If heat gained from the environment exceeds heat loss, body temperature will rise. In addition, physiological adjustments will occur to reduce metabolic heat gain. These physiological adjustments result in reduced productivity. Also, the stress response (Section 22–1) and increased body temperature will lessen the likelihood of gestation with its associated increment of metabolic heat. To maximize reproductive efficiency during the summer, measures must be taken to reduce heat gain and/or facilitate heat loss to the environment.

22–4 MODIFICATION OF SUMMER ENVIRONMENTS TO REDUCE STRESS

During the day, most of the heat gained from the environment comes directly or indirectly from solar radiation. Solar radiation is absorbed when animals are exposed to direct sunlight. Indirect radiation comes from objects that absorb and reemit radiation (e.g., metal buildings or paved lots) and reflected radiation from light-colored surfaces and clouds. Radiation that strikes objects on the earth is either absorbed or reflected. Much of that which is reflected will be lost to a clear sky. If the skies are partly cloudy, clouds will deflect some of the reflected radiation back to the earth, adding to the radiation problem.

Shades provide protection from solar radiation and reduce daytime heat stress during the summer. Both natural shading provided by trees and artificial shades constructed from a variety of materials are beneficial. The efficiency of metal roofs as *radiation*

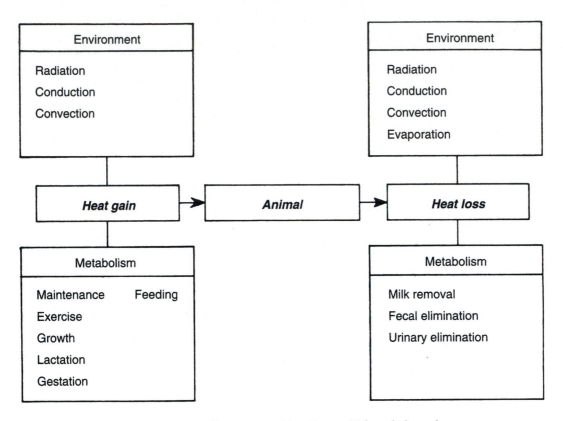

Figure 22–4   Increments of heat gain and heat loss, which are balanced to contribute to thermoregulation in an animal. (From Fuquay. 1981. *J. Anim. Sci.*, 52:164.)

Table 22–1   *Options available to animal managers to reduce heat stress and that are likely to be economically feasible during the summer*

*Radiation shields**	Natural shade
	Artificial shade
Mechanical cooling	Fans and/or sprinklers
	Evaporative coolers (arid regions)
Dietary changes	Low-fiber diets (ruminants)
	Cooled water (ruminants)

*Radiation shields are only protective during the day. At night, radiation shields inhibit radiational cooling.

shields can be improved by painting them white, insulating the underside, or using a sprinkler system to keep them wet (Table 22–1).

Most of the heat loss during the summer is from evaporation of moisture from skin or lungs. Even though cows and sheep are not considered sweating animals, evaporation of natural secretions from their skin surfaces is a major avenue of heat loss during the summer. Pigs are less efficient sweaters but compensate by lying in water to keep skin surfaces wet, if given the opportunity.

Cooling by evaporation is facilitated by reducing the dew point temperature around the animals. This can be accomplished by either lowering the relative humidity or the air temperature. Reduction of relative humidity is quite costly, but use of the evaporative cooler to lower the air temperature has proven to be economically feasible for dairy farms in hot, arid regions and has improved reproductive efficiency. Increasing the movement of air around animals will greatly enhance cooling by evaporation if the dew point temperature of the air is lower than that of the skin. Increased air movement can facilitate heat loss by evaporation during both the day and night. Further, increased air movement will be of benefit in humid regions where mechanical evaporative coolers are inefficient. Direct sprinkling of cattle and pigs has been beneficial in arid regions. Although less efficient in humid regions, intermittent sprinkling in combination with use of fans will increase daytime cooling of animals.

Radiational cooling is an important means of heat loss at night. Animals will radiate to the cooler night sky and lose body heat. The same radiation shields that reduce radiant heat gain during the day will inhibit radiant heat loss at night. During summer nights, animals need to have access to comfortable areas that are not covered by radiation shields.

The economic benefit from environmental modifications in terms of reproduction and meat and/or milk production must be balanced with the cost of providing the added comfort. Shades with natural cross-ventilation provide sufficient comfort and can be justified in most hot environments. Shades modified by fans or a combination of sprinklers and fans have resulted in lower rectal temperature, increased luteal progesterone secretion, improved body condition, strengthened expression of estrus, and improved summer fertility in lactating dairy cows. Some farm managers have limited the use of artificially cooled environments to the time between parturition and first insemination with good results. Cooling for this period has reduced postpartum interval to resumption of the estrous cycle and improved conception rate. If natural mating systems are being used, both males and females should be cooled.

22–5 OTHER MANAGEMENT CONSIDERATIONS IN HOT ENVIRONMENTS

One means of avoiding reduced conception rates during the summer is to breed animals during other seasons. This is done to a large degree in beef herds, with spring as the heavy breeding season, and dairy herds, when most cows are bred in late fall and early winter. This avoids the most troublesome reproductive period as related to heat stress but does not deal with the problem of heat stress on fetal growth. The breeding season of sheep starts during the summer, and marketing systems for swine favor farrowing at a uniform rate throughout the year. For sheep and pigs, the alternative of avoiding the summer breeding season is not desirable.

Part of the reduced conception associated with summer breeding can be avoided through artificial insemination by using frozen semen collected from males during other seasons. This alternative is available only in those species where use of frozen semen has reached commercial practicability. It is not yet available in some species where there is great need.

Providing cooled water for drinking has benefited ruminants. This can be accomplished by placing blocks of ice in watering tanks one or two times daily. Providing low-fiber, high-energy diets during the summer will also benefit ruminants. The heat of digestion of such diets is lower than for high-fiber diets, thus reducing metabolic heat production.

When compared with cool seasons, lactating dairy cows have shorter, less intense periods of estrus during the summer. Early reports indicated that the length of estrus was reduced by 6 to 8 hours with less mounting activity. This makes more frequent checks for estrus as well as use of mount detectors and other aids for detecting estrus (Section 20–2.2a) more critical during the summer. However, even with these measures, there are reports of estrus being detected in only 35% to 40% of the estrous cycles during the summer. Since most cows start estrus and show more mounting activity at night, especially during the summer, the period from midnight until dawn should be the optimum time for observation for estrus. However, the combination of low detection of estrus and low fertility provide little incentive to make this effort. Because cows appear to remain cyclic with a low expression of estrus during the summer, managed breeding programs (Section 18–1.1d) should be effective and result in a higher detection rate. Likewise, use of GnRH and $PGF_{2\alpha}$ to synchronize the time of ovulation (Section 18–1.1d) should result in more cows becoming pregnant. The percentage of cows conceiving to a single service would not be higher. However, the fact that all cows are inseminated a few hours before ovulation, rather than just those observed in estrus, should result in more total pregnancies. With the latter procedure, no other hormone therapy for control of estrus can be administered until they recycle or are diagnosed open, because of the risk of causing abortion.

SUGGESTED READING

AX, R. L., G. R. GILBERT, and G. E. SHOOK. 1987. Sperm in poor quality semen from bulls during heat stress have a lower affinity for binding hydrogen-3 heparin. *J. Dairy Sci.,* 70:195.

BADINGA, L., R. J. COLLIER, W. W. THATCHER, and C. J. WILCOX. 1985. Effects of climatic and management factors on conception rate of dairy cattle in subtropical environment. *J. Dairy Sci.,* 68:78.

CHRISTENSON, R. K. 1981. Influence of confinement and season of the year on puberty and estrous activity in sows. *J. Anim. Sci.,* 52:821.

DREILING, C. E., F. S. CARMEN III, and D. E. BROWN. 1991. Maternal endocrine and fetal metabolic responses to heat stress. *J. Dairy Sci.,* 74:312.

FUQUAY, J. W. 2002. Stress-heat in dairy cattle—Effect on reproduction. *Encyclopedia of Dairy Sciences.* H. Roginski, J. W. Fuquay, and P. F. Fox, Academic Press, an imprint of Elsevier Science.

FUQUAY, J. W., M. YOUNAS, R. V. GONZALEZ, W. R. HEARNE, and A. E. SMITH. 1993. Productive and reproductive responses of cows to fans in a hot, humid environment. *Proc. of Fourth Int. Livestock Envir. Symp.,* Coventry, England.

GANGWAR, P. C., C. BRANTON, and D. L. EVANS. 1965. Reproductive and physiological response of Holstein heifers to controlled and natural climatic conditions. *J. Dairy Sci.,* 48:222.

GWASDAUSKAS, F. C., C. J. WILCOX, and W. W. THATCHER. 1975. Environmental and management factors affecting conception rate in a subtropical climate. *J. Dairy Sci.,* 58:88.

HALL, J. G., C. BRANTON, and E. J. STONE. 1959. Estrus, estrous cycles, ovulation time, time of service and fertility of dairy cows in Louisiana. *J. Dairy Sci.,* 42:1086.

HANSEN, P. J. and C. F. ARECHIGA. 2002. Strategies for managing reproduction in heat-stressed dairy cows. *J. Dairy Sci.,* 82(Suppl. 2):36.

HOWELL, J. L., J. W. FUQUAY, and A. E. SMITH. 1994. Corpus luteum growth and function in lactating Holsteins during spring and summer. *J. Dairy Sci.,* 77:735.

IMTIAZ-HUSSAIN, S. M., J. W. FUQUAY, and M. YOUNAS. 1992. Estrous cyclicity in nonlactating and lactating Holsteins and Jerseys during a Pakistani summer. *J. Dairy Sci.,* 75:2968.

INGRAHAM, R. H., R. W. STANLEY, and W. C. WAGNER. 1976. Relationship of temperature and humidity to conception rate of Holstein cows in Hawaii. *J. Dairy Sci.,* 59:2086.

LUCY, M. C., H. A. GARVERICK, and D. E. SPIERS. 2002. Stress, management induced in dairy cattle— Effect on reproduction. *Encyclopedia of Dairy Sciences.* eds. H. Roginski, J. W. Fuquay, and P. F. Fox, Academic Press, an imprint of Elsevier Science.

PUTNEY, D. J., S. MULLINS, W. W. THATCHER, M. DROST, and T. S. GROSS. 1989. Embryonic development in superovulated dairy cattle exposed to elevated ambient temperatures between the onset of estrus and insemination. *Anim. Reprod. Sci.,* 19:37.

STOEBEL, D. and G. P. MOBERG. 1982. Repeated acute stress during the follicular phase and luteinizing hormone surge of dairy heifers. *J. Dairy Sci.,* 65:92.

ULBERG, L. C. and P. J. BURFENING. 1967. Embryo death resulting from adverse environment on spermatozoa or ova. *J. Anim. Sci.,* 26:571.

YOUNAS, M., J. W. FUQUAY, and A. B. MOORE. 1993. Estrous and endocrine response of lactating Holsteins to forced ventilation during the summer. *J. Dairy Sci.,* 76:430.

23

Nutritional Management

Lack of proper nutrition can reduce reproductive efficiency (Table 23–1). Gross deficiencies or excesses can be easily recognized and steps taken to correct the problem. Other imbalance in nutrition can be subtle and difficult to recognize. Diagnosis is sometimes difficult because reproductive symptoms associated with many deficiencies in nutrition are similar to symptoms caused by other disorders. It should also be recognized that nutrition is often a scapegoat, being falsely blamed for problems in reproduction that are caused by infectious organisms or deficiencies in management.

There are no magic nutritional formulae that ensure efficient reproduction. If diets for animals are sufficient to meet their requirements as established by the National Research Council, nutrition is not likely to limit reproduction. Most nutrition-related reproductive problems result from either neglect or an overestimation of the nutritional value of the feedstuffs used in formulating diets.

Nutrition is of concern in developing countries when programs to upgrade the genetic capabilities of their livestock are employed. This can be done through importation of semen or importation of frozen embryos without the concerns of disease transmission associated with importation of live animals and at lower cost. Many of these countries have limited resources for upgrading nutritional regimens to complement the improved genetics. If in hot climates, production of high-quality forage is very difficult and adds to the problem. Animals with genetic potential for production that exceeds the level of nutrition provided become thin and have low reproductive efficiency. Nutrition can be of concern for range animals in developed countries. Reduced reproductive efficiency has been reported for beef cattle and sheep during drought years when forage is scarce.

The objectives of this chapter are to discuss those dietary components that may reduce reproductive efficiency and to give general guidelines on the nutritional management of animals during different phases of reproduction.

23–1 NUTRITIVE COMPONENTS

Nutritional factors needed for successful reproduction are the same as those needed for maintenance, growth, and lactation (Figure 23–1). They include energy, protein, vitamins, and minerals. A deficiency or an excess of any of these components which is serious enough to affect reproduction will also affect other physiological functions.

Table 23–1 *Nutrient-related abnormalities in reproduction*

Nutrient	Reproductive disorder
Energy excess	Low conception, abortion, dystocia, retained placentae, reduced libido
Energy deficiency	Delayed puberty, suppressed estrus and ovulation, suppressed libido and spermatozoa production
Protein excess	Low conception rate
Protein deficiency	Suppressed estrus, low conception, fetal resorption, premature parturition, weak offspring
Vitamin A deficiency	Impaired spermatogenesis, anestrus, low conception, abortion, weak or dead offspring, retained placentae
Vitamin D deficiency	Defective skeletal development, rickets
Calcium deficiency	Skeletal defects, reduced viable young
Phosphorus deficiency	Anestrus, irregular estrus
Iodine deficiency	Impaired fetal growth, irregular estrus, retained placentae
Selenium deficiency	Retained placentae

Source: Compiled from literature.

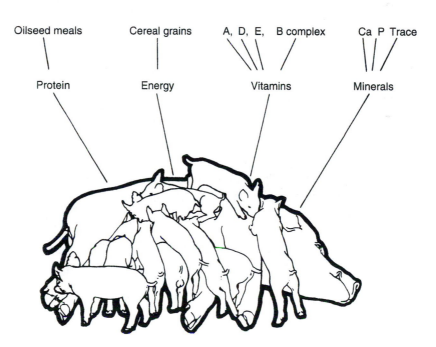

Figure 23–1 Balanced nutrition is needed for good reproductive efficiency.

23–1.1 *Energy*

Many nutrition-related problems in reproduction are due to either underfeeding or overfeeding energy. Energy is unique because, in terms of length of reproductive life, overfeeding is more detrimental than underfeeding. Overfeeding results in excess fatness with fat infiltrating the liver and sometimes the reproductive organs. Such animals have less resistance to infectious diseases and other stressors. Also, lower conception rate, abortion, dystocia, and more frequent retention of the placenta have been reported. Overconditioned males are more likely to have foot and leg problems, which reduce libido (Chapter 7). Extreme fatness is more likely to occur in dairy cows that are fed too liberally during late lactation and in meat animals that have been fattened for livestock shows.

While overfeeding may be more serious, underfeeding occurs more frequently. Underfeeding of energy will delay puberty in both sexes, reduce production of spermatozoa in growing males after puberty, reduce ovulations per estrus in growing polytocous females, cause weak estrus and quiet ovulation, cause or extend periods of anestrus, and reduce libido in males. Some have reported lower conception rates in underfed cattle, but the primary cause of lower calf crops for underfed beef cattle appears to be an extended postpartum anestrus rather than low fertilization rate. These responses likely result from the reduced LH pulsatility that is caused by a negative energy balance. A similar response is seen in early postpartum dairy cows that are in a negative energy balance because of high milk production rather than a limited availability of high-energy feeds (Section 23–3.2).

The data in Table 23–2 show the effects of low, medium, and high levels of nutrition on the age and weight at first calving, services per conception, birth weight of calves, and calving difficulty for Holstein heifers. The medium level of nutrition was recommended. Even though these heifers were $3\frac{1}{2}$ months younger than the low group at calving, they

Table 23–2   *Influence of plane of nutrition on reproductive performance of Holsteins*

	TDN intake (percent of normal)		
Measure	62	100	146
Number of heifers	33	34	34
Age at first estrus, months	20.2	11.2	9.2
Weight at first estrus, kg	303	265	277
Conceived to first mating, %	79	68	58
Matings per first conception, no.	1.55	1.41	1.48
Age at first calving, months	32.0	28.5	27.9
Weight at first calving, kg	384	483	548
Weight of first calf, kg	36	39	41
Requiring help at calving, %	45	26	24
Delivering living calves, %	87	88	94
Matings per second conception, no.	1.71	1.76	2.09
Matings per third conception, no.	1.90	1.64	1.90
Culled for sterility, %	6	12	20

From Maynard and Loosli. *Animal Nutrition.* McGraw-Hill Book Co. 1969.

weighed 99 kg more and experienced approximately half the calving difficulty. Birth weights of calves were not greatly affected by weight of dams. Services per conception were similar for all groups. The medium-level group could have been bred 3 months earlier without additional energy intake.

Major sources of energy include cereal grains, grain by-products, and high-quality forages. For ruminants, legume hay, corn silage, summer and winter annual grasses (grazed or fed fresh), and perennial grass-legume pastures during the spring are good sources of energy. Perennial grasses are frequently overrated during the summer. This is particularly true in subtropic and tropic regions. These grasses remain green, but growth rate and soluble carbohydrates are reduced while the fibrous, structural portion increases. They cannot be digested quickly enough to meet the energy requirements of growing or lactating ruminants. This deficiency may not be readily apparent to a casual observer but can result in delayed puberty or extended postpartum anestrus. Sorghum silage is also frequently overrated as an energy source. Most of the carbohydrate in green sorghum plants is in the form of soluble sugars. When grazed or fed freshly cut, it is a good source of energy. When ensiled, the soluble sugars are lost during fermentation in the silo. By contrast, most of the carbohydrate in corn silage is starch, which is not lost during fermentation.

23–1.2 *Protein*

Feeding excess protein has in some cases resulted in increased milk production in dairy cows. However, feeding protein to excess has lowered first service conception rate while increasing services per conception and days open in lactating dairy cows. On the basis of a limited number of observations, it appears that feeding a total diet containing more than 13% crude protein will result in lower reproductive efficiency.

Lower reproductive efficiency in beef and dairy cows has been related to grazing lush ryegrass pastures that have a high soluble nitrogen concentration. Also, low reproductive efficiency may occur in well-managed dairy herds when herd managers are striving for high milk production through feeding of extra protein to their cows.

For range animals, diets deficient in protein are more common. Diets deficient in protein have resulted in weak expression of estrus, cessation of estrus, repeat breeding, fetal resorption, and birth of premature and/or weak offspring. In practice, diets low in protein are also frequently low in energy. For pigs, the quality of the protein must be considered, since adverse effects have been observed when one or more amino acids are limited. Diets deficient in a single amino acid have slowed growth rate, resulted in delayed puberty, extended postpartum anestrus, and caused abnormal fetal growth patterns.

The best sources of protein are high protein concentrates such as soybean, cottonseed, and peanut meals and legumes such as alfalfa or clover. Both annual and perennial grasses can provide a good source of dietary protein with adequate moisture and liberal fertilization with nitrogen at earlier stages of maturity. Haylage and low moisture silage are frequently overrated because the protein digestibility is decreased by excess heating in the silo. A similar problem exists for heat-damaged hay.

Use of urea and other sources of nonprotein nitrogen in diets of ruminants will not adversely affect reproduction if fed as recommended.

23–1.3 *Vitamins*

It is likely that all vitamins needed for growth and maintenance are also needed for reproduction. However, because of the availability in the usual animal feedstuffs, few have become sufficiently deficient to adversely affect reproduction.

A deficiency in vitamin A can adversely affect reproduction in both males and females. It is necessary for the integrity of the germ cells in the seminiferous tubules in males. A deficiency can reduce or even stop spermatogenesis. In females, a deficiency of vitamin A has resulted in an array of problems, including anestrus, repeat breeding, abortions, weak or dead offspring, and retained placentae. Vitamin A can be stored in the liver. Therefore, a body reserve is available to prevent problems during short periods when the diet is deficient.

Research evidence for a specific role for β-carotene in reproduction remains inconclusive. β-carotene, the plant source of vitamin A, is converted to active forms of vitamin A in the intestine and liver. The corpus luteum has a high concentration of β-carotene and *in vitro* studies have supported the hypothesis that dietary β-carotene is related to corpus luteum function. Some researchers have reported impaired fertility in dairy cows and heifers on diets deficient in β-carotene even if the vitamin A status of these animals is normal. Other researchers in similar experiments have seen no effect from diets devoid of β-carotene. Likewise, supplementation of diets with β-carotene has improved fertility in some cows but not in others. While there may be a specific function for β-carotene in reproduction other than its role as a precursor for vitamin A, conditions for a response need to be better defined before a general recommendation can be made.

Fresh green forages, air-cured alfalfa hay, green silage, and purchased supplements are the best dietary sources of vitamin A (β-carotene). Vitamin A is destroyed by high temperature and by sunlight. Therefore, haylage, low moisture silage, heat-damaged hay, and sun-cured hay are not good sources. Most vitamin A deficiencies in ruminants occur when the forage is from one of those sources. When the vitamin A content of the forage is in doubt, addition of a vitamin A supplement to the concentrate is simple and secure insurance against a vitamin A deficiency.

As a result of early research in rats, vitamin E was called the "antisterility vitamin." In female rats, a deficiency resulted in death and resorption of fetuses. In male rats, degeneration of the testes sometimes resulted in permanent sterility. Efforts to demonstrate a need for supplemental vitamin E for reproduction in other species have not been successful. The availability of vitamin E in cereal grains and forages makes a deficiency of this vitamin unlikely. Salespeople have promoted the use of vitamin E and wheat germ oil, which is high in vitamin E, as a cure for both real and imagined reproductive problems. However, the need for this vitamin as a supplement has not been demonstrated.

Vitamin D is of interest in reproduction because of its role in absorption and retention of calcium and phosphorus. Principal effects of vitamin D deficiency have been related to development of the skeletal system of the fetus. Rickets are common when a deficiency has existed during gestation. Vitamin D may influence the time of first postpartum estrus and calving interval, also. Vitamin D deficiencies do not occur unless animals are deprived of sunlight. Sun-cured hay and supplements which can be added to concentrate feeds will also provide this vitamin. Care must be exercised when supplementing diets with vitamin D, especially when animals are exposed to adequate sunlight. Vitamin D toxicity has occurred in both humans and farm animals from an excess of the vitamin.

Most other vitamins are either synthesized by the animals or are available in adequate quantities in the usual feedstuff to prevent deficiencies. Although vitamin C is synthesized in the body and not required in the diet, supplemental doses have been beneficial in reducing infertility in males and females in some cases. Further research is needed on the mechanisms of action and on the conditions that suggest that this therapy may be beneficial. Vitamin B_{12} is not available from plant sources. It is synthesized in the rumen of ruminants and provided through the addition of B_{12} supplement or meat products to the diet of simple stomached animals.

23–1.4 *Minerals*

Requirements of most minerals are increased per unit of body weight by gestation, lactation, and growth. While gross deficiencies may reduce efficiency of reproduction, such deficiencies seldom occur in field conditions. Mineral mixes containing calcium, phosphorus, iodized salt, and trace minerals are recommended in the nutritional management of animals for meat and milk production. If these minerals are supplied in sufficient quantities and ratios to meet the requirements for meat and milk production, it is doubtful that reproduction will be affected. If mineral mixes are not provided, the mineral content of natural feedstuffs must supply mineral needs. Reproductive problems have resulted in areas where deficiencies of specific minerals in the soil have reduced that found in natural feedstuffs.

Reduced calf crops have been reported in phosphorus-deficient areas of the world. In a phosphorus-deficient region of South Africa, supplementation with bone meal to provide phosphorus resulted in a 29 percentage units improvement of calf crop (80% vs. 51%). Low calf crop in phosphorus-deficient cows appears due to irregular estrous patterns and periods of anestrus. Diets deficient in phosphorus will depress appetite, which could contribute to anestrus and delayed puberty.

Calcium deficiency is seldom a problem in ruminants. Legumes are high in calcium. In addition, animals have physiological control over both absorption and excretion of calcium. Calcium-deficient swine rations have reduced the number of viable young per litter and in some cases caused intrauterine death. The effect of calcium deficiency on the development of the fetal skeletal system might be more severe, except that the fetus can draw minerals from the skeletal system of the mother for development of its own system. If the calcium reserves of the mother are not replenished between gestations, skeletal defects may occur in later gestations. This is a potential problem but seldom occurs. Most defects in the development of the skeletal system of the fetus are due to a lack of vitamin D, which has been discussed.

Iodine deficiency has been reported to cause a number of disorders in reproduction. They include delayed development of the reproductive tract, irregular estrus, impaired fetal growth, and retained placentae. In males, iodine deficiency has been associated with low libido and poor semen quality. Certain regions are deficient in iodine. In such regions, allowing animals to have access to iodized salt provides sufficient protection. Toxic effects from too much iodine supplementation have been associated with abortion and fetal deformities.

A higher than normal incidence of retained placentae has been reported in cows in selenium-deficient regions. An injection of selenium and vitamin E about 2 weeks before expected parturition will reduce the incidence of retained placentae. Vitamin E is needed for efficient utilization of selenium. High levels of selenium can be toxic, but specific adverse effects on reproduction have not been reported.

Deficiencies or toxicities of other minerals have been reported to affect reproduction but their specific roles in the reproductive processes are not clear. Copper and cobalt deficiencies have been associated with depressed estrus, low fertility, and abnormal fetal development. Deficiency of magnesium has been associated with low fertility. A deficiency of manganese is rare but has been associated with irregular estrous cycles and anestrus. Deficiencies of zinc in males have resulted in impaired spermatogenesis and testosterone production. Such deficiencies are not likely if trace mineralized salt is included in the diet or is available free choice. Cattle that are grazing on lands high in molybdenum may show toxicity, with delayed puberty and anestrus being among the symptoms noted.

23–2 GROWING ANIMALS

The primary nutritional concern in females between birth and maturity is to maintain a level of intake and thus growth that will (1) not delay puberty; (2) ensure that adequate size be attained at the desired breeding age; and (3) maintain growth during gestation so that parturition is not made more difficult by the impaired size of the mother (Chapters 5 and 20). In growing males, the nutritional regimen should be sufficient to (1) not delay puberty and (2) not reduce libido and spermatozoa production after puberty (Chapter 7). The nutritional program is controlled by the animal manager and if not managed properly will extend rather than shorten generation interval. Through nutritional management, the animal manager probably has the greatest control over generation interval.

During periods of growth, animals should be maintained on a moderate to heavy plane of nutrition. The goal is to maintain an adequate and steady rate of growth until mature size is reached. The dairy heifer can be used as a model for discussing nutritional needs during growth. The dairy heifer will reach puberty at 8 to 13 months of age at a weight of 160 kg to 270 kg. Both age and weight vary among breeds. If she is to calve at 24 months of age (the optimum age), she will need to reach her minimum recommended breeding weight (Table 20–1) by 15 months of age. To reach this goal, the dairy heifer should gain approximately 0.7 kg per day from birth to 15 months of age. A similar pattern of growth should continue through gestation. A heifer on native forage will not be able to maintain the desired growth rate without supplemental feeding during most of the year. As mentioned previously, young, succulent plants are high in soluble carbohydrates and proteins and will meet these requirements for growing animals. As these plants become more mature, there will be proportionately less soluble carbohydrate and protein with more structural carbohydrates in these plants. Ruminants can digest structural carbohydrates, but the rate of digestion is not fast enough to meet the animal's energy requirements for growth plus maintenance. During late gestation, the additional requirement to account for the growing fetus must be added to requirements for growth and maintenance.

To assure that the nutritive requirements of the growing animal are met, one must know the requirements for energy, protein, vitamins, and minerals. These have been published by the National Research Council (NRC) for dairy cattle, beef cattle, pigs, sheep, and horses. In addition, one must know the nutritive value of the components of the animal's diet. Forages vary greatly in nutritive value depending on amount and kind of fertilization, stage of maturity, season, and methods used in storing and preserving. Therefore, forages used in the diets of ruminants should be subjected to laboratory analysis so that intelligent supplementation can be implemented to meet the nutritive requirements of growing animals. When comparing a maintenance diet with one that is designed for growth, several differences will be noted. Principally, the diet of growing animals will need to be richer in energy, protein, calcium, and phosphorus, since growth involves development of muscles and the skeletal system. Requirements of vitamins and other minerals will be higher, also.

23–3 MAINTAINING REPRODUCTIVE EFFICIENCY

The importance of nutrition in maintaining reproductive efficiency varies with species. Nutrition seldom limits reproduction in mature, lactating dairy cows. In other farm species, where the management systems frequently result in animals receiving marginal or sub-maintenance diets during part of the year, limited reproduction related to dietary deficiencies is not uncommon. It is important to remember that nutritive requirements increase during gestation. This is especially true during the last quarter of gestation, when supplementation is needed to prevent fetal depletion of maternal nutrient reserves. Depletion of nutrient reserves may not interfere with the ongoing gestation unless the deficiencies are severe. Depletion of maternal reserves is more likely to reduce the number of offspring born to future gestations or delay postpartum estrus and the next gestation.

23–3.1 *Flushing*

Low nutrition will sometimes cause anestrus in cows and reduce ovulation rate in ewes and sows. Conversely, animals in good condition and on a high plane of nutrition will have more offspring on a herd or flock basis than animals in poor condition. It has also been demonstrated that, if animals are in a poor nutritional state and thin condition, supplementing their diet so that they are gaining in weight at time of breeding will increase piglets per litter, multiple births in sheep, and percentage of calf crop in beef cows. Even when gilts are in a good nutritional state, increasing their energy level for 8 to 12 days before estrus will increase their ovulation rate (Table 23–3). Supplementing the diet to have animals in a gaining state at time of breeding is called *flushing*. Flushing results in an increase in insulin and insulin-like growth factor in the ovary (Section 4–3.1a). This results in increased ovarian responsiveness to FSH and LH and reduced follicular atresia. The flushing effect in pigs may be offset by higher embryo mortality if heavy supplementation is continued after

Table 23–3 *Effect of dietary energy on ovulation rate in cycling gilts*

| Energy (kcal ME/day)[a] | Ovulation rate | | |
	Mean	Standard error	Range
5,700	14.2	.7	10–17
9,600	18.6	1.1	10–22

Courtesy of N. M. Cox, Department of Animal Science, Mississippi State University, 1983.

[a]During approximately 10 days (range 8 to 12) before estrus.

breeding. In beef cows, the principal effect of flushing appears to be that of bringing animals out of anestrus, so that more have the opportunity to conceive during the next breeding season. To better relate body composition to performance criteria, a 9-point body condition scoring system has been developed for beef cows with a score from 1 (emaciated) to 9 (obese). Using this system, it has been demonstrated that cows calving with a body condition score of 5 to 7 have higher subsequent pregnancy rates than those calving with a score less than 5. Postpartum estrous cycles are resumed earlier when body condition scores are over 5 at calving.

23–3.2 *Dairy Cows*

It has been demonstrated in other species that having animals in a gaining state at time of breeding will improve reproductive efficiency. If dairy cows are to maintain a 12-month calving interval, they must be bred at a time when most are losing weight. They are losing weight because the energy and protein output through milk in early lactation exceeds the energy and protein that can be consumed and utilized from their diet. The period of negative energy balance will be extended if cows are injected with growth hormone starting the ninth week after calving, as is recommended for increased milk production. However, the effects on reproduction will be minimal if these animals have started cycling before growth hormone treatment begins. Management of the dairy cow during the last 2 months of the gestation is critical. She will not be lactating during that 2-month period. It is recommended that dairy cows be "turned dry" (milking stopped) 60 days prepartum. Her nutrient needs are those for maintenance and her fetus. The manager should feed her to meet her nutrient requirements and to store reserves for early lactation, while guarding against overconditioning. As a means of quantifying nutritional status, a 5-point body condition scoring system has been developed for dairy cows (1 = emaciated; 5 = obese), with some further dividing this scale into as little as 0.25 increments. When evaluated using this scale, cows with body condition scores of 2 to 3 at breeding have conceived in a shorter interval after parturition than cows with scores under 2 or over 3. Since dairy cows are in a negative energy balance for at least 60 days postpartum, they should calve with a body condition score of 3.5 to 4 if they are to be in the desired range at breeding. Nutritional adjustments during the dry period will ensure that they achieve proper body condition at calving. Managing the nutrition of the dairy cow during the last one-third of lactation so that a body condition score of 3.5 to 4 is achieved at dry-off will minimize the severity of fatty liver and associated metabolic problems that occur around the time of calving. In turn, this will reduce the negative effects of these on reproduction.

The manager should also be aware that changing the diet from that needed during the 60-day nonlactating period before parturition to that desired during early lactation places great stress on the digestive system. During the nonlactating period, the diet is typically greater than 95% forage, with the remainder concentrate. During early lactation, this changes to 60% to 70% concentrate. This change should not be made suddenly. It should be started during the last week of the gestation, with daily concentrate gradually increased so that the rumen can adjust to higher concentrate before parturition. Having her on a high level of concentrate as lactation starts will reduce the depletion of nutrient reserves from her body and reduce digestive disturbances that could lead to ketosis or other disorders. The cow that comes through parturition without sickness will be more likely to maintain the desired efficiency in reproduction.

23–3.3 *Males*

Nutritional recommendations for growing males are similar to those for growing females. Moderate to heavy feeding is recommended. Underfeeding will delay puberty. After puberty, underfeeding will reduce libido and spermatozoa production in growing males. The principal concern is to provide enough energy and protein, but vitamins and minerals cannot be overlooked.

The mature male should be restricted to a maintenance diet. Underfeeding for an extended period will reduce libido, which effectually reduces spermatozoa production. However, feeding above the recommended diet for maintenance will not further increase libido or spermatozoa production. It may shorten the reproductive life of the male (Chapter 7).

SUGGESTED READING

ASCARELLI, I., Z. EDELMAN, M. ROSENBERG, and Y. FOLMAN. 1985. Effect of dietary carotene on fertility of high-yielding dairy cows. *Anim. Prod.,* 40:195.

BUTLER, W. R. and R. O. SMITH. 1989. Interrelationships between energy balance and postpartum reproductive function in dairy cattle. *J. Dairy Sci.,* 72:767.

DEROUEN, S. M., D. E. FRANKS, D. G. MORRISON, W. E. WYATT, D. F. COMBS, T. W. WHITE, P. E. HUMES, and B. B. GREENE. 1994. Prepartum body condition and weight influences on reproductive performance of first-calf beef cows. *J. Anim. Sci.,* 72:1119.

FERGUSON, J. O. and W. CHALUPA. 1989. Impact of protein nutrition on reproduction in dairy cows. *J. Dairy Sci.,* 72:746.

FOOTE, W. C., A. L. POPE, A. B. CHAPMAN, and L. E. CASIDA. 1959. Reproduction in the yearling ewe as affected by breed and sequence of feeding levels. I. Effect on ovulation rate and embryo survival. *J. Anim. Sci.,* 18:453.

HEMKIN, R. W. and D. H. BREMEL. 1982. Possible role of beta-carotene in improving fertility in dairy cattle. *J. Dairy Sci.,* 65:1069.

HURLEY, W. L. and R. M. DOANE. 1989. Recent developments in the roles of vitamins and minerals in reproduction. *J. Dairy Sci.,* 72:784.

JORDAN, E. R. and L. V. SWANSON. 1979. Effect of crude protein on reproductive efficiency, serum total proteins and albumin in high producing dairy cows. *J. Dairy Sci.,* 62:58.

JOUBERT, D. M. 1954. The influence of high and low nutritional planes on the estrous cycle and conception rate of heifers. *J. Agric. Sci.,* 45:164.

JULIEN, W. E., H. R. CONRAD, J. E. JONES, and A. L. MOXON. 1976. Selenium and vitamin E and incidence of retained placenta in parturient dairy cows. *J. Dairy Sci.,* 59:1954.

MCNAMARA, J. P. 2002. Body condition score—Effects on health, milk production, and reproduction. *Encyclopedia of Dairy Sciences,* eds. H. Roginski, J. W. Fuquay, and P. F. Fox. Academic Press, an imprint of Elsevier Science.

REID, J. T. 1960. Effect of energy intake upon reproduction in farm animals. *J. Dairy Sci.* 43(Suppl.):103.

SELF, H. L., R. H. GRUMMER, and L. E. CASIDA. 1955. The effect of various sequences of full and limited feeding on the reproductive phenomena of Chester White and Poland China gilts. *J. Anim. Sci.,* 14:573.

SMITH, T. R. 2002. Ration formulation—Dry period and transition rations in cows. *Encyclopedia of Dairy Sciences.* eds. H. Roginski. J. W. Fuquay, and P. F. Fox. Academic Press, an imprint of Elsevier Science.

WILDMAN, E. E., G. M. JONES, P. E. WAGNER, R. L. BOWMAN, H. F. TROUTT, JR., and T. N. LESCH. 1982. A dairy cow body condition scoring system and relationship to selected production characteristics. *J. Dairy Sci.,* 65:495.

WILTBANK, J. N., W. W. ROWDEN, J. E. INGALLS, and D. R. ZIMMERMAN. 1962. Effect of energy level on reproductive phenomena of mature Hereford cows. *J. Anim. Sci.,* 21:219.

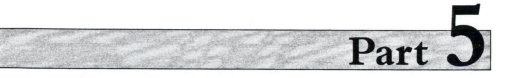

Part 5

Causes of Reproductive Failure

There are many causes of reproductive failure. Although some are congenital and cannot be treated, most others can be minimized through proper management and appropriate treatment. With a goal of culling less than 5% for reproductive failure in a 12-month period, application of the information provided in the next three chapters is important to reaching that goal.

24

Anatomical and Inherited Causes
of Reproductive Failure

24–1 FREEMARTIN

The *freemartin* condition is considered to be a problem in cattle. The condition occurs in the female member of heterosexual twins in which the allanto-chorionic membranes of the twins fuse early during embryonic development (Color Plate 31). This fusion allows an exchange of blood between the twins. In order for the freemartin condition to develop, fusion of the embryonic membranes must occur during the embryonic period prior to the development of the reproductive organs. Between 5% and 10% of the female members of heterosexual twins are not freemartins, presumably because the chorionic membranes fail to fuse or fuse after the reproductive organs differentiate. Freemartin-like conditions have been reported in sheep, goats, and swine. Even though multiple births are much more common in these species, the phenomenon is not considered to be a serious problem.

The freemartin is sterile. The gonads vary widely in appearance and in histological makeup. Some have almost normal ovaries, while others resemble small testes complete with epididymides. The oviducts, uterus, cervix, and most of the vagina fail to develop as tubular structures (Figure 24–1). They often appear as bands of tissue, with various abnormal deviations in shape. Varying degrees of development of both the Müllerian and Wolffian ducts contribute to these deviations. The presence of some degree of development of vesicular glands has been frequently reported. The external genitalia generally appear normal. Occasionally, the clitoris is enlarged and the tuft of hairs at the tip of the vulva is more prominent. The mammary gland remains rudimentary and frequently can be distinguished from a normal mammary gland by 1 to 2 months of age.

The cause of the freemartin condition is still not fully understood. As early as 1916, a hormonal theory was presented. The male gonads develop earlier than female gonads (Chapter 9). This is related to the fact that the testes originate from the primary sex cords, while in the female the primary sex cords give way to the development of the secondary sex cords, which in turn develop into ovaries. According to the hormonal theory, the developing male testes produce hormones, presumably androgens, which interfere with the development of the female reproductive organs. More recent knowledge casts serious doubt on the hormonal theory. Androgens do not appear to have the ability to interfere with the development of the reproductive system. They also do not appear to have the ability to cause the regression of the Müllerian ducts, which frequently occurs in the

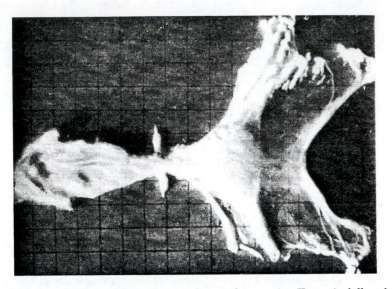

Figure 24–1   Reproductive organs from a freemartin. (From Asdell and Bearden. 1959. *Cornell Ext. Bull.* 737.)

freemartin. Also, the external genitalia which are most sensitive to masculinization generally remain normal.

Current thoughts on the subject relate to the exchange of cells between the twins. Blood cells, blood-forming cells, and perhaps other cells are exchanged through the fused chorionic blood vessels. Evidence has been presented supporting a theory that X chromosomes carry genes for both male and female organ development but that, in the absence of Y chromosomes, the expression of genes for male development is suppressed. When Y chromosomes are present, the inhibition of the genes for male development is removed and the genes for female development are suppressed. Each twin contains two genetic populations of cells, one representing its own genotype and one like its twin's. The presence of the Y chromosome may interfere with or suppress to varying degrees the genes for female development. (Section 9–2.4).

The male member of heterosexual twins has generally been thought to be normal in every respect. Based on either theory described here, one would suspect this to be true. There is increasing evidence, however, that such male twins may also experience reduced reproductive efficiency.

The freemartin condition can be diagnosed in newborn calves by inserting a suitable instrument into the vagina. A sterile plastic inseminating catheter may be used if proper precautions are taken. The vagina of a normal heifer is 12 cm to 15 cm long, while the vagina of the freemartin is only 5 cm or 6 cm long. Care should be taken not to allow the catheter to enter the suburethral diverticulum in a normal heifer, thus indicating a freemartin. Some individuals prefer to use a 16 mm by 125 mm test tube for this test. In a normal heifer, the entire test tube can be inserted into the vagina.

Single birth freemartinism has been reported also. It may result from loss of one embryo from a double ovulation and fertilization after differentiation of sex organs.

24–2 Infantile Reproductive System

An infantile or underdeveloped reproductive system is not usually a permanent cause of reproductive failure (Figure 24–2). It is most frequently found in underfed heifers as characterized by small inactive ovaries, the absence of estrus, and lack of growth of the uterus and vagina. The problem can be corrected by increasing the energy intake, such as turning out to lush spring grazing or by liberal feeding of a good concentrate mixture containing 16% protein. Hormone treatments such as PMSG may be effective, but improved nutrition would be preferred.

Genetically related infantile ovaries that cannot be corrected by hormone treatment or nutrition have been reported. Fortunately, the frequency of this condition is low.

24–3 Incomplete Structures— Oviduct, Uterus, Cervix, or Vagina

Occasionally, females have incomplete oviducts, malformed uteri, blind cervixes, blind vaginas, and the like (Figure 24–3). Usually, these defects cannot be repaired and are difficult to detect without slaughter of the female. These animals come into estrus regularly because the ovaries are functional but are sterile because the defects prevent sperm and egg from meeting. Some of these defects are inherited and would be expected to occur more frequently if inbreeding were practiced. In fact, some defects are never suspected until they are uncovered by inbreeding. In a normal outcross population, the frequency of these structural abnormalities is not great. Even in subfertile dairy heifers, the frequency of incomplete structures is only 3.9%.

Bulls may have similar abnormalities. Most frequently, they take the form of incomplete union of the testes with the ducts that transport spermatozoa or of malformations of the penis. The latter condition may prevent copulation.

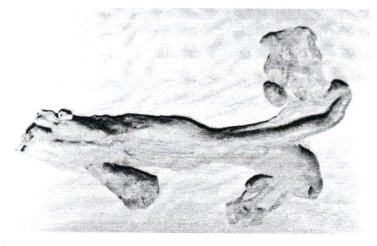

Figure 24–2 Infantile reproductive tract from 2-year-old heifer. Note small uterine horns and small, inactive ovaries.

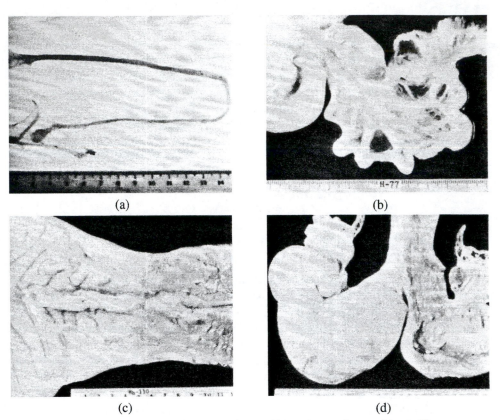

(a)   (b)

(c)   (d)

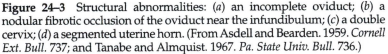

Figure 24–3 Structural abnormalities: (*a*) an incomplete oviduct; (*b*) a nodular fibrotic occlusion of the oviduct near the infundibulum; (*c*) a double cervix; (*d*) a segmented uterine horn. (From Asdell and Bearden. 1959. *Cornell Ext. Bull.* 737; and Tanabe and Almquist. 1967. *Pa. State Univ. Bull.* 736.)

24–4 HERMAPHRODITE

The phenomenon described by the term *hermaphrodite (intersex)* is a situation in which the sexuality of an individual is confused by the presence of anatomical structures of both sexes. Hermaphrodites are classified as either true hermaphrodites or pseudohermaphrodites. A true hermaphrodite has both male and female gonads. These may be either separate or combined as ovo-testes. The pseudohermaphrodite has either testes or ovaries, but the remainder of the reproductive system has parts representing both sexes. Pseudohermaphrodites are usually classified male or female according to the type of gonads present. The male pseudohermaphrodite has testes but otherwise may be largely female in makeup (Figure 24–4).

Genetic sex is determined by the pairing of sex chromosomes. Normal females have an XX pairing; normal males an XY pairing. Deviations can result from abnormalities of either or both of the sex chromosomes, by increases (XXY) or decreases (XO) in the number of sex chromosomes, or by a chimerism of male (XY) and female (XX) cells in the same individual. All of these abnormal sex chromosome combinations have been reported in farm animals. True hermaphroditism with varying combinations of ovaries, testes, and ovo-testes

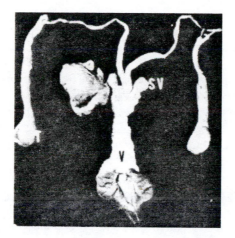

Figure 24–4 Internal genitalia of a male bovine pseudohermaphrodite. (From Hafez. 1974. *Reproduction in Farm Animals.* (3rd ed.) Lea and Febiger.)

has been described in the horse, goat, cow, and pig. They occur much more frequently in goats and pigs than in the other species. Pseudohermaphrodites are more common than true hermaphrodites.

In the case of pseudohermaphrodites, genetic and gonadal sex develops sequentially, but there are discrepancies in the development of structures arising from the Wolffian or Müllerian ducts, the urogenital sinus, and external genitalia. In the normal male, the development of these structures appears to be dependent on androgen or other substances needed for normal expression (Section 9–5). In the male hermaphrodite, either the gonads do not produce androgens or the target cells do not respond to them. In the human female pseudohermaphrodite, a deficiency of an enzyme in the metabolic pathway in the adrenal gland causes cortisone not to be produced. This is accompanied by an increase in the production of androgens by the adrenal gland. This syndrome has not been well documented in livestock.

24–5 CRYPTORCHID

Cryptorchidism is a condition in which the testes fail to pass through the inguinal canal into the scrotum. It may be unilateral (one testis remaining in the abdomen and one passing into the scrotum) or bilateral (both testes remaining in the abdomen). The bilateral cryptorchid is sterile, since spermatogenesis in mammals cannot occur normally at body temperature (Section 3–2.1). The germinal epithelium of the seminiferous tubules in these males is unaffected until puberty, but if the condition is not corrected by surgery, the spermatogonia degenerate and the male will be permanently sterile. The unilateral cryptorchid produces normal, viable, and fertile spermatozoa from the testis that descended into the scrotum. The testis that remained in the body cavity experiences the same fate as the testes of the bilateral cryptorchid.

The interstitial cells of the cryptorchid testes are not affected by the higher temperature. These males, even though sterile, develop normal secondary sex characteristics and normal sexual behavior. The testes of the cryptorchid are smaller than normal for the species. This is presumably due to the failure of the seminiferous tubules to develop normally or to the degeneration of the germinal epithelium after puberty.

Cryptorchidism occurs in most mammalian species. It occurs in humans and most domestic animals but is more common in stallions, bucks, and boars than in bulls. The cause of the phenomenon is not fully understood. It may be related to hormonal deficiencies in some cases. In other cases, anatomical obstruction of the inguinal canal or shortness of the ligaments that connect the testes to the body wall may cause the condition. Androgens administered to the foal shortly after birth have resulted in descent of the testes to the scrotum. The other causes require surgery for correction. Whatever the causes, most agree that they are genetically related and therefore the cryptorchid condition occurring in any livestock species should not be corrected by surgery or hormone treatment. Likewise, unilateral cryptorchids should not be used for breeding, since both unilateral and bilateral offspring are likely. All cryptorchids, both unilateral and bilateral, should be destroyed, with the possible exception of horses, and these should not be used for breeding. Cryptorchid pigs should be destroyed as soon as discovered. If they are reared for meat, they will have the characteristic of boars and produce undesirable meat. Cryptorchid bulls and rams may be reared for meat purposes only.

24–6 INJURIES

Injury to the reproductive organs is the cause of significant reproductive failure in both males and females. Some injuries occur spontaneously, but a greater percentage results from human-made causes.

The most common spontaneous injuries to the female reproductive tract occur during parturition. The fetus becomes hyperactive during parturition due to varying degrees of anoxia (Chapter 10). The thrashing of the feet of the fetus has been known to tear the uterus (Figure 24–5). Such injuries may heal without residual effects but may also contribute to breeding failure. Injuries to the vagina may occur during the mating act when males are too vigorous or the penis too large for the female. This is especially a problem with thoroughbred horses.

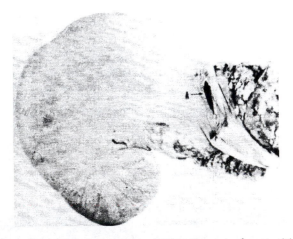

Figure 24–5 Uterus that was torn during the act of parturition. Note point A. (From Asdell and Bearden. 1959. *Cornell Ext. Bull.* 737.)

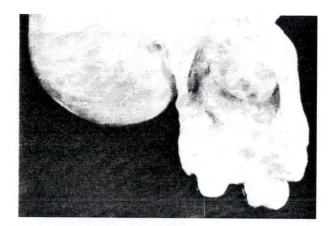

Figure 24–6 Obstructive ovarian and infundibular adhesions: partial envelopment of ovary and total incorporation and incapacitation of infundibulum. (From Tanabe and Almquist. 1967. *Pa. State Univ. Bull.* 736.)

The most common, and by far the most serious, injuries to the female reproductive tract are human-made. These injuries are primarily inflicted on the cow, but some may also occur in the mare. Perhaps the most common relate to adhesions which involve the ovaries and upper portion of the oviducts, particularly the infundibulum (Figure 24–6). They are caused by malpractice of the livestock manager or veterinarian. The injury occurs most commonly during the process of expressing the corpus luteum from the ovary. This is done by placing the end of the thumb against the ovary at the base of the corpus luteum and applying sufficient pressure to expel the corpus luteum from the ovary. Before the development of $PGF_{2\alpha}$ as an injectable compound, this was a favorite treatment of many individuals for the so-called retained corpus luteum. In reality a retained corpus luteum may not exist (Chapter 25). In addition to the damage that might be done to the ovary while expressing a corpus luteum, it is impossible to determine whether the infundibulum or the oviduct is between the thumb and the ovary when the pressure is applied. If the serosa of these delicate structures is broken, the injured area will grow to any surface that comes in contact with it during the healing process. Thus, many oviducts are permanently blocked and infundibula are injured to the point that they may be unable to function normally in capturing the oocytes as they are released from the ovary. A corpus luteum, retained or not, should never be expressed from an ovary. In one group of 180 subfertile dairy heifers, 6.1% had been injured sufficiently to obstruct conception. An additional 26.1% showed injuries to the ovaries, infundibula, and oviducts that were not sufficiently serious to obstruct conception. Adhesions may also occur as a result of injury caused by manual rupture of follicular cysts in the same manner as described for CL expression. With the availability of commercial $PGF_{2\alpha}$ products at a low cost, there is no reason for this to be done.

Other injuries to the reproductive tract usually occur during or immediately following parturition. Too much force used to pull the fetus may result in injury to the uterus, cervix, vagina, or vulva. A high percentage of cows experiencing dystocia also experience breeding problems and many become permanently sterile. When a female must be given assistance during parturition and the fetus cannot be pulled with relative ease, the livestock manager is advised to enlist the service of a veterinarian unless adequately qualified through experience and training.

Injuries to the uterine mucosa are frequently inflicted during manual removal of a retained placenta. Any attempt to disconnect the chorionic villi from the caruncles in the cow's uterus will result in injury. Some individuals unfamiliar with the anatomy of the cow's uterus have been known to tear one or more caruncles loose from the uterus. In view of the possible injury that may occur, the manual removal of the placenta is ill advised. The student is referred to Section 10–6 for management practices related to retained placentae.

Injuries to the reproductive system of the male may also occur. Perforating wounds to the scrotum or the sheath may in themselves cause inflammation or may lead to the introduction of harmful microorganisms that can produce inflammatory conditions. Injuries to the penis have occurred during natural mating and during collection of semen for use in artificial insemination. The most common is the "broken penis." This usually occurs when the penis is bent at a sharp angle during the ejaculatory thrust, resulting in a rupture of the corpus cavernosum penis. These males may retain their ability for erection but, due to the ruptured area, the distal portion of the penis cannot be raised to horizontal position (Figure 24–7). Venous outlets develop during healing which allow the pressure to bleed off, preventing erection in some cases. Such males may be collected by use of the electroejaculator. A few bulls have had their penises amputated by tight rubber bands lost from the artificial vagina during collection. These accidents have occurred infrequently, but anyone who collects semen with the artificial vagina is advised to count the rubber bands used both before and after collection.

24–7 PROLAPSE OF VAGINA AND UTERUS

A slight prolapse or protrusion of the vagina through the vulva during late gestation is not uncommon in older cows and in ewes. It is presumably caused by an excessive relaxation of the pelvic ligaments brought about by relaxin. The condition is not serious.

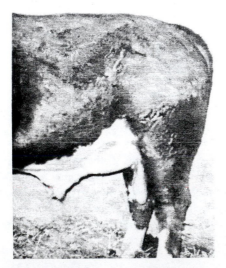

Figure 24–7 Bull with a broken penis. Note swelling between sheath opening and testes. (Courtesy of Dr. Leslie Johnson, College of Veterinary Medicine, Oklahoma State University.)

Prolapse of the uterus (turned inside out) occurs shortly after parturition. The incidence of prolapsed uterus is much less common than prolapsed vagina. It occurs more frequently in cows and ewes than in sows and mares. The condition is associated with dystocia and retained placenta. Pastures rich in estrogenic compounds have been cited as a cause in ewes.

When uterine prolapse occurs, it is necessary to clean the surface and sanitize it as completely as possible before pushing it back into place. The female is usually straining to the point that suturing the lips of the vulva together is necessary to prevent recurrence. Repeat prolapses are sufficiently common to warrant culling the females unless they are very valuable.

24–8 GENETIC ABNORMALITIES

Mulefoot (syndactylism—Holstein and Aberdeen Angus breeds), Bull-Dog (achondoplasia—Holstein breed), weaver condition (bovine progressive degenerative myeloencephalopathy—Brown Swiss breed), limber leg (Jersey breed), spinal muscular atrophy (SMA—Brown Swiss breed), rectovaginal constriction (RVC—Jersey breed), Bovine leucocyte adhesion deficiency (BLAD—Holstein breed), deficiency of uridine monophosphate synthase (DUMPS—Holstein breed) have been identified.

SUGGESTED READING

ASDELL, S. A. 1955. *Cattle Fertility and Sterility.* Little, Brown and Co.

FAULKNER, L. C. and E. J. CARROLL. 1974. Reproductive failure in males. *Reproduction in Farm Animals.* (3rd ed.) ed. E. S. E. Hafez. Lea and Febiger.

FUNK, D. A. 2002. Genetic defects in cattle. *Encyclopedia of Dairy Science.* eds. H. Roginski, J. W. Fuquay, and P. F. Fox. Academic Press, an imprint of Elsevier Science.

HAFEZ, E. S. E. and M. R. JAINUDEEN. 1974. Reproductive failure in females. *Reproduction in Farm Animals.* (3rd ed.) ed. E.S.E. Hafez. Lea and Febiger.

MILNE, F. J. 1954. Penile and preputial problems in the bull. *J. Amer. Vet. Med. Assn.,* 124:6.

OLDS, D. 1978. Inherited, anatomical and pathological causes of lowered reproductive efficiency. *Physiology of Reproduction and Artificial Insemination of Cattle.* (2nd ed.) eds. G. W. Salisbury, N. L. VanDemark, and J. R. Lodge. W. H. Freeman and Co.

ROBERTS, S. L. 1986. *Veterinary Obstetrics and Genital Diseases.* (3rd ed.) Published by the author.

TANABE, T. Y. and J. O. ALMQUIST. 1967. The nature of subfertility in the dairy heifer. III. Gross genital abnormalities. *Pa. State Univ. Bull.* 736.

25

Physiological, Toxicological, and Psychological Causes of Reproductive Failure

Normal reproduction is a complex series of events which must occur at precisely the right time. The timing mechanism is almost totally dependent on the endocrine system. Disturbances of the endocrine system may induce either temporary or permanent sterility. The disturbance may be the breakage of a link in the total chain and may be temporary or permanent. The total system may be influenced by age, environment, or other factors. The more recently developed techniques for studying the endocrine system have been used primarily to develop a better understanding of normal functions. The application of these techniques to the abnormal situation should make them better understood and provide clues for more effective treatment.

25–1 CYSTIC OVARIES

Cystic ovaries are probably among the more perplexing causes of reproductive failure. No treatment can be prescribed that will be effective in all cases. In fact, spontaneous recovery has been almost equal to the effect of treatment in some experiments. This is probably related to the fact that different types of cysts occur in the ovaries. Ovulatory failure may result in a thin-walled cyst (follicular cyst) or a thick-walled cyst (luteinized follicle) in which layers of luteal tissue cover the follicular membrane. A third type of cyst is the cystic corpus luteum. Ovulatory failure without the development of cysts has been reported for all farm species but is much more common in horses and swine than in cattle and sheep. The follicles become partially luteinized and then regress during the estrous cycle in much the same manner as a normal corpus luteum.

25–1.1 *Follicular Cysts*

The usual incidence of follicular cysts in cows is 10% to 15%, but incidences as high as 30% have been reported and confirmed by ultrasonography. Some remain as thin-walled and produce estrogens primarily, along with a higher concentration of androgens (Figures 25–1 and 25–2 and Color Plate 32). The result is usually continuous or chronic estrus (3 to 10 days between heats), a condition referred to as nymphomania. If the condition continues for an extended period of time, the cow develops an apparent high tail head caused by the relaxation of the pelvic ligaments permitting the pelvis to tilt forward and develops a masculine neck, and the cow may bellow like a bull. The cause of cystic ovaries is not known.

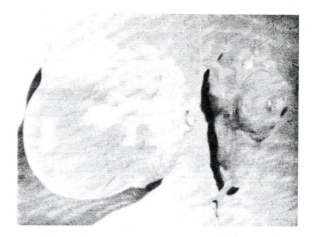

Figure 25–1 Ovary with a large, thin-walled follicular cyst on left. Normal ovary on right. (From Asdell and Bearden. 1959. *Cornell Ext. Bull.* 737.)

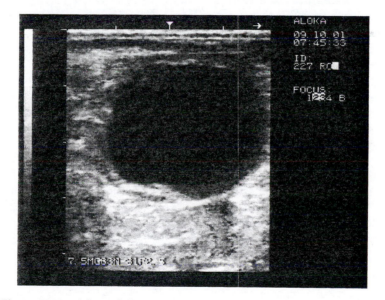

Figure 25–2 A large follicular cyst on the ovary of a cow, as viewed using ultrasonography.

However, some evidence indicates a deficiency of luteinizing hormone or its receptors in the ovarian follicle.

Early diagnosis and treatment enhance success. Large doses of LH, hCG, and GnRH have been used intravenously and intramuscularly to initiate rupture of these cysts. Both LH and hCG act directly on the cysts, while GnRH produces an LH surge similar to a preovulatory surge and causes the cysts to rupture, followed by normal estrous cycles in cows with cysts. Progesterone given subcutaneously daily for 15 days has also been used successfully. The cyst regresses and presumably the progesterone causes a buildup of LH in the pituitary.

When treatment is terminated and a new follicle develops, sufficient LH is released to cause ovulation and CL formation.

The preferred treatment is an injection of GnRH, followed in 10 to 14 days with an injection of $PGF_{2\alpha}$. This regimen has shown the shortest interval between treatment and first estrus and offers the best chance for pregnancy. A small peptide molecule, GnRH, is less antigenic than LH or hCG, which are large protein molecules. Cows are less likely to produce antibodies against GnRH, and it remains effective on repeated use. Both LH and hCG may lose effectiveness by second or third treatment if the cow continues to be a problem.

Follicular cysts are most common in dairy cattle and in swine but rarely occur in beef cattle, sheep, and horses. Sows almost always develop luteal cysts and stop cycling.

25–1.2 *Luteinized Follicles*

A high percentage of thin-walled cysts become luteinized. The luteal tissue produces progesterone and the follicular fluid is usually high in progesterone. Multiple cysts are common, resulting in a greatly enlarged ovary (Figure 25–3). The condition is usually characterized by long periods of anestrus. The preferred treatment for luteal cysts is GnRH, followed in 10 to 14 days with $PGF_{2\alpha}$. If GnRH is not effective in regressing the cyst, $PGF_{2\alpha}$ should lyse the luteal tissue, while LH is not effective as a treatment due to the thickness of the follicular wall. Oral progestins have been used and are usually effective in causing the regression of the luteinized follicles. The material must be fed for 2 to 3 weeks or until the cyst has regressed as determined by rectal palpation. Use of $PGF_{2\alpha}$ may prove to be an effective treatment.

25–1.3 *Cystic Corpus Luteum*

The cystic CL differs from the luteinized follicle even though some similarities exist. While the cystic CL contains a cavity which is usually filled with fluid, its origin is the same as that of a normal corpus luteum. In the early stages of development of the CL, the theca interna of the follicular membrane proliferates rapidly and folds into the crater left by the ruptured follicle, thus creating a small cavity. Some reports indicate that 25% of these cavities

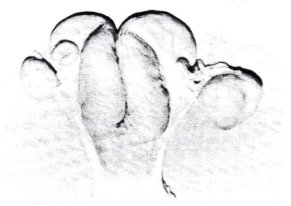

Figure 25–3 Ovary on right has multiple large luteinized follicles. Ovary on left is normal.

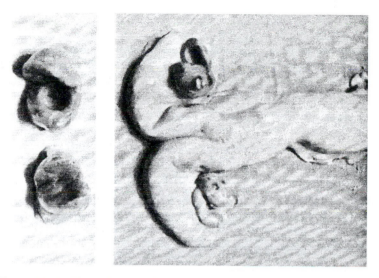

Figure 25–4 The right ovary *(top)* contains a cystic corpus luteum. A normal corpus luteum is shown at bottom left.

are never completely filled with granulosa cells growing from beneath and a small cavity persists throughout the life of the CL. The question arises as to which of the cavities are pathological and which are normal. Some workers have set arbitrary maximum sizes for normal cavities, usually 7 mm or 8 mm in diameter. Larger cavities are considered cysts and pathological (Figure 25–4). The cystic corpus luteum is considered to contribute to early embryonic mortality. In one large study, no pregnancies were observed with cysts larger than 7 mm in diameter. In another study, of aged infertile cows, a high percentage had cystic CL, whereas none were seen in aged fertile cows. Nonpregnant animals with cystic corpora lutea exhibit essentially normal cycles, but abnormal estrus periods have been reported. Based on physiological evidence, it has been postulated that three types of ovulatory dysfunction—delayed ovulation, follicular cysts, and cystic CL—stem from the same basic inadequacy of luteinizing hormone but reflect different degrees of insufficiency.

25–2 Retained Corpus Luteum

Much has been said and written concerning the retained (persistent) corpus luteum. Many cows have been treated and mistreated because of this elusive phenomenon. In the authors' opinion, the corpus luteum probably is retained only in association with some pathological condition of the uterus. Pyometra, mummified fetus, or other conditions which cause the uterus to react as a pregnant uterus can cause the retention of the corpus luteum, resulting in suppression of the estrous cycle. The persistence of the corpus luteum in these cases is due to an interference of the uterine luteolytic mechanism (release of $PGF_{2\alpha}$, Chapter 5). The corpus luteum of the preceding pregnancy is probably never retained, since luteolysis is a normal part of parturition initiation (Chapter 10).

Many cows have been diagnosed as having retained CL that were simply between periods of estrus. Either these cows ovulated without overt symptoms of estrus or estrus was undetected. It is impossible for a veterinarian or a livestock manager to differentiate between a normal CL and the "retained CL" by rectal palpation. The only way to be sure that the CL is not normal would be by repeated palpations at 3- or 4-day intervals for a period of 2 weeks. If the cow does not return to estrus and the CL does not regress, then a retained CL exists. For practical purposes, if the uterus is found to be empty (not pregnant and does not contain a mummified fetus, pus, or other fluids) and a corpus luteum is detected on an ovary, it is safe to assume that the animal is cycling.

Some cows exhibit long estrous cycles due to embryonic mortality. If the embryo death occurs by 12 days postbreeding, the cow will return to estrus in the usual length of time. When death occurs later than this, the return to estrus is delayed depending on when the death occurs. The later the death occurs, the longer the interval between death and return to estrus. Some of these cows have also been classified as having retained CL. In reality, these are cases of corpora lutea of pregnancy and do not fit the classical definition of a retained corpus luteum. The sow and doe both have corpora lutea that are lysed as part of the parturition process, also. The mare's CL and accessory corpora lutea regress between 150 and 180 days of gestation. It appears that in these species, in addition to the cow, the CL of pregnancy can not be retained into the next postpartum period.

25–3 ANESTRUS

Anestrus is defined as the absence of estrus. There are several causes of anestrus but the most common one is pregnancy. In cows and mares that can be rectally palpated for pregnancy, no female should be treated for anestrus until she is checked for pregnancy. Most cows exhibit a period of anestrus following parturition. In dairy cows, this period lasts from 20 to 40 days, but in beef cows that are suckling calves the anestrus period may be greatly extended. The sow usually has a period of estrus a few days after parturition but will not cycle again until the piglets are weaned. She usually will cycle 5 to 7 days after the piglets are removed. Sows that wean pigs in late fall and winter tend to go into temporary anestrus. They can be treated with PG600 (400 IU of PMSG and 200 IU of hCG) to return them to cycling. The mare usually exhibits a foal heat 9 or 10 days postparturition, and most will cycle again about 30 days postpartum. Most mares are seasonal breeders and are stimulated to sexual activity by increasing day length, with some coming into estrus as early as February. Most begin cycling by April. They will usually cycle through November and, if they do not become pregnant, will go into anestrus until the following spring.

Most breeds of sheep and goats are also seasonal breeders and are stimulated to sexual activity by decreasing day lengths. Most ewes will exhibit one or more quiet ovulations at the beginning of the breeding season. Some flocks have had their breeding season extended by selection and management to the extent that three lamb crops can be obtained in a 2-year period.

Low energy intake levels have been shown to delay puberty in all species. This results in anestrus at a time when these females are old enough for the first breeding. Low energy levels have also caused anestrus and particularly have contributed to prolonged anestrus following parturition in beef cattle. This topic is more thoroughly discussed in Chapter 23. About 3% of the cows in dairy herds where nutrition should not be a factor have been found to be in anestrus. The major difference between dairy and beef cattle would appear to be the calf suckling the beef cow. Marginal management which contributes to low energy intake obviously aggravates the situation.

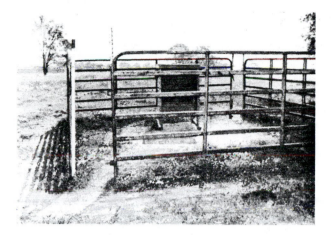

Figure 25–5 Calves allowed access to a creep feeder tend to nurse less often.

Beef cows can be managed to reduce the pospartum anestrus. After about 40 days postpartum, calves will start eating at a creep feeder if available (Figure 25–5), as well as nibbling on hay and grass. Having a creep feeder available will reduce suckling activity, a major cause of extended postpartum anestrus (Section 10–7.1). Research has shown that calves can be limited to one 30-minute suckling period per day without reducing weaning weights if they have creep feeders available. This does require additional labor, but the reduced suckling activity will shorten pospartum anestrus. If postpartum cows have a low body condition score, flushing (Section 23–3.1) will enhance return to estrus and fertility in beef cows. Use of progestin implants for 8 to 20 days followed by calf removal for 48 hours has stimulated return to estrus in postpartum cows. Also, injection of GnRH followed by $PGF_{2\alpha}$ 10 days later will induce cycling in many cases. These procedures are more effective in cows that are in a gaining state and if measures have been taken to limit suckling prior to treatment.

25–4 IRREGULAR ESTROUS CYCLES

The normal estrous cycle length in the cow has been accepted as 18 to 25 days. Similar variations for the other species would also be expected as a normal range. The data in Table 25–1 show the distribution of estrous cycle lengths for 200 cows through 500 cycles. The ovaries of these cows were palpated at least once weekly so that accurate determinations were made relative to cycle length and ovarian involvement. It is interesting that only 60.4% of the cows had normal length cycles. An additional 29% had either short (1.4%) or long (27.6%) cycles. Most of the remaining cows (9.8%) ovulated without demonstrating estrus previous to the first postpartum estrus. Four cows (0.8%) demonstrated estrus but either failed to develop a follicle and/or failed to develop a corpus luteum. Of the 27.6% that had long estrous cycles, 8.8% were long because of quiet ovulations following a normal estrous cycle. An additional 3.6% returned to anestrus following a normal postpartum estrus. The remaining 15.2% were reported as having retained corpora lutea. The researchers did not report the condition of the uterus in cows diagnosed to have retained

Table 25–1   *Number and percentage of normal and abnormal intervals between heats, as determined from ovarian examination of 200 cows through 500 cycles*

	Intervals	
Condition	Number	Percentage
Normal estrous cycles—18–25 days	302	60.4
Estrous cycles < 18 days—not cystic	7	1.4
False estrus < 18 days	4	.8
Quiet ovulations previous to first postpartum estrus	49	9.8
Estrous cycles > 25 days	138	27.6
Quiet ovulations after the first postpartum estrus	44	8.8
Persistent corpus luteum	76	15.2
Anestrus—smooth ovaries	18	3.6
Total	500	100.0

Adapted from Trimberger and Fincher. *Cornell Exp. Sta. Bull.* 911, 1956.

corpora lutea, nor did they mention the probability of embryonic mortality as a cause of delayed return.

Other researchers have reported from 16% to 44% of the estrous cycles occurring shorter or longer than 17 to 24 days. The higher figures were reported for large-scale studies using nonreturns to artificial insemination. These studies were also made during a time when the disease vibriosis was being transmitted through AI, and a major symptom of this disease is embryonic mortality. A high percentage of cows infected with vibriosis return to estrus between 27 and 55 days postbreeding. Other factors that may have contributed to these high figures are quiet ovulation, undiagnosed estrus, and one or more natural services (information not available to the researchers) between the AI services.

The conception rate for cows bred during the period of estrus following short estrous cycles is much lower than when breeding follows a normal-length cycle. Conception is also lower following cystic ovaries. However, when cows are bred at the first estrus following long cycles, quiet ovulations, and anestrus, the conception rate is equal to that attained for cows bred following normal cycles, as shown by the data in Table 25–2. This could be expected, since short cycles and cystic ovaries are indicative of endocrine imbalances. The periods of estrus following quiet ovulations and anestrus were normal from an endocrine standpoint. The same can be said for those periods of estrus following a retained corpus luteum, since there is a good possibility that the delayed regression of the corpus luteum was related to embryonic mortality rather than endocrine imbalance.

25–5   QUIET OVULATION

The term *quiet ovulation* is defined as ovulation without behavioral manifestation of estrus. The data in Table 25–1 show that 9.8% of the cows had a quiet ovulation preceding the first observable estrus following parturition. An additional 8.8% had a quiet ovulation after the first observable estrus following parturition. Of the 500 estrous cycles detected by palpation, 18.6% involved quiet ovulations. The cows in this study were observed twice daily

Table 25–2 *Conception rates in cows bred during and following various ovarian conditions*

Estrus and ovarian conditions	Cows bred	Conception to one service
Cows bred in control group*	200	60.0
Cows bred in experimental groups†	200	65.0
Artificially bred during quiet ovulation	20	65.0
Normal estrus after quiet ovulation	48	62.5
Estrus after persistent corpus luteum	46	65.2
Estrus after anestrus—smooth ovaries	15	80.0
Service after recovery from cystic ovaries	34	41.2
Service following short cycles—< 18 days	36	33.3

Adapted from Trimberger and Fincher. *Cornell Exp. Sta. Bull.* 911, 1956.

*Not palpated, bred at observed estrus.

†Palpated regularly to determine condition of ovaries.

with other cows in an exercise yard. In addition, they would not stand to be mounted by "indicator" cows (cows treated with diethylstilbestrol) or by a teaser bull when checked at 2- to 4-hour intervals. They were also tried for natural breeding without success. The only sign of estrus was the characteristic mucous discharge and the presence of a follicle on the ovary. Other reports have shown the incidence of quiet ovulation to be as high as 27.3%. Twenty cows were artificially inseminated during quiet ovulation, during which they would not stand for natural mating. Of these, 65% conceived. Inseminations were timed by frequent palpations of the ovary to determine when the follicle was reaching maturity. The follicle bulges beyond the contour of the surface and is more turgid during the last several hours before ovulation than it is previously.

No treatment or corrective measure is known for quiet ovulation. The physiological cause is not known, but subthreshold hormone production or balance between hormones may be factors. The intervals preceding and following quiet ovulation are usually normal. Since ovulation occurs followed by a normal corpus luteum, no disturbance from a functional standpoint is indicated. Usually, the estrus following a quiet ovulation will be indicated by normal symptoms but occasionally two or three quiet ovulation periods occur in succession.

Ovulation without manifested estrus probably occurs in other species. However, it is difficult if not impossible to diagnose in ewes, does, and sows, since palpation of the ovaries cannot be accomplished.

25–6 AGE

The effect of age on reproductive efficiency is difficult to measure in farm animals. The selection pressures for both producing ability and reproductive ability eliminate many animals from the herds and flocks at relatively early ages. Additional environmental factors that affect reproductive efficiency also tend to mask the effects of age. A number of studies in cattle have shown that heifers have a lower reproductive efficiency than cows. It is true that most anatomical abnormalities that interfere with normal reproduction are discovered in heifers and eliminated. When these are eliminated, the remaining heifers under excellent

Table 25–3   *Percent conception for cows by age groups, compared with cows more than 36 months of age*

Age (months)	Average percentage unit		
	1st service	2nd service	3rd service
36–47	1.0	.9	1.9
48–59	−1.9	−3.8	1.2
60–84	−6.2	−3.1	−6.4
> 84	−14.8	−12.7	−6.9

Adapted from Spalding et al. *J. Dairy Sci.,* 58:718, 1975.

management conditions should have a higher reproductive efficiency than cows. Unfortunately, the managers of many herds do not spend adequate time checking heifers for estrus so that inseminations can be properly timed. Many heifers will show symptoms of estrus for 6 to 12 hours before standing when mounted. Cows will usually only show estrual symptoms for 2 to 4 hours before standing. These factors probably contribute to the lowered reproductive efficiency reported for heifers.

The data in Table 25–3 indicate that reproductive efficiency is highest for dairy cows 3 to 4 years of age. Conception began decreasing in the 5- to 7-year age group and a marked decrease in reproductive efficiency occurred in cows over 7 years of age. Studies with beef cattle show considerably more variation, but generally the highest level of reproductive efficiency is seen between 4 and 9 years of age. Similar effects of age in the other species can be expected.

Reproductive efficiency in the male is also affected by advancing age. Studies have shown that the fertility of bulls used in artificial insemination reaches a peak between 2 and 4 years of age. The fertility peak may occur prior to the peak in sperm production. The percentage of motile sperm after freezing and thawing and the percentage of morphologically normal sperm at the time of collection are lower for older bulls than for younger ones. Even though these statements are generally true, there is considerable individual variation. There are many older bulls being used in artificial insemination that produce semen with fertilizing capabilities as high as that of the younger bulls.

The cause of lowered reproductive efficiency with advancing age is not known. It may be due to hormonal imbalance or a deficiency, which contributes to reduced ovulation rate or abnormal spermatogenesis. It may also be related to a deterioration of the gametes, which in turn may affect fertilization rate or contribute to an increased embryonic mortality rate.

25–7   REPRODUCTIVE TOXICOLOGY

A number of chemical compounds in the environment can adversely affect reproductive function in livestock. Most are naturally produced compounds that are a component of various feedstuffs and forages, whereas others are introduced synthetic compounds that can act as endocrine disrupters, mimicking endogenous hormone actions. While toxicities of various nutritional components (e.g., mineral toxicities) were addressed in Chapter 23, this section will focus on the specific chemical compounds present in nature that can interact directly with the reproductive system in males and females, resulting in reduced reproductive efficiency. In addition to these chemical compounds, there are a myriad of other factors that can result in reproductive failure (e.g., mare reproductive loss syndrome—MRLS) above and beyond those produced by infectious diseases (Chapter 26).

25–7.1 *Toxic Feedstuffs, Forages, and Plants*

Toxicities beyond those seen as a result of an excessive ingestion of various nutritive components (e.g., vitamins, minerals) are observed when livestock consume specific types of forages and other feedstuffs. This can result when cattle and sheep maintained on rangelands come in contact with plants that contain noxious compounds or in intensive livestock production operations when mismanagement in the preparation, handling, and storage of feed occurs.

25–7.1a Mycotoxins Mycotoxins are toxins produced by molds, which are a type of fungus. Extremes in weather conditions resulting in plant stress can result in the occurrence of mycotoxins preharvest; however, the most common cause is poor feed storage and handling practices. The presence of fungal spores and physical damage to the feedstuff in combination with the right moisture, oxygen, and temperature conditions can precipitate mold growth and mycotoxin build-up. *Aspergillus, Fusarium,* and *Penicillium* molds are the primary molds that produce mycotoxins detrimental to cattle following storage. Molds often have symbiotic relationships with the forages they infect, including tall fescue, ryegrass, and some cereal grains, which imparts hardiness to the plant in the form of drought and insect resistance. Livestock intensively grazing these infected forages can develop a toxicosis from the compounds produced by the molds (e.g., ergot alkaloids), which can have severe consequences to reproductive efficiency and productivity.

Fescue toxicosis in cattle grazing fungal-infected tall fescue (*Neotyphodium coenophialum*), referred to as endophyte-infected, can result in decreased weight gains and direct effects on reproductive performance, including delayed onset of puberty, impaired luteal function, and decreased calving rates. Reproduction in cattle grazing endophyte-infected tall fescue may be further compromised during periods of high temperatures, as cattle may retain their winter coats, experience elevated body temperatures, and a reduced tolerance to heat stress as consequences of fescue toxicosis. Sheep also exhibit reduced reproductive efficiency during fescue toxicosis; however, sheep are not as severely affected as cattle and exhibit normal feed intake and weight gain patterns while consuming fescue. In mares, fescue toxicosis can result in prolonged gestation intervals and an increased incidence of dystocia and retained or thickened placentae in addition to agalactia. Foals born to mares on fescue-infected pastures are usually immature and weak due to placental insufficiency during gestation. Reductions in circulating concentrations of serum prolactin, melatonin, and progesterone are common in infected animals. The ergot peptide alkaloids (primarily ergovaline) produced by the endophyte is the primary toxic agent which causes vasoconstriction, an inhibition of implantation, embryotoxic effects, spontaneous abortion, and decreased lactation. These negative implications for grazing endophyte-infected tall fescue have greatly hampered the use of this forage in some regions, as there is no practical method to detoxify affected forages. Management strategies for control and alleviation of fescue toxicity in mares include the removal of pregnant mares from fescue pastures 60 to 90 days before anticipated foaling dates and the medication of pregnant mares with D_2 receptor (dopamine) antagonist drugs (domperidone or fluphenazine), although these drugs are still in experimental stages of development. New strains of novel, nontoxic endophyte-infected fescue are also becoming available for grazing which do not produce the toxic effects but still maintain the positive symbiotic relationships gained by the plant from endophyte presence.

Zearalenone is an estrogenic mycotoxin produced by *Fusarium* that can elicit an estrogenic response in monogastrics and ruminants. Concentrations of zearalenone above 400 ppb have been associated with poor reproductive performance, including reduced testis weight, lower conception rates, persistent CLs in swine, irregular periods of estrus, estrus in pregnant animals, early embryonic mortality, and mammary gland development in virgin heifers. High levels above 1,000 ppb have been associated with abortions in livestock in some studies. Field surveys and assessments of samples submitted for analysis have revealed that zearalenone may be found in 10% to 20% of feeds analyzed.

Aflatoxin produced by *Aspergillus flavus* is a mycotoxin of great concern, since it has been shown to be carcinogenic and is commonly found in crops in the southern United States. The FDA limits aflatoxin in feedstuffs to 200 ppb in breeding cattle rations and 20 ppb in lactating dairy cattle rations, given the public health concern regarding the potential for aflatoxin residues in milk and meat products. These are below levels considered toxic to cattle, which occurs at concentrations greater than 300 to 700 ppb. While aflatoxins in cereal grains can cause reduced feed efficiency and growth rates, which could delay puberty, regulatory aspects for controlling aflatoxin exposure in livestock likely prevent such levels from becoming high enough to produce a directed effect on reproductive processes, although this cannot be discounted completely.

25–7.1b Gossypol Toxicosis

Gossypol is a naturally occurring plant compound found in the pigment glands of seeds, roots, and leaves of cotton plants (*Gossypium* spp.). Originally, the processing of cottonseed meals, which are used in livestock rations as a protein supplement, by the screw-press method produced cottonseed meal that was relatively low in gossypol content due to the heat that was produced when using this method. The added heat increases protein binding, converting more free gossypol (the toxic form) to the bound form (nontoxic form). However, when processing procedures changed to a direct-solvent extraction procedure for the extraction of cottonseed oils, the residual free gossypol content of cottonseed meal increased considerably. This higher free gossypol content of processed cottonseed meal resulted in an increased incidence of detrimental physiological and reproductive effects directly related to cottonseed meal (gossypol) ingestion. Unprocessed, whole cottonseed with a high gossypol content can similarly cause adverse effects in livestock if consumed in excess. The toxic effects of gossypol are greater in non-ruminants and young ruminants, as a functional rumen can detoxify gossypol to some extent. However, even in mature ruminants, excessive ingestion of meals containing a high free gossypol content can overwhelm the detoxifying capabilities of the rumen and cause a gossypol toxicosis.

Gossypol can affect the heart, kidneys, liver, and reproductive system. A hallmark of gossypol toxicity, which has also been used as a test for gossypol toxicosis, is erythrocyte fragility. In bulls, the effects of gossypol on reproduction are well characterized, with observed effects on testicular tissue morphology, ejaculated sperm quality, and spermatogenesis. Some studies have shown direct effects on the ultrastructure of spermatozoa, with increases in mid-piece abnormalities of the mitochondrial sheath. At one time, gossypol was considered as a potential male contraceptive agent in humans; however, adverse side effects (renal damage) from the gossypol administration have not permitted its widespread use outside of clinical research trials. In female rodents, swine, and other monogastrics, the effects of gossypol on reducing litter sizes and increases in the number of stillborn offspring have been reported. In contrast, few overt effects have been observed with respect to reproduction and estrous cyclicity in cows consuming cottonseed feedstuffs. However, an increased number of degenerative embryos were collected from superovulated Brangus heifers consuming cottonseed meal in one study, and *in vitro* effects of gossypol on oocyte and embryo development have been reported, including decreased rates of nuclear maturation of cultured bovine oocytes.

The deleterious effects of gossypol (*in vivo* and *in vitro*) are thought to involve the generation of free radicals. Recent work suggests that dietary supplementation with antioxidants (free radical–reducing agents) such as vitamin E may provide some protection against the manifestation of a gossypol toxicosis. Other management recommendations when feeding gossypol-containing feedstuffs include limiting the feeding of whole cottonseed to less than 10% of the total diet in young bulls, and only 15 to 20% of the total diet in mature bulls. Mechanically extracted cottonseed meals can be fed up to 15% of the total diet, whereas solvent-extracted cottonseed meal should be limited to 5% or less of the total diet in bulls to prevent fertility problems. Testing the cottonseed for gossypol content can also aid in determining how much may be tolerated in the diet. Swine, calf, and lamb rations should not contain more than 0.01%, or 100 ppm gossypol. In adult ruminants, the tolerance to gossypol can be highly variable and is dependent on rumen function, age, and amount and type of the gossypol-containing feed that is consumed. Gossypol levels of 800 ppm fed over long periods of time have produced toxicities in adult ruminants. New "glandless" varieties of cotton have been developed which have very low levels of gossypol. However, these varieties of cotton plants need high levels of insecticides to achieve acceptable cotton yields, since gossypol acts as a natural insecticide as part of the cotton plant's defense mechanisms. Therefore, the use of "glandless" cotton plants as a means for reducing gossypol content in whole cottonseed and cottonseed meal may be limited.

25–7.1c Pine Needle Abortion

In areas where cattle are grazed within or around stands of ponderosa pine trees *(Pinus ponderosa)* in the western United States, pine needle abortion can be a severe problem. When cows consume the pine needles, premature parturition can result. Abortions can occur as early as 24 hours to as long as 3 weeks after ingestion. As few as one pine tree per 3 acres is enough to cause pine needle abortion in a group of grazing cows. Other effects have been seen in addition to late-term abortion, including postpartum retention of the placenta, metritis, peritonitis, and cow mortality. The stage of pregnancy affected is the last third of gestation in which blood flow to the fetus may be reduced by up to 60%. It is believed that the reduced blood flow stresses the fetus, causing premature parturition (see Section 10–3 on the role of the fetal stress on induction of parturition). The compound in pine needles responsible for the reduced blood flow and etiology of pine needle abortion is isocupressic acid. Calves born early as a result of pine needle abortion may be viable if caught shortly after birth, since calves are usually born prematurely but not dead. However, calves born before 250 days of gestation have a much lower chance of survival than those born after 250 days of gestation. The only management strategies to prevent pine needle abortion are to remove ponderosa pine trees from grazing areas, to fence cattle away from pine stands, and to prune trees and gather any pine needles that have fallen from the trees to prevent consumption.

25–7.1d Teratogenic Plant Toxins   A whole host of noxious forages and weeds contain compounds which can affect embryo survival and fetal development, some producing severe teratogenic-like deformities (i.e., birth defects). For some of these plant compounds, the time period when the embryo or fetus is vulnerable has been identified; in others, the critical period of exposure is poorly understood.

False hellebore *(Veratum californicum)* grows on moist meadows and hillsides at elevations of 1,500 to 4,000 meters from south-central Alaska to California and throughout the western states. Sheep grazing pastures contaminated with false hellebore on days 14 to 21 of gestation can result in a high incidence of embryonic mortality, whereas grazing from days 27 to 32 results in abnormal skeletal development. Later exposure from days 31 to 33 results in abnormal development of the trachea, leading to neonatal suffocation. The compounds in the plant responsible for these effects are steroidal alkaloids (jervine, cyclopamine, cycloposine) produced by *Veratum*, with similar developmental abnormalities as those described for sheep observed in goats and cattle grazing this plant.

Toxins found in a number of plant species, such as the *Lupinus* (lupins; western North America), *Conium* (hemlocks; found throughout North America), and *Nicotiana* (tree tobaccos; found in low elevations in California and Arizona) have also been known to have detrimental effects on reproduction in livestock. Cattle grazing pastures contaminated with lupins between days 40 and 70 of gestation experience an increased incidence of cleft palate formation in calves. Similar abnormalities were seen in piglets born to sows fed hemlock and tree tobacco by-products between days 30 and 45 and days 18 and 68 of gestation, respectively. Locoweeds (*Astragalus;* western rangelands of North America and western Australia), which contain an indolizidine alkaloid called swainsonine, cause similar skeletal defects in fetuses of pregnant ewes as well as fetal edema of the heart, leading to congestive heart failure. In some cases, ultrasonography has been used to detect toxic plant–induced skeletal and related developmental abnormalities in livestock consuming plants that can cause these effects. Limiting grazing in areas with known infestations of these plants can reduce the potential for exposure and manifestation of toxic effects; however, this may be impractical in large-acreage rangeland grazing systems.

25–7.1e Phytoestrogens   Many plants produce naturally estrogenic compounds, called phytoestrogens, which aid in plant metabolic and defense mechanisms. When consumed by herbivores, they can exhibit both agonistic and antagonistic effects on estrogen-sensitive pathways in mammalian systems, including the reproductive and endocrine systems. Plant species such as subterranean clovers (*Trifolium* spp.) and alfalfa *(Medicago sativa)* have been shown to have estrogenic properties that may reduce fertility in both sheep and cattle. Soybeans also contain estrogenic compounds, which can carry over into soybean meal and other soy-based by-products to produce an estrogenic effect. Isoflavones are the most common naturally occurring phytoestrogens and include the compounds diadzein, genistein, biochanin A, and formononetin. Formononetin and diadzein can be further metabolized to equol, a potent estrogenically active compound. A second class of plant compounds that possesses estrogenic activity is the coumestans, with coumestrol being the dominant compound found in both alfalfa and clovers. Coumestrol has been estimated to be 30 to 100 times more estrogenically active than any of the isoflavones. The affinity of coumestrol for the estrogen receptor is only 10 to 20 times lower than the affinity of estradiol. Phytoestrogens may alter reproductive and endocrine processes by binding directly with the estrogen receptor; by competing with estrogen for estrogen receptors (antiestrogenic actions—blocking estrogen); by inhibiting enzymatic activity related to estrogen processing, such as uterine peroxidases and aromatase; and by having synergistic effects with estrogen itself or other hormones, including growth factors (Section 4–7).

The consumption of phytoestrogenic forages can cause a number of reproductive disturbances in sheep and cattle, including weak or prolonged estrus, lack of estrus, irregular estrous cycle lengths, cystic ovaries, endometrial hypertrophy, and abortion. In ovariectomized heifers grazing red clover pastures, uterine and cervical weights have been observed to increase almost 70%, compared with animals on nonestrogenic pastures. Some heifers on estrogenic pastures have also been known to exhibit an increase in udder development. Infertility related to phytoestrogen ingestion in sheep and cattle may be brought about by a combination of factors, including interference with sperm or ova transport and implantation as a result of a thickening of the uterine endometrium and/or cervical and vaginal epithelium. Effects of phytoestrogens on male reproduction have not been well characterized but may be similar to the types of problems encountered when males are exposed to introduced environmental endocrine disrupters (Section 25–7.3).

Management of large and small ruminants on estrogenic pastures, or when fed rations with large quantities of soybean meal or other estrogenic feeds, should be done with some caution to prevent unnecessary losses in fertility and production. In Australia, agronomic measures have been aimed in some cases at replacing estrogenic clover pastures with other types of plants. In other areas, producers may be unable to change pasture systems due to soil conditions, climatic considerations, and costs associated with changing management systems. Animal husbandry procedures can be adopted which can reduce the risks of phytoestrogen-induced effects on reproductive efficiency. Preventing sudden shifts from nonestrogenic to estrogenic pastures or limiting grazing of estrogenic pastures can prevent such effects. Recent data suggest the incidences of hyperestrogenism in cattle fed alfalfa may also be attributed to alfalfa that has been irrigated with treated sewage water. When estrogen content of the sewage water was examined in one study, it contained 16.7 ng of steroidal estrogen per 100 ml. Alfalfa grown with the addition of 50 ng per day was observed to increase its coumestrol concentration by four-fold over plants not receiving estrogen-containing water. While some systems using irrigation with wastewater may not reach these specific levels, any added exposure may contribute to the problems of infertility in animals grazing phytoestrogen-containing pastures.

In swine, recent research using soy phytoestrogens has been directed toward potential benefits from phytoestrogen exposure. Positive effects on growth and metabolism in prepubertal gilts have been attributed to a phytoestrogenic effect from soy feeding. Investigations are currently determining whether soy phytoestrogens may reduce follicular atresia and lead to more follicles recruited for ovulation to increase litter sizes. However, more research is needed to substantiate these results and the use of soy phytoestrogens in this manner.

25–7.2 *Mare Reproductive Loss Syndrome*

Mare reproductive loss syndrome (MRLS) is complex and is characterized by epidemic early fetal loss, late fetal loss and neonatal foal losses, as well as other equine health problems (e.g., pericarditis). During the spring of 2001 and 2002, the Central Ohio Valley region and neighboring states (Kentucky, Ohio, Virginia, and Tennessee) experienced a high incidence of MRLS. In 2001, 3,500 cases of early fetal loss were reported, with approximately 1,166 cases in 2002. The causative agents contributing to MRLS have been the subject of continuing investigation. A number of theories have been put forward, including viruses, mycotoxin contamination, fescue toxicity, cyanide poisoning from wild cherry tree seedlings in pastures, and an infestation of the eastern tent caterpillar, which feeds on wild cherry tree leaves.

Early fetal loss from MRLS is associated with embryonic loss between days 35 and 100 of gestation, and late fetal loss is associated in most instances with late-term abortion, although some foals may be born alive. Mares that experience late fetal loss exhibit symptoms of restlessness, discomfort, and sweating, followed by an intense and explosive presentation to deliver their foals. In most instances, expulsion of the fetus is associated with premature placental separation and engorged allantochorionic membranes ("red bag syndrome"). Foals born alive are usually immature and require aggressive therapeutic intervention to help them survive.

Recent studies have provided convincing evidence that the causative agent of MRLS may, in fact, be the eastern tent caterpillar, since mares consuming eastern tent caterpillars have resulted in specific effects on the feto-placental unit. Insects, including caterpillars, are known to secrete and/or regurgitate compounds that act as predatory deterrents. Moreover, eastern tent caterpillars secrete steroids from their integuments that may have hormonal or antihormonal effects detrimental to equine pregnancy. Studies have demonstrated that the ingestion of eastern tent caterpillars by mares during early pregnancy (38 to 88 days of gestation) results in early fetal losses within 8 to 13 days after the onset of treatment. Although this and other studies provide convincing evidence of the association between eastern tent caterpillar ingestion and MRLS, the nature of the toxic factor(s) produced by the eastern tent caterpillars responsible for pregnancy loss remains unknown.

25–7.3 *Other Disrupters of Endocrine and Reproductive Processes*

In addition to naturally occurring toxins and plant compounds, synthetic compounds introduced into the environment in the form of pesticides and herbicides are also of concern to livestock, wildlife, and human health. The most widely studied class of compounds is the xenoestrogens, or estrogen mimics, which can have profound effects on reproductive processes following long-term exposure in some species. In livestock, the effects of xenoestrogens are less well characterized than in laboratory animal models or wildlife examples of environmental endocrine disrupter exposure. Nevertheless, the application of pesticides and herbicides to crops that may be grazed by livestock would suggest that exposure can occur, yet specific adverse effects on livestock or on milk/meat residues from a risk assessment perspective have not been examined extensively.

Compounds such as dichlorodiphenyltrichloroethane (DDT), which was widely used for mosquito and agricultural pest control and is now banned, among other synthetic compounds which are by-products of agricultural and industrial mechanization, including polychlorinated biphenyls (PCB), octylphenol, nonylphenol, and bisphenol A, have all been shown to elicit an estrogenic response in biological systems. Disruption of sexual differentiation *in utero* and in neonates through altered urogenital development, delayed puberty, decreased sperm production in males, and irregular estrous cycles in females are the consequences of xenoestrogen exposure. However, the affinity of these compounds for the estrogen receptor can be quite low, indicating that a significant exposure must occur before an estrogenic response above and beyond what might be produced naturally is observed. What constitutes a "significant" exposure is debatable and depends greatly on the species, stage of development, compound, dose, and duration of exposure. Many of these compounds are derived from the petrochemical industry and, like steroid hormones, can be fat-soluble, leading to an accumulation of these compounds in body fat reserves. Therefore, even low-dose exposure may lead to adverse effects on reproduction if the exposure is long-term. Of increasing concern is the role of these xenoestrogens in the development of endocrine-related cancers in humans. The occurrence of similar pathologies in livestock would be expected to be low, since most livestock production systems cull or harvest animals at relatively young ages before such pathologies would be expected to occur. However, for animals in the wild, the potential impact of environmental endocrine disrupters on the life cycle and reproductive success of insects, birds, reptiles, and mammals in environmentally sensitive areas should not be discounted. In addition to xenoestrogens, some fungicides have recently been identified as xenoandrogens, which may have similar adverse effects on male reproduction, acting through androgen receptors. Further research should reveal whether synthetic environmental endocrine disrupters, xenoestrogens and xenoandrogens, from pesticide and/or herbicide use on pastures grazed by livestock are of concern with respect to reproductive processes in livestock, as has been suggested for various species of wildlife and humans.

25–8 PSYCHOLOGICAL DISTURBANCES

The relationship between psychological phenomena and reproduction has been researched but is not well understood. This research along with observations by alert managers and data gleaned from unrelated research have led to the general conclusion that handling animals gently aids both production and reproduction (Section 22–2).

25–8.1 *Females*

Two extensive studies involving dairy and beef cattle have shown that cows that were extremely nervous or excited at the time of insemination had a lower conception rate. The degree of nervousness may have been an indication of the amount of adrenalin released. Adrenalin is known to interfere with contractions of muscles normally stimulated by oxytocin. Contractions of the muscles of the uterus and oviduct are involved in the transport of sperm to the site of fertilization. Therefore, it is conceivable that the adrenalin released by these nervous cows may have interfered with sperm transport. Release of ACTH and glucocorticoids which suppress LH may also be a factor.

Both dairy and beef cows isolated from the herd at the beginning of estrus and confined until the time of insemination showed lower conception rates than cows left with the herd until time for insemination. Conception rate was affected more in the beef cows than in the dairy cows. The confinement apparently caused stress, which resulted in lower conception rate. Confinement of the cows after insemination lowered conception rate in beef cows, but dairy cows were not affected. The probable reason that dairy cows were less affected when confined both before and after insemination is that dairy cows are more accustomed to being handled and confined than are beef cows. Driving cows from the pasture and separating them from the rest of the herd at the time of insemination had no effect on conception. This management practice appears to create less trauma than confining the estrous cow before or after insemination.

Cows that are difficult to inseminate have shown lower conception than those in which insemination is accomplished more easily. This may be caused by extra excitement or trauma on the part of the cow. Admittedly, it may also be caused by inseminators not properly placing the semen. Lower nonreturn rates are reported for inexperienced AI technicians for the first 3 months (Table 25–4). Part of this may be related to the extra time required to pass the catheter through the cervix and the resulting excitement and trauma.

The sow's reproductive performance is also affected by psychological factors. The overt signs of estrus are more clearly demonstrated when boars are within hearing and smelling range. Recordings of boars' mating noises or pheromones isolated from the boar have been shown to be stimulating in the absence of boars. The effect of these factors on conception and litter size has not been reported.

Gilts reared in confinement have suppressed estrus as long as they remain in the same pen. Moving them to an adjacent pen has some stimulating effect, but moving them to a pasture area has a greater effect. Many gilts will come into estrus within 2 to 3 days after being moved. Even gilts reared on pasture are stimulated by movement to new quarters. Gilts have shown response from being moved out of a pen for a few minutes and put back into the same pen.

Gilts not moved to a different pen or location will fight a boar that is put in with them for mating. If the boar is of similar age and size, he may be seriously injured or even killed. The boar can be introduced at the same time the gilts are moved to a new location and little animosity is shown by the gilts. Anestrus, pubertal gilts thus introduced to a boar will begin cycling in a synchronized fashion.

Table 25–4   *Breeding efficiency of inexperienced inseminators in areas where AI was new and in areas where AI had previously been established*

Month of operation	New areas		Old areas	
	Number of areas	Percentage of 60-day nonreturn	Number of areas	Percentage of 60-day nonreturn
1st	29	49.0	14	57.0
2nd	26	52.0	14	62.8
3rd	24	61.0	12	64.8
4th	22	64.5	12	65.4

From Olds and Seath. *Ky. Agr. Exp. Sta. Bull.* 605, 1954.

Ewes show no overt symptoms of estrus in the absence of the ram even though ovulation occurs. Ewes appear to be stimulated to start cycling earlier at the beginning of the breeding season when rams are running with them (Section 5–5 and Section 7–1.2).

25–8.2 *Males*

Bulls in AI centers have demonstrated several psychological effects on performance. Some bulls develop inhibitions about certain teaser animals or a particular collection area. These can be overcome by changing the teaser animal and/or collecting the bull at a different location.

Pain or discomfort related to copulation or AI collection has caused loss of libido in bulls. An artificial vagina with too high a temperature will cause a bull to be reluctant to mount for ejaculation. If the AV is not held at the proper angle, the resulting pain may have similar results. No data seem to be available on the effect of mistreatment prior to or at the time of collection on quality or quantity of semen produced.

Simulated mistreatment by daily injections of adrenalin for 10 weeks has shown a marked decrease in sperm output by bulls, compared with control bulls. Daily shocking of bulls with an electric cattle prod did not reduce sperm production. However, any stress or change in routine causes an increase in abnormal sperm in some bulls. All types of abnormalities increase, but cytoplasmic droplets appear first and are last to disappear.

Based on what is known for both males and females, animals should be handled in a manner that produces the least amount of stress possible. Treatment resulting in undue excitement or pain should be avoided. Both reproduction and production will be enhanced.

SUGGESTED READING

BISHOP, M. W. H. 1970. Aging and reproduction in males. *J. Reprod. Fert.* 12(Suppl.):65.

BUNCH, T. D., K. E. PANTER, and L. F. JAMES. 1992. Ultrasound studies of the effects of certain poisonous plants on uterine function and fetal development in livestock. *J. Anim. Sci.,* 70:1639.

CARPENTER, L. M. 1976. A study of management factors as they relate to conception rate in cattle artificially inseminated. Ph.D. dissertation, Miss. State Univ.

CROSS, D. L. 2000. Toxic effects of *Neotyphodium coenophialum* in cattle and horses. *Proc 4th International Neothyphodium/Grass Interacations Symposium.* Soest, Germany.

DAY, N. 1991. The treatment and prevention of cystic ovarian follicles. *Vet. Med.,* 86:761.

DIEKMAN, M. A. and M. L. GREEN. 1992. Mycotoxins and reproduction in domestic livestock. *J. Anim. Sci.,* 70:1615.

GILMORE, L. O. 1949. The inheritance of functional causes of reproductive inefficiency: A review. *J. Dairy Sci.,* 32:71.

JAMES, L. F., K. E. PANTER, D. B. NIELSEN, and R. J. MOLYNEUX. 1992. The effects of natural toxins on reproduction in livestock. *J. Anim. Sci.,* 70:1573.

MCENTEE, K. 1958. Cystic corpora lutea in cattle. *Internat. J. Fert.,* 3:120.

MORGAN, S. E. 1989. Gossypol as a toxicant in livestock. *The Veterinary Clinics of North America: Food Animal Practice.* ed. G. E. Burrows. W. B. Saunders.

OLDS, D. and D. M. SEATH. 1954. Factors affecting reproductive efficiency in dairy cattle. *Ky. Agr. Exp. Sta. Bull.* 605.

PANTER, K. E., L. F. JAMES, and R. J. MOLYNEUX. 1992. Ponderosa pine needle–induced parturition in cattle. *J. Anim. Sci.,* 70:1604.

PANTER, K. E., R. F. KEELER, L. F. JAMES, and T. D. BUNCH. 1992. Impact of plant toxins on fetal and neonatal development: A review. *J. Range Manage.,* 45:52.

PORTER, J. K. and F. N. THOMPSON. 1992. Effects of fescue toxicosis on reproduction in livestock. *J. Anim. Sci.,* 70:1594.

RANDEL, R. D., C. C. CHASE, JR., and S. J. WYSE. 1992. Effects of gossypol and cottonseed products on reproduction of mammals. *J. Anim. Sci.,* 70:1628.

ROBERTS, S. J. 1986. *Veterinary Obstetrics and Genital Diseases.* (3rd ed.) Published by the author.

RYAN, P. L. 2001. Relaxin, fescue toxicosis and placental insufficiency in the mare. *Proc. Ann. Conf. Soc. Theriogenology (Equine Symposium),* Vancouver, BC, Canada.

SALISBURY, G. W., N. L. VANDEMARK, and J. R. LODGE. 1978. *Physiology of Reproduction and Artificial Insemination of Cattle.* (2nd ed.) W. H. Freeman and Co.

SHUTT, D. A. and R. I. COX. 1976. The effects of plant oestrogens on animals reproduction. *Endeavour,* 35:110.

SPALDING, R. W., R. W. EVERETT, and R. H. FOOTE. 1975. Fertility in New York artificially inseminated Holstein herds in dairy herd improvement. *J. Dairy Sci.,* 58:718.

TANABE, T. Y. and J. O. ALMQUIST. 1967. The nature of subfertility in the dairy heifer. III. Gross genital abnormalities. *Pa. State Univ. Bull.* 736.

TRIMBERGER, G. W. and M. G. FINCHER. 1956. Regularity of estrus, ovarian function, and conception rates in dairy cattle. *Cornell Exp. Sta. Bull.* 911.

WHITMORE, H. L., W. J. TYLER, and L. E. CASIDA. 1974. Incidence of cystic ovaries in Holstein-Friesian cows. *J. Amer. Vet. Med. Assoc.,* 165:693.

26

Infectious Diseases That Cause Reproductive Failure

The material presented in this chapter will deal with those diseases that contribute to reduced reproductive efficiency, cause abortions, or adversely affect the offspring that are carried to term. Some are venereal diseases, affecting only the reproductive processes, while others are general systemic diseases with the effects on reproduction being secondary. Some of the diseases have public health significance and this will be alluded to. This presentation will be limited to those diseases that have economic significance to the livestock producer. Some of the diseases may strike suddenly and cause extensive losses in production and reproduction in a very short period of time. Others are more chronic and may not be recognized but cause significant economic loss over a long period of time.

This chapter is not intended to train students in the field of veterinary medicine but, rather, to make them aware of the diseases that cause reproductive failure and to acquaint them with symptoms, methods of transmission, and methods of control so that they can be better livestock managers and presumably avoid many disease problems through these management techniques. Table 26–1 summarizes the diseases that will be covered in this chapter from the standpoint of affected species, causative organisms, method of transmission, major effects on reproduction, and control measures.

26–1 BACTERIAL DISEASES

26–1.1 *Vibriosis*

Vibriosis (Campylobacteriosis) affects both cattle and sheep. The causative organism for cattle is *Campylobacter fetus venerealis* (previously listed as *Vibrio fetus venerealis*), while *Campylobacter fetus fetus* (previously listed as *Vibrio fetus venerealis* and *Vibrio fetus intestinalis*) causes the disease in sheep (Figure 26–1). The distribution of the disease is worldwide and is found throughout the United States.

26–1.1a Methods of Transmission *Campylobacter fetus venerealis* in cattle is a venereal disease organism. Transmission other than by natural mating and through infected semen has not been reported. Even when experimentally infected cows are confined with noninfected cows, the disease is apparently not transmitted. Figure 26–2 shows how highly contagious the disease can be when introduced into herds practicing natural mating.

Table 26–1   *Summary of diseases affecting reproduction in farm species*

Disease	Affected species	Causative organism(s)	Effects on reproduction	Method of transmission	Control measures
Bacterial Diseases					
Vibriosis	Cattle	*Campylobacter fetus venerealis*	Embryonic mortality Early abortion	Sexual contact Contaminated semen	Vaccination Breed AI
	Sheep	*Campylobacter fetus fetus*	Abortion last trimester	Contaminated feed and water	Vaccination
Leptospirosis	Cattle	*L. pomona* *L. canicola* *L. grippotyphosa* *L. icterohemor-rhagiae* *L. hardjo* *L. sejroe*	Abortion last trimester Infertility Weak calves	Urine-contaminated feed, water, and air Contaminated semen Wildlife	Annual vaccination Antibiotic therapy of acute cases Sanitation
	Swine	*L. pomona* *L. hardjo* *L. bratislava* *L. icterohemor-rhagiae*	Late abortions Weak pigs	Same	Same
	Horses	Same as swine	Late abortion	Same	Same
Brucellosis	Cattle	*Brucella abortus*	Premature births Abortions Weak calves Retained placentae Reduced breeding efficiency	Contaminated feed and water from aborted material and at calving Contaminated semen	Calfhood vaccination Test and slaughter Prevent exposure
	Sheep, Goats	*Brucella melitensis*	Abortion	Same	Vaccination Test and slaughter
	Swine	*Brucella suis*	Abortion Weak pigs	Same	Test and slaughter
Listeriosis	Cattle, Sheep	*Listeria monocy-togenes*	Late abortion Retained placentae Metritis	Contaminated environment Poor-quality silage	Sanitation Antibiotic therapy
Nonspecific uterine infections	Cattle	Variety of bacterial organisms	Extended anestrus Reduced breeding efficiency	Contaminated calving area Introduced with treatments, etc.	Sanitation
Contagious equine metritis	Horses	*Taylorella equigenitalis*	Endometritis, cervicitis, vaginitis	Natural mating Contaminated equip.	Sanitation Antibiotic therapy

Table 26–1   *(Continued)*

Disease	Affected species	Causative organism(s)	Effects on reproduction	Method of transmission	Control measures
Protozoan Diseases					
Bovine trichomoniasis	Cattle	*Trichomonas fetus*	Early abortion Pyometra Sterility	Sexual contact	Sexual rest Breed AI Slaughter infected bulls Vaccination
Toxoplasmosis	Sheep, cattle, swine	*Toxoplasma gondii*	Late abortions Weak young Stillbirths Retained placentae	Ingestion of oocysts from contaminated environment	Prevent ingesting oocysts and contaminated carcasses
Neosporosis	Cattle	*Neospora caninum*	Abortion—all stages of gestation	Mainly congenital Ingestion of oocyst Oral or nasal exposure to trachyzoites Oral exposure to bradyzoites	Test aborting cows and cull those positive Eliminate exposure?
Viral Diseases					
Bovine viral diarrhea	Cattle	BVD virus	Abortion Fetal abnormalities	Contaminated environment Virus comes in contact with mucous membranes Infected semen	Vaccination Booster vaccination may be desirable
Infectious bovine rhinotracheitis or pustular vulvovaginitis	Cattle	IBR-IPV virus	Abortion in 2nd half of gestation Temporary infertility	Contaminated environment Virus comes in contact with mucous membranes Infected semen	Vaccination (IM or nasal) Booster vaccination with nasal preparation desirable
Equine rhinopneumonitis	Horses	Equine herpes virus I	Abortion last trimester	Virus comes in contact with mucous membranes by aerosols	Vaccination
Equine viral arteritis	Horses	Equine arteritis virus	Abortion in 2nd half of gestation	Virus comes in contact with mucous membranes by aerosols Infected semen	Isolation of apparently infected mares during abortion and parturition Don't use infected stallion
Bluetongue	Sheep, cattle	Bluetongue virus	Damage to central nervous system of fetus	*Culicoides* gnat, sheep ked Possibly by infected semen	Vaccination of nonpregnant animals

Table 26–1   *(Continued)*

Disease	Affected species	Causative organism(s)	Effects on reproduction	Method of transmission	Control measures
Viral Diseases					
Pseudorabies	Swine	Pseudorabies virus	Embryonic mortality Mummified fetuses Abortion Stillbirth	Virus comes in contact with mucous membranes Oral exposure	Vaccination Test and slaughter
Porcine Reproductive and respiratory syndrome	Swine	PRRS single-stranded DNA virus	Stillbirths Mummified fetuses Abortions Premature farrowing Respiratory disease in neonates, nursery, and finisher pigs	Pig to pig contact Aerosols inhaled Virus comes in contact with mucous membranes Infected semen	Eliminate exposure Nursery depopulation Vaccination Management changes to reduce exposure and eliminate losses

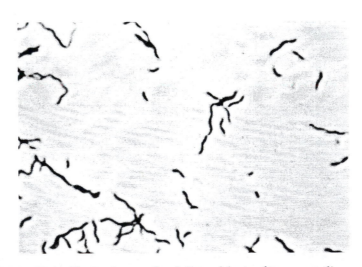

Figure 26–1   Photomicrograph of *Campylobacter fetus venerealis* organisms. (Courtesy of R. Hidalgo. College of Vet. Med., Miss. State Univ.)

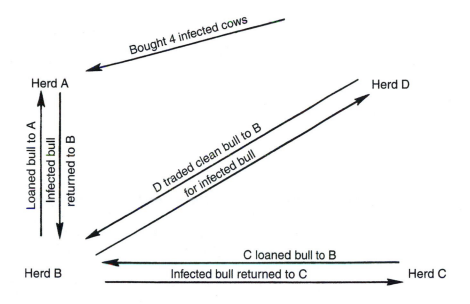

Figure 26–2 Diagram of vibriosis transmission in a case study in New York State.

The four herds involved were grade Holstein herds in western New York. The owner of Herd A bought four cows from a fifth herd, which was infected with vibriosis. In the process of trying to get the cows pregnant, the owner's four bulls became infected. In turn, these bulls transmitted the disease throughout the herd. The owner thought that the problem of low fertility in his herd was due to his bulls, so he borrowed a bull from herd B. After finding that cows did not settle when bred to this bull, either, he was returned to herd B and eventually infected that entire herd. The owner of herd C felt sorry for the owner of herd B because his bulls were sterile, so he loaned him a young bull that had been very fertile in his own herd. The cows did not settle to the bull from herd C, either, so he was returned. The first 19 cows serviced by this bull after returning to herd C all failed to conceive. Vibriosis was transmitted to other bulls in the herd and eventually to the entire herd. Herd D was a small herd of only 30 cows and 1 bull. The owner had two calf crops from the bull he was using and did not want to breed the bull's daughters back to him, so the owner arranged to trade his bull for a bull that had been used and infected in herd B. His herd became infected, also.

Vibriosis can be transmitted between bulls in AI situations. When the same teaser animals are used for both infected and noninfected bulls, it is difficult to prevent the infected bull from leaving organisms on the teaser animals. If the clean bull touches the same area with his glans penis and picks up the organism, he becomes infected. Fortunately, the commercial AI organizations are now maintaining vibriosis-free studs. The *Campylobacter fetus venerealis* organism is shed in the semen of infected bulls. If this semen is not properly treated with antibiotics (Section 16–3), vibriosis will be transmitted to the cows bred. The organism will survive freezing and thawing, so it is essential that semen to be used for artificial insemination comes from bulls free of vibriosis or that it be properly treated with antibiotics to kill the *Campylobacter fetus venerealis* organism. Commercial semen producers endeavor to maintain disease-free stud, but they also use recommended antibiotic treatment in their semen processing.

In sheep vibriosis, the *Campylobacter fetus fetus* organism may be ingested with feed and water contaminated by fluids and discharges from aborting ewes. The infection may persist for some time in the gallbladder of infected animals, and the organisms shed may continue to contaminate the environment.

26–1.1b Symptoms in Cattle

1. The most common symptom is repeat breedings. The average number of natural matings required for conception is 5, with a range from 2 to 25.
2. The estrous cycles are long and irregular, ranging from 25 to 55 days in length. These long cycles are caused by early embryonic mortality. The death of the embryo occurs late enough to postpone the return to estrus.
3. The estrual mucus will be cloudy. This cloudiness is caused by pus, and flakes of pus may be observed in the mucus.
4. Cows usually develop sufficient immunity after several services to carry a calf to term.
5. About 10% of the infected cows will have noticeable abortions. Most of these will occur at 2 to 3 months of gestation.

The bull demonstrates no clinical symptoms of the disease, even though the organism may persist in the reproductive tract for an extended period of time. Spontaneous recovery by bulls has been reported.

26–1.1c Symptoms in Sheep   The effect of vibriosis in sheep is usually much more dramatic than in cattle. In order for the disease to exhibit reproductive symptoms, it must occur 4 to 6 weeks prior to lambing. Abortion rates up to 70% have been reported. The disease is fatal to a small percentage of ewes, and these show significant necrosis of the caruncles.

26–1.1d Diagnostic Procedures   The symptoms of vibriosis are not different enough from the symptoms of other diseases in either cattle or sheep to be relied on as a diagnostic procedure. In herds where breeding dates are kept and close observations are made at the time of estrus, one can strongly suspect vibriosis from the symptoms. In beef herds in which the bulls run with cows, vibriosis should be suspected with prolonged breeding and calving seasons. In either case, a positive laboratory diagnosis is desirable to rule out the possibility of other diseases.

Isolation and identification of the organism is the most definitive test used. However, *Campylobacter* organisms are very difficult to isolate, because they grow slowly. Most samples available for culturing are contaminated with large numbers of fast-growing organisms that rapidly overgrow the culture media. Stomach fluid from aborted fetuses, estrous mucus, and semen from bulls are preferred materials for culture. A diagnosis should not be made based on a single negative culture. Several negative cultures on the same animal or negative cultures on several problem animals make a diagnosis more reliable. Selected antibiotics in the culture media, to control contaminants but allow the *Campylobacter* organism to grow, are helpful.

Antibodies appear in the female reproductive tract. Cervicovaginal mucus can be tested for the presence of these antibodies. The test is usually considered to be a herd test, and samples of mucus should be taken from six to eight problem cows during diestrus about 60 days after first breeding. A positive agglutination test results when *Campylobacter* organisms added to the antibody preparation form clumps. A more sensitive procedure is obtained when soluble antigens from the organism are adsorbed onto red blood cells or latex particles. These cells or particles agglutinate in a positive test.

Bulls are sometimes tested for vibriosis by breeding virgin heifers negative to vibriosis naturally or with untreated semen and testing the heifers. In some cases where large numbers of bulls are to be tested, preputial scrapings are pooled from a few bulls and deposited in test heifers. In the case of a positive test, the individual bulls in the small group would have to be tested.

In sheep, the diagnosis may be made by direct microscopic observation or by the culture of the *Campylobacter fetus fetus* organism from the placenta or from the aborted fetus.

26–1.1e Control Measures Prevention is preferable to treatment. Vibriosis is virtually unheard of in dairy herds practicing 100% AI and using semen from commercial semen-producing organizations. If natural mating is to be utilized, maintaining a closed herd has a lot of merit in preventing several diseases, including vibriosis. When male or female replacements must be purchased, it is much safer to buy prepubertal animals. If postpubertal females are purchased, heifers in late pregnancy are safer than cows. Purchased postpubertal animals should be isolated and adequately tested before they are added to the breeding herd.

Cows infected with vibriosis will develop immunity and/or experience spontaneous recovery from the disease if allowed 60 to 90 days sexual rest. Intrauterine infusion with 0.5 gm to 1 gm of streptomycin 24 hours after insemination or one estrus period prior to insemination will restore fertility. Bulls have been successfully treated with large subcutaneous doses of streptomycin accompanied by local treatment of the sheath and glans penis with the same material. Because of the elusiveness of the organism, it is difficult to know without exhaustive testing when a bull is free of the organism.

Vaccination with a bacterin prepared from respective subspecies is available for both cattle and sheep. Cattle should be vaccinated approximately 2 months prior to breeding and annual vaccination may be indicated. Sheep may be vaccinated prior to the breeding season or during early pregnancy.

26–1.2 *Leptospirosis*

Leptospirosis, caused by several serovars of *Leptospira interrogens,* has long been considered a serious disease only in animals (both wild and domestic). Occasional cases have been reported in humans but not traced to farm animals. However, human health outlook changed when an outbreak of illness in milk hands working in three large Florida dairy herds was traced to exposure to *Leptospira* organisms related to leptospirosis outbreaks in the herds. Eleven of 17 milk hands became infected and exhibited the following symptoms: fever, malaise, nausea and vomiting, myalgia and coryza, chills, enlarged lymph glands, pharyngitis, anorexia, stiff neck, photophobia, arthralgia, diarrhea, conjunctival

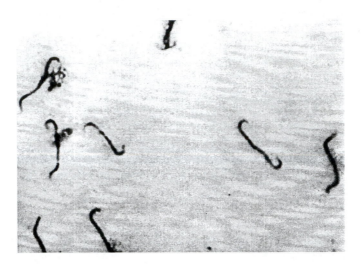

Figure 26–3   Photomicrograph of *Leptospira* organisms. (Courtesy of R. Hidalgo. College of Vet. Med., Miss. State Univ.)

suffusion, and skin rashes. Serologic evidence incriminated *L. hardjo* in 9 and *L. pomona* in 2 of the 11 patients. The *seiroe* serovar is currently causing even more public health concern.

Leptospirosis is not a venereal disease, although it does seriously affect the reproductive processes in cattle, horses, and swine. The disease also causes many symptoms totally unrelated to reproduction. There are many serovars of the genus *Leptospira* which cause leptospirosis in wild animals, domestic animals, and humans. Seven serovars have been associated with leptospirosis in farm animals.

26–1.2a Causative Organisms

The serovars responsible for leptospirosis in cattle are *L. pomona, L. hardjo, L. grippotyphosa, L. canicola, L. icterohemorrhagiae,* and *L. sejroe* (Figure 26–3). Swine and horses are affected by *L. pomona, L. hardjo, L. bratislava,* and *L. icterohemorrhagiae.*

26–1.2b Methods of Transmission

The most common method of transmission is by ingesting or inhaling the organisms from a contaminated environment. Urine from infected animals, both wild and domestic, is the most common means of contaminating the environment. Once in the body, the organisms find their way into the circulatory system and affect many parts of the body. The kidneys become a reservoir for collection and reproduction of the *Leptospira* organisms and serve as the principal means for eliminating the organisms from the body along with urine. Each drop of urine can contain millions of organisms. The amount of damage done to the kidneys is related to the severity of the infection.

The high-density management systems usually practiced with dairy cattle provide an ideal exposure system. When infected cows urinate on concrete pads, a tremendous numbers of water particles (aerosols) are produced, each containing many organisms for all of the cows to inhale. In turn, splashing urine and aerosols contaminate both the feed and water available to the cows. One infected cow can expose an entire herd in a very short period of time. Cows recovering from the disease continue to shed organisms in their urine for 2 to 3 months or longer. There is evidence that swine and some species of wild animals may become permanent vectors.

The principal vector for introducing *Leptospira* organisms into a herd that is free of leptospirosis is wild animals. The list of animals is almost limitless when both active and passive contamination is considered. Visiting humans, domestic cats, and even blackbirds at dairy facilities are examples of passive vectors. Wild animals ranging from skunks and opossums to white-tailed deer are examples of active vectors. Visits by neighboring livestock also have to be considered as possible vectors.

The survival of the organisms left by vectors in the environment depends on several factors. Pastures with wet areas and pastures that are frequently flooded will retain viable organisms longer than well-drained pastures. Farm ponds and natural water holes appear to be reservoirs for *Leptospira* organisms. Fencing the areas and providing a source of fresh water for farm animals is recommended.

Leptospirosis is not classified as a venereal disease; however, it is possible for an infected bull to transmit *Leptospira* organisms to cows during natural mating. Commercial artificial breeding organizations do not process semen from bulls that are shedding *Leptospira* organisms in their semen.

It is impossible to prevent livestock from being exposed to *Leptospira* organisms. Therefore, other control measures are of utmost importance.

26–1.2c Symptoms   Several symptoms have been described for leptospirosis in cattle. Depending on the severity of the disease, some or all of the symptoms may be observed in the same animal. This variation is probably related to the level of exposure to the antigen and to the level of the individual's immunity (from prior exposure or vaccination). The incubation period is usually 7 to 9 days. However, longer periods are possible. Following are the symptoms to watch for:

1. *Sudden onset with loss of appetite.* In acute cases, animals lose interest in water and feed.
2. *Rapid loss of body weight.* In acute cases in mature dairy cows, body weight losses up to 136 kg in 3 days have been reported. Some of this weight loss is due to shrinkage due to decreased feed and water intake. However, much of it is true weight loss. They do not return to their former weight after they resume eating and drinking.
3. *Drop in milk production.* The effect on milk production will vary with the severity of the disease. In severe cases in high producing dairy cows, the level of production may drop almost to zero. The little milk obtained from these cows usually is abnormal, is thick and dark yellow in color, or may contain some blood cells. Because of the abnormal udder secretion, some have suggested that the *Leptospira* organism causes mastitis. However, it is more probable that the abnormal secretion is due to abnormal body metabolism rather than an invasion of the mammary gland by the organism.
4. *Elevated body temperature.* Most infected animals of various ages will have elevated body temperatures as high as 40.5°C to 41.7°C.
5. *Blood in the urine.* The urine of some animals will have a red tint. The color results from damage caused to the kidney tissue by the invasive organisms. The blood cells are hemolyzed so that the hemoglobin is released from the cells and does not settle on standing.

6. *Abortions.* The incidence of abortion in a herd infected with leptospirosis varies from a few to as high as 40%. The incidence depends on the stage of pregnancy of the herd as a whole. Most lepto-initiated abortions occur during the latter third of pregnancy, 7 to 10 days after the onset of the disease. For example, a herd owner in western New York had 10 Holstein heifers in a pasture that was isolated from all other domestic animals. The heifers were between 210 and 260 days of gestation. They were checked daily, and the pasture provided adequate nutrients. In a 14-day period, 8 of the 10 heifers aborted. A diagnostic laboratory confirmed that the heifers were infected with *L. pomona.* The vector in this case was presumed to be white-tailed deer, which also frequented the pasture. Early on, it was thought that the high body temperature caused the death of the fetus. Later data have shown that the organisms have the ability to cross the placental barrier from the maternal circulation to invade the fetus. Presumably, this passage is made easier during advanced stages of pregnancy when some hemorrhage occurs at the hylus of the placentome. This concept is supported by the fact that aborted fetuses are extensively autolyzed (enzymatic degeneration of cells). In some herd outbreaks, abortion without apparent illness may be the only sign of the disease. Some calves carried full-term are weak and have low viability.

7. *Reduced breeding efficiency.* There is little experimental evidence to indicate that cows recovering from leptospirosis continue to experience reduced breeding efficiency. However, many astute managers report that reproductive problems do continue up to 1 year in the form of increased services per conception and retained placentae. These problems seem to be more pronounced with *L. hardjo* than with the other serovars. Animals recovering from severe leptospirosis frequently have a slow and prolonged convalescence.

In swine, leptospirosis not only causes abortions but also often infects pigs that are carried to term so that they are weak at birth and die in a few days. Mummified fetuses may also be seen, along with weak pigs. The disease has been reported to result in abortion and premature births in mares. The clinical disease and abortion occur less frequently in horses than in cattle and swine. The *bratislava* serovar has been reported to cause extended periods of reduced breeding efficiency in both swine and horses.

26–1.2d Diagnostic Procedures   The serum agglutination test using the tube or plate procedures is the most common diagnostic method used for leptospirosis. A positive titer does not necessarily mean that an animal is currently infected with leptospirosis. It may mean that the animal has previously had the disease or that it has been vaccinated. There is value in repeating the tests in 2 or 3 weeks and comparing the two. Animals negative to the first test and positive to the second test, or rising titers in animals that were positive on the first test, would indicate active disease. Testing for all serovars is recommended when leptospirosis is suspected.

Isolation and identification of the organism is a more positive diagnostic procedure. However, there are some problems associated with culturing *Leptospira* organisms, in that *Leptospira* do not grow well on most artificial culture media. The samples, whether urine or blood, must be taken at a time when the disease is active. Aborted fetuses are not usually a good source of material for culturing *Leptospira.* These organisms are very delicate and die readily outside of the host.

26–1.2e Control Measures   There is very little that can be done to prevent animals from being exposed to *Leptospira* organisms. The wide variety of susceptible animals in both wild and domesticated species makes the exposure to *Leptospira* organisms a continuous threat. Preventing access to farm ponds and slow-moving streams may be helpful. Vaccination of cattle, horses, and swine annually is the best option for preventing the disease. Multivalent bacterins (a preparation of killed organisms) are available for cattle containing five serovars, but not containing *L. sejroe.* Under the lowest exposure conditions, cattle should be vaccinated every 6 months, but, under high exposure conditions, vaccination should be repeated every 3 to 4 months. All animals over 2 months of age should be vaccinated. *L. bratislava* bacterin should be added to *L. pomona, L. hadjo,* and *L. icterohemorrhagiae* to the vaccination program for horses and swine. Horses should be vaccinated every 6 months, and for management reasons swine should be vaccinated before each breeding period. Isolation and vaccination of newly purchased animals are recommended.

Leptospirosis is a serious disease that affects all farm livestock as well as humans. Since it is impossible to prevent exposure to the six serovars involved, good management practices, including a vigilant vaccination program, are an absolute necessity. A good relationship between the herd manager and a practicing veterinarian is highly recommended.

26–1.3 *Brucellosis*

Brucellosis is a worldwide problem with both public health and economic importance. The disease may be caused by three major and one minor species of the genus *Brucella.* Each is specific for a species of farm animals but all are contagious to humans.

Most human cases of brucellosis (also called undulant fever) are contracted from exposure in slaughterhouses, with infection largely traced to sows. Some cases have been traced to cattle both in the slaughterhouse and on farms. At one time, most human brucellosis was due to the consumption of raw milk. This is no longer true, since very little raw milk is consumed. More important, however, brucellosis has essentially been eliminated from dairy cattle in the United States.

Young animals apparently carry a rather strong passive immunity to the *Brucella* organism. Offspring from infected females usually are infected at the time of birth, and they consume many organisms while nursing their dams. These organisms apparently do not cause any ill effects and usually are eliminated within a few weeks. If an adult nonpregnant cow becomes infected, the organisms localize in the mammary gland and later spread to the uterus during pregnancy. The organisms invade the pregnant uterus, placenta, and fetus.

26–1.3a Causative Organisms   In cattle, *B. abortus* is the organism responsible for the disease. *B. melitensis* is the major species causing brucellosis in sheep, but *B. ovis* also causes a problem, especially in rams. *B. suis* is responsible for swine brucellosis.

26–1.3b Symptoms of *Brucella abortus*   The most prominent clinical sign of brucellosis in cattle is abortion after the fourth or fifth month of gestation. Subsequent pregnancies may result in a normal calf carried to term but two or three abortions may occur in the same animal. Some full-term calves are weak and may not survive. Retained placentae and uterine infections are both common after-effects of brucellosis and may be related to infection dose and stage of gestation. In severe cases of uterine infection, sterility may occur. The testes of the bull may become infected, and this orchitis can result in sterility. In the acute phase of the infection, semen may contain large numbers of organisms. Infected bulls should not be used for natural mating, and semen should not be used for AI.

Brucella melitensis causes abortions in the ewe and doe and probably other symptoms similar to those in cattle. Abortions usually occur in the third or fourth month of gestation and retained placentae may not occur. *B. ovis* infections are more serious in the ram, causing epididymitis, which causes lesions in the epididymis, and, if the lesions are bilateral, sterility may result. Ewes may abort late in gestation, but this is not common.The prevalence of brucellosis in goats is negligible or nonexistent in the United States.

The most common symptom of brucellosis in swine is abortion and the birth of weak pigs. Sows may have a slight uterine discharge, indicating a uterine infection that persists for an extended period of time. Such uterine infections result in temporary, if not permanent, sterility. Sows that abort following the onset of the disease usually carry litters to term thereafter. The testes of the male may become infected and result in sterility.

26–1.3c Methods of Transmission
The primary methods of transmission are contact with aborted fetuses and fluid from the uterus that contain high concentrations of *Brucella* organisms or ingesting feed, including grass and water, contaminated by the products of the abortion. Females that carry their offspring to term have a buildup of organisms in the reproductive tract and the fluids and discharges during and following parturition contaminate the environment. While the disease may be transmitted at other times, the most contagious period certainly is during and immediately following abortion or parturition.

The disease can also be transmitted through the semen from infected males. Bulls used for semen production for AI use are tested frequently for brucellosis to be sure that no semen is processed from bulls infected with brucellosis.

26–1.3d Diagnostic Procedures
The most common test procedure for brucellosis is the serum agglutination test utilizing blood serum (SAT). The plate, tube, and card tests are variations that are used. The card test is the most sensitive and is still being used as a field test, but its use has been restricted to state and federal personnel working with the brucellosis eradication program. Because of its level of sensitivity, one of the other tests should be utilized to confirm positive card tests. Until recently, it has not been possible to differentiate between positive titers caused by vaccination and those caused by the field strain of the *Brucella* organism. The Rivanol and complement fixation tests (CFT) have been adapted to supplement the serum agglutination test and, with these, field strain antibody titers can be differentiated from vaccination antibody titers. The Cite test is a newer test that is capable of differentiating between Strain 19 blood titers and field strain titers with about 95% accuracy.

The brucellosis ring test (BRT) is used as a screening test for dairy herds. A bulk milk sample from an entire herd can be tested for the presence of antibodies. The test is sensitive enough to detect the presence of 1 infected cow in a herd of 200 or more cows. When a positive BRT occurs, each cow in the herd must be blood tested to determine which are infected.

26–1.3e Control Measures
A nonpathogenic strain of *Brucella abortus*, known as Strain 19, has been used to produce a live organism vaccine to evoke immunity in cattle since its discovery circa 1930. Even though it provided excellent protection, it also

had an undesirable feature. Its use was restricted to prepubertal female calves. When used in older animals, they retained a titer that for many years could not be distinguished from field strain titers. A new vaccine made from another mutant strain of *Brucella* (*B. abortus* strain 2308) that has been designated RB 51 is being used exclusively for cattle in the United States. The efficacy of this vaccine is about the same as the Strain 19 vaccine, but its advantage is that it leaves no residual titers.

The United States has had a state-federal cooperative eradication program in effect since 1955. Progress has been slow, but much of the country is virtually free of cattle brucellosis. All but two states have been declared brucellosis-free and those two states have depopulated their last known infected herd. They will have to remain free of brucellosis for 12 months before they can be certified free of brucellosis. There is still some concern about *B. abortus* in wild species such as bison and the reintroduction of *B. abortus* into the cattle population.

The use of Strain 19 vaccine plus test and slaughter of infected cows have been the principal tools used to bring about the near eradication of brucellosis. The RB 51 vaccine is still being recommended even in many states that have achieved brucellosis-free status and will continue to be used in the foreseeable future. However, the federal disease control officials are in favor of discontinuing all vaccinations.

Vaccination plus test and slaughter are used to control brucellosis in sheep. Rams with epididymitis should be slaughtered. Immature rams may be vaccinated with two doses of a killed *B. ovis* vaccine.

The control of brucellosis in swine is based on test and slaughter. In many cases, an entire herd may need to be slaughtered. There is no commercial vaccine available to evoke immunity in swine. Feral and other wild swine may pose a brucellosis exposure threat to domestic swine in some states. Managers need to assess their situation and decide whether a swine proof buffer zone is justified around their swine facilities.

26–1.4 *Listeriosis*

This disease occurs in many species of mammals and birds. While not especially common in domestic livestock, listeriosis is increasingly recognized as a severe disease in dairy animals, including cattle, sheep, and goats. It also has significance in that it causes similar disease symptoms in humans, especially in those with compromised immune systems (the very young and older individuals, etc). Listeriosis can be contracted from contact with sick animals, especially at the time of abortions, and from raw milk from infected cows. However, most cases have been traced to food sources. The disease is estimated to be responsible for 2,500 cases in humans annually in the United States. While the number of human cases of listeriosis is small when compared with other food-borne diseases, listeriosis has a much higher case mortality rate (20%), accounting for an estimated 500 deaths annually in the United States alone. Faulty valves in dairy processing plants, which allowed small quantities of raw milk to contaminant pasteurized milk, have resulted in outbreaks covering several states. Deaths are caused by the bacterium *Listeria monocytogenes,* which commonly invades the brain and meninges (membranes covering the brain) resulting in encephalitis.

The genus *Listeria* contains five serovars—*L. monocytogenes, L. ivanovii, L. innocua, L. seeligeri,* and *L. welshimeri. L. monocytogenes* causes disease in humans and animals, while *L. ivanovii* is predominantly a disease (specifically abortions) in sheep. The other three serovars are nonpathogenic. *L. monocytogenes* predominantly affects the central nervous system, causing encephalitis, but also causes septicemia, as well as uterine infections in ruminants, which may lead to abortions or to weak offspring. Less common symptoms are mastitis, iritis, and keratoconjunctivitis. A significant number of animals may remain asymptomatic carriers, often shedding *L. monocytogenes* organisms in fecal material.

The primary method of transmission is the ingestion of contaminated feed and water. Poor-quality silage is the most common feedstuff to contain large numbers of *L. monocytogenes* organisms. The organisms are common throughout plant material; fortunately, they are unable to multiply and survive at a pH below 5.0 to 5.5. Even with good-quality silage, there may be pockets of improperly ensiled material containing viable organisms. Birds and rodents are also sources of contamination. Carrier cows expose other animals in the herd by fecal contamination of feed and water. Once the organisms are in the gut, they find their way into the circulatory system and are transported to the sites where the damage is done.

Isolation and identification of the organism by culture is the best means of diagnosis. Very early treatment is essential for recovery. Ampicillin, amoxicillin, oxytetracyline, and penicillin G have all been used successfully in treating listeriosis. However, extremely high dose levels are necessary for good results. Natural immunity to *Listeria* probably provides protection for most animals exposed to *L. monocytogenes*. Only attenuated live organism vaccine is effective in providing further protection, but none have been licensed for use in the United States. The abortions usually occur between the fourth and seventh month of gestation. Encephalitis and abortion may occur in the same animal, but outbreaks in herds usually result in either encephalitis or abortions. The abortion rate in sheep may be more common than in cattle, with reported rates ranging to 50%. The abortions in sheep are usually near term.

26–1.5 *Nonspecific Uterine Infections*

Many studies have been conducted on the microorganisms in the uterus of repeat breeder cows compared with normal cows in an attempt to determine the cause of reduced fertility. These studies have revealed very little, since most uteri contain organisms capable of causing infections. Inoculations of the uterus with organisms capable of pathogenicity have shown little effect on breeding efficiency. It appears that the uterus has a good defense mechanism and becomes infected only when this mechanism is interrupted. It is generally agreed that the uterine defense is much greater during estrus than it is during the luteal phase of the estrous cycle.

Most serious uterine infections occur at the time of, or immediately following, parturition. Many are associated with retained placentae. *Metritis* is described as an infection of the endometrium of the uterus and is characterized by the elimination of pus. The endometrium thickens and the myometrium loses its tone. The total uterine wall is spongy and unresponsive.

No particular pattern as to causative organisms has been established. *Streptococci, Staphylococci, Diplococci,* and *Escherichia coli* are examples of isolations from the uteri of cows with metritis. Control measures involve sanitation during parturition, proper treatment of retained placentae (Chapter 10), and treatment with broad-spectrum antibiotics.

26–1.6 *Contagious Equine Metritis*

Contagious equine metritis (CEM) is a highly contagious acute venereal disease of horses. The disease was first officially reported in the United Kingdom during the summer of 1977.

Later reports reveal that CEM occurred on at least four stud farms in Ireland in 1976. Unconfirmed reports indicate that CEM may have occurred in France before 1976. Contagious equine metritis was diagnosed in Kentucky in the spring of 1978 and in Missouri in 1979 but was confined to a few stud farms. The disease has been reported only in Thoroughbred horses.

The causative organism is a bacterium, *Taylorella equigenitalis*. Transmission has been primarily, if not entirely, by natural mating. AI has not been allowed in the Thoroughbred ranks. It is conceivable that the organism may be transferred by humans using contaminated equipment.

Symptoms of the disease are metritis associated with cervicitis and vaginitis. A copious mucopurulent discharge from the vulva may occur. The severity varies from mares that have an almost complete sloughing of the endometrium to mares that appear almost clinically normal but fail to conceive. All infected mares are at least temporarily sterile.

The stallion shows no clinical symptoms of the disease yet remains a carrier and transmits the disease for an extended period of time. The stallion with CEM appears to play the same role in the spread of the disease that the bull does in spreading trichomoniasis.

Diagnosis is presumptive when several mares bred to a particular stallion come back into estrus and show other clinical symptoms. Cervical and clitoral swabs may be taken for bacteriological culture. Swabs should be taken from the penile sheath and the urethral fossa and the urethra of the stallion for culture. There is no serologic test available to date.

Control measures include quarantine of infected animals. The United States and Canada have placed a ban on importation of all equidae except geldings, weanlings, and yearlings from Ireland and the United Kingdom, France, and Australia. Strict sanitation should be practiced when working with the breeding herd.

Treatment of infected mares involves several days of systematic treatment with large doses of antibiotics along with intrauterine infusions. Less intense therapy appears to induce a carrier state in some mares. Treating the stallion includes cleansing the penis and prepuce thoroughly with chlorhexidine and topical treatment with nitrofurazone daily for at least 3 days or with three treatments over a 5-day period. In addition, intramuscular treatment with antibiotics for 5 to 10 days is desirable. Further treatment may be necessary, depending on the results of bacteriological tests or trial breedings. Economics must be considered in the treatment of mares and stallions.

26–2 PROTOZOAN DISEASES

26–2.1 *Bovine Trichomoniasis*

Trichomoniasis is a venereal disease of cattle caused by a protozoan, *Trichomonas fetus*. The organism is 10 μ to 25 μ in length and has three anterior flagella and an undulating membrane with one posterior flagellum (Figure 26–4).

26–2.1a Method of Transmission Since trichomoniasis is a venereal disease, it is mainly transmitted by sexual contact. Sexual contact in this case includes artificial insemination. There is no satisfactory way to treat semen from infected bulls to make it safe for use in AI.

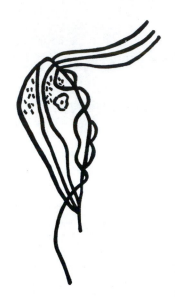

Figure 26–4   *Trichomonas fetus* protozoan. (From Asdell and Beareden. 1959. Cornell Ext. Bull. 737.)

26–2.1b Symptoms   The symptoms of trichomoniasis are similar to those of *Campylobacter fetus* infection. Many cows conceive, but the organism kills the embryo and causes the cow to return to estrus at irregular, long intervals. A major difference between the two diseases is the development of pyometra in trichomoniasis, characterized by the accumulation of pus along with the degeneration of a fetus in the uterus. The liquefaction necrosis of the fetus in the pus may continue for an extended period of time. Herds infected with trichomoniasis will have a high incidence of discharge containing pus from the reproductive tract.

26–2.1c Diagnosis   Diagnosis is made by direct microscopic examination of exudates from the female or preputial washings from the male. It is a tedious process, and negative results should not be considered proof of freedom from infection. Further testing may be needed. A field kit with a contained culture medium is available for diagnosing this disease. A preputial sample from the bull is used to inoculate the medium and the pouch is sent to the manufacturer's laboratory for diagnosis.

26–2.1d Control Measures   When the disease is diagnosed in a herd, a period of sexual rest for the females is the only treatment. A rectal examination may be performed to determine those having pyometra. These animals should be selectively treated with antibiotics. The cervical plug may be broken to allow the exudate to drain from the uterus. Prostaglandin $F_{2\alpha}$ may be injected to lyse the CL, which in turn should eliminate the cervical plug. Approximately 90 days will be required for the cows to recover and to eliminate the organisms from their reproductive tracts. In most cases, bulls should be slaughtered. Success in eliminating the organisms from bulls with topical applications of sodium iodide, acroflavin, and bovoflavin ointment has been reported. The time and expense of the treatment and the testing procedures to determine whether the bull is free of the organism can be justified only in the very valuable bulls. Sexual rest for cows followed by at least 1 year of artificial insemination is recommended. A vaccine for *Trichomonas fetus* is available that will provide some protection in herds using natural mating. It is doubtful that the vaccine will be beneficial for infected cows or bulls.

26–2.2 *Toxoplasmosis*

This organism causes disease in sheep, cattle, swine, and humans. The causative organism is *Toxoplasma gondii,* a small, elongated organism frequently observed in compact masses. Transmission is by ingestion of sporulated oocysts, from either cat feces or the flesh of infected animals.

The symptoms associated with reproduction are abortion, premature births, and stillbirths. Some full-term offspring appear to be infected as a result of intrauterine transmission resulting in high mortality. Abortions in sheep occur during the last 4 to 6 weeks of gestation.

Diagnosis is based on the isolation of the organism or by serologic tests. Microscopic examination of necrotic areas of the placentome, or impression smears of the necrotic area, may reveal the organism. The Sabin-Feldman dye test is a valuable serologic test for the organism.

Control measures depend on breaking the infection cycle. Further studies concerning the role of the cat in transmission may be helpful. No vaccine is commercially available.

26–2.3 *Neosporosis*

Neosporosis was first recognized in California in the mid-1980s but since then has been found to be the causative organism for abortion in cattle throughout most of the United States. *Neospora caninum* is a single-celled protozoal parasite closely related to *Toxoplasma gondii.* Infection of the fetus with *N. caninum* can result in abortion, but many infected calves are normal and symptom-free. A few live-born calves have clinical symptoms ranging from paralysis and stunting to mild proprioceptive deficits. Infected heifers will subsequently pass the disease on to most of their offspring. Congenital infection has been found in 78% to 88% of calves born to seropositive cows, and this accounts for most infections in herds examined. The only scientifically documented natural route of infection in cattle is by transplacental infection of the fetus from an infected dam.

Because some infected cows are offspring of seronegative dams, there has to be other means of transmission. Canines, both domestic and wild, seem to be the primary host for *N. caninum.* Therefore, it seems probable that they shed oocysts in their feces that are ingested by cattle, which accounts for at least a portion of infected cows.

Neospora abortions can be diagnosed by histologic and immunohistochemical tests on the brain of aborted fetuses. Currently, available serologic tests include indirect fluorescent antibody test and ELISA.

No known definitive control programs have been published. However, because most transmission occurs *in utero,* it seems logical that aborting cows should be serotested in addition to submitting the fetus for tests. Positive cows should be culled and preferably slaughtered, since their future offspring will have a high probability of being infected.

Additionally, reducing exposure by keeping canines out of the feeding areas should be beneficial.

26–3 VIRAL DISEASES

26–3.1 *Bovine Viral Diarrhea (BVD)*

The bovine viral diarrhea virus affects a high percentage of the cattle in the United States. In many herds where no clinical symptoms of the disease have been observed, as high as 50% of tested cattle exhibit antibodies against the virus. Four clinical forms of the disease have been described. (1) A subclinical form with which no symptoms are observed is perhaps the most common. (2) Chronic viral diarrhea may occur insidiously and not be recognized for some time. Loss of appetite, emaciation, mild diarrhea, and subnormal growth rate are symptoms that accompany this form. (3) Acute viral diarrhea is characterized by profuse diarrhea, elevated body temperature, and erosion of the gastrointestinal tract. Herd outbreaks have been reported in which essentially 100% of the animals were infected and in other cases where only a few individuals were affected. In the latter case, it is probable that the remainder of the animals were immune from previous infection. (4) The mucosal disease form is the most severe and is characterized by all of the symptoms described for the acute form plus an ulceration of the oral cavity and the mucous membranes of the digestive tract. The animals die in about 14 days without developing immunity. This form of the disease is seen more frequently in animals from 8 to 18 months of age.

In pregnant cows, the virus may invade the fetus, causing death and abortion. The dead fetus is usually held in the uterus for several days before expulsion. Most abortions caused by the BVD virus occur during the first 3 to 4 months of gestation. The incidence of abortion caused by BVD is much lower than early data suggested. Concurrent diseases or the appearance of antibodies against BVD in serum following abortions has been taken as circumstantial evidence that BVD was the cause of the abortions.

BVD infections during the middle third of gestation have resulted in developmental defects of the brain, eye, and hair in calves. Brain and eye defects occur more frequently than hair defects.

The disease is transmitted by the viral agent coming in contact with mucous membranes from a contaminated environment. The virus may be transmitted in the semen from infected bulls either through AI or natural services. It is diagnosed by isolation of the virus or by fluorescent antibody technique, serum neutralization test, and tissue culture procedures. The virus is difficult to isolate from aborted fetuses because of the state of deterioration by the time of expulsion.

Control measures depend entirely on vaccination with either a modified live virus (MLV) or a killed virus vaccine. There are both advantages and disadvantages for both products. The MLV vaccine will induce immunity, which will last at least 1 year with a single dose; with an annual booster, lifetime protection will be provided. With the killed virus vaccine a two-dose priming regimen is required to induce immunity, and at least three vaccinations during the year are required to maintain adequate immunity. The MLV vaccine will cause some pregnant cows to abort and has been associated with the mucosal disease form of BVD infection. The killed virus vaccine can be used on pregnant cows.

The following regimen is recommended for the MLV vaccine. All replacement animals should be vaccinated between 6 and 8 months of age, followed with annual booster vaccinations. All adult female vaccinations, including annual booster shots, must be administered to nonpregnant animals. In herds where the disease has been diagnosed, calves 2 months of age and older should be vaccinated. Any animal vaccinated under 6 months of age should be revaccinated at about 12 months of age. These younger animals usually have some passive immunity from their dams which interferes with the establishment of lasting immunity.

26–3.2 *Infectious Bovine Rhinotracheitis—Infectious Pustular Vulvovaginitis (IBR-IPV)*

The IBR-IPV virus, like others, is transmitted by viral particles from contaminated environments that come in contact with mucous membranes. The symptoms produced depend on the systems affected. As a respiratory ailment, it causes coughing, wheezing, nasal discharge, and fever. As a digestive system ailment, particularly in calves, it causes diarrhea. When the organism invades the reproductive system, a profuse pustular vulvovaginitis results. A discharge containing pus may be observed from the vulva. Temporary infertility is experienced, and it is usually a good idea to suspend breeding during the early phases of the disease. The glans penis of the bull usually develops pustules, and the associated pain may be sufficient to prevent breeding.

Cows with either respiratory or vulvovaginitis forms of the disease may experience viral invasion of the fetus, resulting in abortion. The fetuses are generally aborted from 3 weeks to 3 months after infection of the dam. Retained placentae are commonly associated with the disease.

The disease is diagnosed by isolation of the virus by tissue culture or by serum neutralization tests. Control measures involve vaccination with modified live virus vaccine as a preventive measure. Both intramuscular and nasal spray preparations of the vaccine are available. Replacement animals after 6 months of age and nonpregnant adult females may be vaccinated with the IM preparation. This vaccination may give lifetime immunity, but booster vaccinations with the nasal spray preparation may be advisable. Most nasal vaccines may be used on pregnant cows without fear of abortion. A killed virus vaccine for IBR-IPV is available and is subject to the same limitations as the killed BVD vaccine (Section 26–3.1).

26–3.3 *Equine Viral Rhinopneumonitis*

Equine rhinopneumonitis virus is also known as equine herpes virus I. It causes a respiratory problem in young horses and is a major cause of abortion. Symptoms include nasal discharge, fever, depression, and coughing. The duration of the disease is usually about 4 weeks, followed by spontaneous recovery. The disease is more serious in young animals. Occasionally, the central nervous system is affected, causing paralysis. The disease is transmitted by viral particles coming in contact with mucous membranes, primarily from aerosols. Immunity following the disease is usually transient, and the animals are susceptible again after several months.

The nursing foals that are infected provide massive exposure to the mares, which are usually in midpregnancy. The rate of abortion in mares depends on their susceptibility and has been reported as high as 80% in some outbreaks. The fetus dies *in utero* and is promptly expelled without evidence of autolysis. Most abortions occur from the eighth month to term. Mares usually show no symptoms of the illness, the placentae are not retained, and fertility is normal following abortion.

Diagnosis of the disease is based on viral isolation and identification and from gross and microscopic lesions in the aborted fetus.

Control programs should be based on vaccination. Two vaccination materials are available; one is a killed product and the other is a modified live product. The practicing veterinarian should be relied on to develop a vaccination plan for each farm.

26–3.4 *Equine Viral Arteritis*

A disease that was very common in horses during the early part of the twentieth century was probably caused by equine arteritis virus (EAV). This disease was first officially recognized in the United States in 1950, following an outbreak of abortion and systemic illness at a Standardbred stud farm in Ohio. After the successful control of that outbreak, the disease was not reported again until 1984. Since then, equine viral arteritis has been infrequently diagnosed in the United States, although isolated cases have been documented in several states. One serologic study revealed that 85% of the Standardbred population was positive for the disease, followed by American Saddlebred Horses with 25%, Quarter Horses with 12%, and Thoroughbreds with 2%. The reason for this high prevalence difference is unknown.

The disease presently occurs only sporadically in the United States. As the name implies, the disease causes an inflammatory reaction in the small arteries. Pulmonary edema and edema of the limbs are common. Other symptoms may be elevated body temperature, severe depression, loss of appetite, weight loss, colic, and diarrhea. A brick red mucous membrane protrudes around the eye, with watery and sometimes purulent discharge. Abortions occur in 50% to 80% of the infected mares. Abortions tend to occur in the latter half of gestation. The tissues and fluids associated with the infected aborted fetuses contain large numbers of viral particles. Transmission is primarily by the viral particles coming in contact with the mucous membranes due to inhaling aerosols containing these particles. Venereal transmission occurs when carrier stallions are used to breed mares. Experimentally, EAV has been recovered from the nasopharynx, serum, and buffy coat during the first 3 weeks of infection.

Diagnosis is based on clinical symptoms and the elimination of other causes of abortion, such as equine viral rhinopneumonitis. Virus isolations from nasal secretions, semen, urine, and aborted fetuses are more definitive. Failure to isolate the virus is not necessarily a reliable negative test. Several serologic tests are available, including virus neutralization, complement fixation, and enzyme-linked immunosorbent assay. Infected and carrier stallions should not be used to service mares. A modified live virus vaccine has been available since 1985 based on the Ohio strain of EAV that elicited long-lived protective antibodies. It is available commercially, but its use is controlled by state regulatory officials. Disinfection of equipment and facilities can and should be done with antiseptic detergents which dissolve the lipid envelope of the EAV. Control measures include isolation of apparently infected mares, particularly at the time of abortion and parturition because of the large numbers of particles eliminated with the fluids at the time of abortion or parturition.

26–3.5 *Bluetongue*

The virus that causes the disease bluetongue in sheep and cattle (BTV) is transmitted by anthropod-vectors. Until recently, the disease has been considered primarily a problem of the western states. A survey in which blood samples from all 48 contiguous states were shipped to the National Animal Disease Laboratory at Ames, Iowa, and tested for antibodies against the bluetongue virus revealed cattle with antibodies in essentially all states. One area in the Central Atlantic states (Georgia and North and South Carolina) and another near midcontinent (Nebraska to Texas) approached the epizootic stage.

General symptoms of the disease in sheep are elevated temperature, severe depression, and loss of appetite. Erosions occur on the lips, cheeks, and tongue, with the tongue appearing cyanotic (turns blue due to O_2 deficiency), hence the name of the disease.

Reproductive effects are primarily on the fetus. Although lambs are born at full-term, some are stillborn, and others are spastic and lie struggling until death. Some are referred to as "dummy lambs" and are unable to stand or may be uncoordinated and fail to nurse. The most severe effects occur when the disease is contracted while the ewes are in the fourth to eighth week of gestation. Infections at later stages may produce problems but not so severe. Natural BTV infection of cattle is very rarely accompanied by clinical symptoms. When symptoms do occur, they are similar to many of those described for sheep. The first signs of the disease in a dairy herd may be a drop in milk production and either a stiffness of gate or more severe lameness in 10% to 20% of the animals. There are several other diseases that can cause some or all of these symptoms, so a diagnostic workup of outbreaks will be necessary to determine which organism is involved.

Reproductive problems in cattle include abortions, early embryonic deaths, birth of full-term nonviable fetuses, and congenitally abnormal fetuses have been attributed to BTV. Although male reproductive tract damage has been reported once in an experimental infection, the male bovine reproductive tract is not considered highly susceptible to the pathological effects of BTV. However, the virus can be excreted in semen during periods of viremia. This is probably associated with red blood cells or mononuclear cells in the semen that carry the BTV.

Control measures involve vaccination with a modified live virus vaccine, which provides good immunity for a period of 2 to 4 years. Pregnant ewes cannot be vaccinated, because the vaccine produces conditions similar to the disease itself. Ewes should be vaccinated at least 4 weeks prior to the breeding season. Use of bluetongue vaccine may require permission of the state veterinarian. Cost-benefit ratio must be given serious consideration in the control of BTV.

26–3.6 *Pseudorabies*

Pseudorabies, caused by a herpes virus, was a serious disease in swine in the United States and still is in many countries. However, a persistent eradication program between 1995 and 2002 almost eradicated pseudorabies in domestic swine in the United States. Forty-two states are considered free, while 8 states have eradicated the last known infected herds but will have to remain free for 12 months before being declared free. Two states have just recently depopulated their last known herds and are still involved in area testing. If no other infected herds are found, they will begin their 12-month countdown toward being pseudorabies free. Much of the United States has populations of feral and/or wild swine. Those animals will continue to pose serious threats of reinfecting commercial swineherds. Constructing swine-proof buffer fencing around domestic swine facilities may have merit.

Pseudorabies in animal species other than swine is usually a fatal disease. Humans are resistant to this virus. The virus readily crosses the placental barrier in pregnant sows and infects the embryo or fetus. When this occurs prior to day 30 of gestation, the embryos die and are reabsorbed and pregnancy is terminated. If infection occurs later than 30 days but prior to 60 to 80 days of gestation, fetal mummification and maceration of some or all of the fetuses may occur. When infection occurs after 60 to 80 days of gestation, abortion, stillbirth, or weak piglets may occur. Parturition may be delayed 2 or 3 weeks when all fetuses die in late gestation.

Pseudorabies diagnosis can be made by culturing tissue from infected fetuses, by the immunofluorescent antibody (FA) test on fetal tissues, or by serologic test on live pigs or sows. The serologic test includes the virus neutralization test and the enzyme-linked immunosorbent assay (ELISA) test.

Treatment of animals does not significantly alter the course of disease once symptoms are present. Attenuated and inactivated vaccines are available. When properly used before breeding and in young pigs, they will produce good immunity and largely prevent losses due to pseudorabies. Vaccines cause positive serologic titers, but supplemental tests can differentiate between vaccine titers and field strain titers.

26–3.7 *Porcine Reproductive and Respiratory Syndrome*

The first porcine reproductive and respiratory syndrome (PRRS) disease outbreak in the United States was reported in 1987 as undiagnosed acute reproductive failure in herds in North Carolina and Minnesota. A retrospective study of banked swine serum revealed PRRS antibodies as early as March 1986. As of August 1995, the disease had been reported in 19 states. Presently, it is estimated that 40% to 60% of the herds in the major swine producing areas of the Midwest and Southeast are currently endemically infected. In 1994, the disease was officially recognized in 16 countries on at least 3 continents. A new RNA virus was isolated in the Netherlands in 1991 that was later identified as the causative agent of PRRS. The same year, similar viruses were identified in Germany and the United States.

The PRRS virus infection is typified by two distinct phases. The reproductive phase is generally acute in onset and results in significant reproductive losses due to an increase in stillbirths, mummified fetuses, abortions, or premature farrowing. The respiratory phase is usually found in pigs and results in poor performance or death due to severe respiratory disease that remains a problem in a herd for many months. Morbidity may reach 80% in neonatal pigs with mortality being 90% or higher for those showing clinical symptoms. It is a multisystemic disease that has been characterized by profound, prolonged viremia and extensive tissue distribution. Lesions described include interstitial pneumonia, vasculitis, lymphadenopathy, myocarditis, and encephalitis. The PRRS virus infections are frequently followed by secondary bacterial infections presumably due to a compromised immune system. These infections contribute to further reduced performance.

The most commonly used serologic test for PRRS is the ELISA test, which detects antigens to both the United States and European isolates and results are reported as a Sample:Positive (S:P) ratio. The test will begin to detect seropositive pigs on day 7 postinfection when the S:P ratios approach 0.4. Field samples with S:P ratios as high as 6.67 have been reported. The indirect fluorescent antibody test can also detect PRRS virus antigens.

The transmission of PRRS virus appears to be primarily from pig to pig. Aerosols have been suggested as a vehicle for transmission, but this concept has been difficult to prove. Because the virus has been isolated from several body parts and fluids including urine, it is reasonable that particles would find their way into aerosols. The PRRS virus can be transmitted by natural mating and by AI with semen from infected boars. The virus lives for less than 30 minutes on most substrates commonly found around the barn, including urine and feces; however, it has survived for 9 days in well water and water from a municipal system.

Controlling PRRS is a difficult assignment because it has the ability to mutate as readily as the influenza virus. Control measures include the following:

1. *Eliminating exposure* includes within the farm premises as well as from off-farm sources.
2. *Nursery depopulation* provides a strategic and temporary interruption in pig flow to eliminate the spread of the virus from older infected pigs to recently weaned pigs.
3. *Vaccination* using modified live vaccines to induce a protective response in weaned pigs and the breeding herd is safe and efficacious if the infection involves a single strain of the virus. However, when the infection is heterologous (several strains), the degree of protection obtained is unclear. Vaccination also makes interpretation of serology difficult.
4. *McRebel,* an acronym for management changes to reduce exposure to bacteria to eliminate losses, has been adapted to the PRRS virus in an attempt to curtail the spread of the virus and secondary bacterial infections. It consists of the following management modifications:
   Cross-foster only during the first 24 hours of life.
   Do not move sows or piglets between farrowing rooms.
   Eliminate the use of nurse sows.
   Destroy pigs that become sick and are not likely to survive.
   Minimize handling of piglets and stressors, such as antibiotic or extra iron injections.
   Do not transfer undersized piglets back to the rooms containing younger litters.
   Stop all biological feedback programs.
   Adhere to strict all-in/all-out pig flow principles and allow a minimum of 2 days between groups for thorough disinfection.

SUGGESTED READING

BARTLETT, D. E., K. MOIST, and F.A. SPURRELL. 1953. The *Trichomonas fetus*-infected bull in artificial insemination. *J. Amer. Vet. Med. Assoc.,* 122:366.

BEARDEN, H. J. 2002. Diseases of dairy animals, infectious-Leptospirosis. *Encyclopedia of Dairy Sciences.* eds. H. Roginski, J. W. Fuquay, and P. F. Fox. Academic Press, an imprint of Elsevier Science.

BERCOVICH, Z. 2002. Diseases of dairy animals, infectious-Brucellosis. *Encyclopedia of Dairy Sciences.* eds. H. Roginski, J. W. Fuquay, and P. F. Fox. Academic Press, an imprint of Elsevier Science.

BIBERSTEIN, E. L. and Y. C. ZEE, eds. 1990. *Review of Veterinary Microbiology.* Blackwell Scientific Publishers, Inc.

COUTO, M. A. and J. P. HUGHES. 1993. Sexually transmitted (venereal) diseases of horses. *Equine Reproduction.* Lea and Febiger.

DOLL, E. R. and J. T. BRYANS. 1963. A planned infection program for immunizing mares against viral rhinopneumonitis. *Cornell Vet.,* 53:249.

JONES, T. C. 1969. Clinical and pathological features of equine viral arteritis. *J. Amer. Vet. Med. Assoc.,* 155:315.

KAHRS, R. F., F. W. SCOTT, and A. DELAHUNTA. 1970. Bovine viral diarrhea-mucosal disease, abortion and congenital cerebella hypoplasia in a dairy herd. *J. Amer. Vet. Med. Assoc.,* 156:851.

KENDRICK, J. W. and O. C. STRAUB. 1967. Infectious bovine rhinotracheitis-infectious pustular vulvovaginitis virus infection in pregnant cows. *Amer. J. Vet. Res.,* 20:1269.

McENTEE, K., D. W. HUGHES, and W. C. WAGNER. 1959. Failure to produce vibriosis in cattle by vulvar exposure. *Cornell Vet.,* 49:34.

OSEBOLD, J. W. 1977. Infectious diseases influencing reproduction. *Reproduction in Domestic Animals.* (3rd ed.) eds. H. H. Cole and P. T. Cupps. Academic Press.

ROBERTS, S. J. 1986. *Veterinary Obstetrics and Genital Diseases.* (3rd ed.) Published by the author.

SCHARKO, P. and D. MILSCH. 1995. BVD vaccine—MLV or killed? *Herd Health Memo,* Univ. of Ky.

SCHOLL, D. T. 2002. Diseases of dairy animals, infectious-Bluetongue. *Encyclopedia of Dairy Sciences.* eds. H. Roginski, J. W. Fuquay, and P. F. Fox. Academic Press, an imprint of Elsevier Science.

TIMONEY, J. F., J. H. GILLESPIE, F. W. SCOTT, and J. E. BARLOUGH, eds. 1988. *Hagan and Bruner's Microbiology and Infectious Diseases of Domestic Animals.* (8th ed.) Comstock Publishing Associates/Division of Cornell University Press.

VARNER, D. D., J. SCHUMACHER, T. L. BLANCHARD, and L. JOHNSON. 1991. *Diseases and Management of Stallions.* ed. P. W. Pratt. American Veterinary Publications.

WALDNER, C. A., E. D. JANSON, and C. S. RIBBLE. 1998. Determination of the association between *Neospora caninum* infection and reproductive performance in beef herds. *J. Amer. Vet. Med. Assoc.,* 213:685.

WALKER, J. S. 1978. *Contagious Equine Metritis Reference Handbook.* Plum Island Anim. Dis. Ctr., USDA, SEA, FR.

WEDIEMANN, M. and K. G. EVANS. 2002. Diseases of dairy animals-Listeriosis. *Encyclopedia of Dairy Sciences.* eds. H. Roginski, J. W. Fuquay, and P. F. Fox. Academic Press, an imprint of Elsevier Science.

Index

Index

A

Abortion, 18, 125 (*See also* specific diseases)

Acidity-alkalinity (pH), and spermatozoa metabolism, 180

Acrosome, 175, 175i
  damaged, 194–195
  reaction, 85, 103, 262

Activin, 40, 45–46

Adenohypophysis, 38

Adrenal cortex, 48

Adrenocorticotropic hormone (ACTH), 37t, 39t, 40
  in heat stress, 342

Age
  and reproductive efficiency, 292t, 292–293, 377–378
  and semen production, 309, 309t

Alfalfa (*Medicago sativa*), 382

Alflatoxin, carcinogenic mycotoxin, 380

Allanto-chorion membrane, 114, 115i

Allantois, 115, 115i

Alpha-fetoprotein (AFP), 52

Alveoli, 145, 145i

Amnion membrane, 114, 115i

Amplified restriction fragment length polymorphism (AFLP) technique, genetic markers, 283, 284i, 285i, 286t

Ampules, bull semen, 208, 208i, 209

Ampulla, 13, 14i

Ampullary-isthmic junction, 13, 14i

Androgenized heifers, estrus checking, 295

Androgens, 22, 39t, 44t, 47, 76, 361, 365. *See also* Testosterone
  and spermatozoa metabolism, 181

('i' indicates an illustration; 't' indicates a table)

Anestrus, 63, 374–375
  postpartum, 138, 139

Angiogenesis, 51

Animal handling techniques, and stress, 340–341

Annular rings, 18, 18i

Anterior pituitary, 38, 39t, 40, 41, 41i

Antibiotics
  and AI, 159
  semen diluters, 201–202
  and spermatozoa metabolism, 182

"Antisterility vitamin" (vitamin E), 352

Artificial insemination (AI), 3, 101, 105. *See also* Insemination
  advantages/disadvantages, 159
  definition, 155
  deposition sites, 229-230
  estrus synchronization, 237
  handler's experience factors, 386, 386t
  history, 156–159
  restraining facilities, 230
  and superovulation, 249
  techniques, 223–225
  timing of, 298–301

Artificial vagina (AV), 156, 157i
  semen collection, 162–170, 164i, 166i, 167i, 168i

Aspergillus flavus, 380

Aspergillus spp, 411

Atretic follicle, 9, 10

Axial filament, 175i, 176

Assisted reproductive technologies (ART), 261–269

Astragalus (locoweeds), 382

Athetic follicle, 9, 10

Autocrine hormone effects, 36

Axial filament, 175i, 176

415

B

β-endorphin, 42, 138
Bacterial diseases, 389-403, 390t
Beltsville F5 diluter (boar semen), 314t
Beltsville National Research Laboratory, 273
Beta-carotene, 352
Bicarbonate, in seminal plasma, 178
Bicornuate uterus, 14, 15i
Bioinformatics, 288–289
Bilateral cryptorchid, 22
Biotechnology
    definition, 261
    future reproductive tools, 286–289
Bipartite uterus, 14, 15i
Birth position, rotation, 128–131
Blastocoele, 110, 111i
Blastocyst, 110–111, 111i, 112–113, 112t,
        255, 256, 266, 268t
Bluetongue virus (BTV), 391t, 409
Boar
    accessory glands, 32i
    penis, 34i
    reproductive system, 24i
    semen collection, 169-170, 171
    semen composition, 174i
    semen processing, 214–217
    seminiferous epithelial cycle, 84
    sperm cell concentration, 187
    testes, 25
"Boar effect," 89
Body condition scoring, 356
Bovine trichomoniasis, 391t, 403–405
Bovine viral diarrhea (BVD), 391t, 406–407
Breeding fitness tests, 311–313
Briggs and King cloning, 277
Broad ligament, 8i, 19
"Broken penis," 368, 368i
Brucella spp., 399
Brucellosis, 390t, 399-401
Brucellosis ring test (BRT), 400
Buck (goat)
    photoperiod, 71
    semen collection, 168, 171
    semen processing, 221
    sperm cell concentration, 187
    testes, 25
Bulbospongiosus muscle, 33, 93
Bulbourethral glands, 23i, 24i, 31, 32i,
        33, 174t

Bull
    accessory glands, 32i
    breeding fitness tests, 311–313
    glossypol toxicity, 380
    handling techniques, 309-310
    heat stress, 338
    liquid semen, 212–214
    penis, 34i
    psychological disturbances, 387
    reproductive organ injuries, 368
    reproductive system, 23i
    secondary sexual characteristics, 76i
    semen collection, 161, 163–168, 171
    semen composition, 174i
    semen diluters, 202–204
    semen processing, 204–211
    seminiferous epithelial cycle, 84
    sperm cell concentration, 187
    testes, 25
    vibriosis, 393, 394

C

Calcium, dietary, 353
Campylobacter fetus venerealis, 389, 390t,
        393i, 393–395
Capacitation, spermatozoa, 84–85, 261–262
Carbohydrates, 351
Caruncle, 15
Castration, 313i, 313–314, 315i
Catheter, inseminating, 226, 227i
Certified Semen Services (CSS), 198, 199
Cervical fixation insemination, 224
Cervical insemination, 223
Cervical ripening, 133
Cervix, 8i, 17–18
    incomplete, 363, 364i
Cholesterol, steroid precursor, 36
Chorion membrane, 114, 115i
Chorionic villi, 15–16, 16i
Citrate buffer solution, semen diluter, 200
Cleanup natural mating, 240
Cleavage, cell division, 110–112
Clitoris, 8i, 19
Cloning, 261
    embryo splitting, 276–277
    nuclear transfer, 277–278
Cloprostenol, 238
Clovers (*Trifolium* spp.), 382
Cobalt, dietary, 354

Cold shock, semen analysis, 196
Colony stimulating factor (CSF), 52
Colostrum, 136, 151
Complement fixations test (CFT),
        brucellosis, 400
Computer automated semen analyzers
        (CASA), 195–196
Contagious equine metritis (CEM), 390t,
        402–403
Controlled Internal Drug Releasing (CIDR)
        progestin inserts, 239i, 243, 244
Copper, dietary, 354
Corona madiata, 10, 12i, 98i, 103, 104i
Corpus albicans, 10i, 13
Corpus cavernosum penis, 33, 34i, 93
Corpus hemorrhagicum, 10i, 12
Corpus luteum, 10, 10i, 11i, 12, 64, 66, 67,
        121, 122, 123, 238
    cystic, 372–373, 373i
    retained, 373–374
Corpus spongiosum penis, 33, 34i, 93
Cortex, ovaries, 7
Corticotropin-releasing hormone (CRH), 39t, 42
Cortical granules, 98i, 104, 104i
Cortisol, 39t, 48
Cotyledons, 15 16i
Counting slides, 192
Courtship patterns, 92
Cow
    abnormal birth positions, 130i
    cervix, 18i
    conception rates various conditions, 377t
    embryonic development, 111i, 112t
    endocrine glands, 37i
    estrous cycle, 62t, 65i
    estrus, 90–91, 293–296, 298–299, 299i
    estrus synchronization, 237–246
    follicular development, 67–69
    freemartins, 361–362
    gestation, 109, 110t
    in vivo capacitation, 84
    insemination, 85t, 223–230
    mammary glands, 143t
    milk composition, 150t
    milk ejection, 149i
    normal birth position, 129i
    nutrition and reproduction, 350t, 356–357
    organ differentiation, 118t
    ovaries, 7
    oviductal motility, 102i
    parturition stages, 129t
    placentation, 15, 16i
    postpartum recovery, 138–139, 301–302
    pregnancy diagnosis, 318–329
    pregnant weight changes, 120t
    prolapses, 368–369
    psychological disturbances, 385–386
    reproductive organ injuries, 367–368
    reproductive system, 8i
    size and weight at first insemination, 292t
    summer breeding, 339, 345, 346
    superovulation, 249, 250–252
    twinning, 125
    udder, 142–143, 143i
    uterine involution, 139
    uterus, 14
    vibriosis, 393
Cowper's glands, 33
Cryoprotectants, frozen embryos, 257, 258
Cryptorchidism, 22, 365–366
CSS Minimum Requirements for Disease
        Control of Semen Produced for AI, 198
Cumulus, 10, 98i, 103, 104
Cumulus oopherus, 10, 12i
Cyclic adenosine monophosphate (cAMP),
        53, 54i
Cystic corpus luteum, 372–373, 373i
Cystic ovaries, 370–373
Cytokines, 50, 51–52
Cytoplasmic droplet, 81, 84

D

Daily barn sheet, 303, 304i
Dairy Herd Improvement Association (DHIA),
        record program, 306–307
Dairy Herd Monitor, 303, 305i
DDT (dichlorodiphenyltrichloroethane), 384
Defined medium (DM), *in vitro* fertilization,
        262, 262t
Delayed fertilization, 107
Delayed implantation, 111
Demiembryos, 276
Deoxyribonucleic acid (DNA), 54
Detection of estrus
    cow, 293–296, 293t, 294i, 295i
    doe, 296–297
    ewe, 296, 296i
    mare, 297–298, 298i
    sow, 297, 297i

Dictyate oocyte, 96
Diestrus, 64
Differential diagnosis
  cow pregnancy,
  mare pregnancy, 333
Differentiation, cell division, 112–118
Dilution process, semen, 204–205
Dilution rate, 205–206
Direct cell count, sperm cell concentration,
    186–187
Dizygous twins, 125
DNA fingerprinting, 282
DNA microarrays ("DNA chips"), 287–288
DNA microinjection, 278, 279i
Doe (goat)
  estrous cycle, 62t
  estrus, 296–297, 300
  estrus synchronization, 248–249
  gestation, 109, 110t
  insemination, 230–231
  mammary glands, 143t
  milk composition, 150t
  pregnancy diagnosis, 329-331
  superovulation, 252
Dolly lambs, 277, 278
Down-regulation, 52, 53
Duplex uterus, 14, 15i
Dystocia, 135, 367

E

Eastern tent caterpillars, and MRLS, 384
Ectoderm, 113, 114t
Egg-binding proteins (EBPs), 104
Egg yolk, semen diluter, 203t
Ejaculation, 93–94
Electroejaculator, 170–171, 171i
Electronic particle counter (EPC), sperm cell
    concentration, 189-190, 190i
Emasculator, 313i, 314, 315i
Embryo
  development 111i, 112i
  differentiation, 112–118
  female reproductive system origins, 7
  and heat stress, 339
  migration, 109-110
  sexual differentiation, 116–118, 117i
  species comparative, 116i
Embryo transfer
  freezing and thawing, 257–258

  history, 252–253
  recipient selection, 256
  storage, 258
  techniques, 257
Embryonic diapause, 111
Embryonic stem cells, and transgenesis, 280
Endocrine system, 44–43. *See also* Steroid
    hormones
  first experiment with, 2
  glands of, 36, 37i
  and stress, 344–343
  synthetic compound disruption, 384–385
Endoderm, 113, 114t
Endogenous opioids, 42
Endometrium, 15
Energy, nutrition component, 350–351
Environmental stressors, 338–341
Environmental variation, definition, 3
Enzyme-linked immunosorbent assay (ELISA),
    56–57
Eosin, differential stain, 192
Epididymis, 23i, 24i, 29-30, 29i
Epigenesis, theory of, 2
Equilibration
  frozen embryos, 258
  semen processing, 208
Equine arteritis virus (EAV), 391t, 408–409
Equine chorionic gonadotropin (eCG), 49
Equine viral rhinopneumonitis, 391t,
    407–408
Erection, 93
Estradiol, 39t, 44, 67
  and mating behavior, 87, 88
Estrogens, 39t, 44t
  and mammary gland development, 147
  and mating behavior, 87
  in pregnancy maintenance, 121
Estrous cycle
  definition, 61
  hormonal control, 64–67
  periods of, 63–64
Estrus, 63
  behavioral characteristics, 90–91
  detection of, 293–298
  expectancy lists, cows, 293
  and heat stress, 339
  irregular cycles, 375–376
  postpartum, 138–139
Estrus, synchronization
  in cows, 237–246

in does, 248–249
in ewes, 247–248
in mares, 246–247
in sows, 247
Ewe
  embryonic development, 112t
  estrous cycle, 62t, 65i
  estrus, 91, 296, 299-300
  estrus synchronization, 247–248
  gestation, 109, 110t
  insemination, 230–231
  mammary glands, 143t
  milk composition, 150t
  parturition stages, 129t
  placentation, 15
  pregnancy diagnosis, 329-331
  and ram's presence, 387
  summer breeding, 339
  superovulation, 252
  twinning, 124
  uterus, 14
  vibriosis, 394
External cremaster, 28
Extraembryonic membranes, 114–115, 115i

F

Fallopian tubes, 1. *See also* Oviducts
False hellebore (*Veratum californicum*), 382
"Farrowing estrus," 137
Feeding, and age at puberty, 63
Feedstuffs, toxicities, 379, 380
Female reproduction system, 8i, 9t
  cervix, 17–18
  embryonic differentiation, 116–118, 117i
  embryonic origins, 7
  estrous cycle, 63t, 63–64
  ovaries, 7–13, 8i, 11i
  oviducts, 8i, 13, 14i
  puberty, 61–62, 62t
  steroid hormones, 44–47
  support structures, 19-21
  uterus, 8i, 13–17
  vagina, 19
Fertilization, 103–105
Fescue toxicosis, 379
Fetal calf, 119i
Fetal calf serum (FCS), and IVF, 266
Fetal growth, 119-120
Fetal motility, at parturition, 134

First polar body, 98
Flow cytometric analysis, sperm DNA, 273, 275i, 276i, 276t
Flushing, diet supplementing, 355–356
"Foaling estrus," 138
Foley catheter flush, embryo transfer, 253–254, 254i
Follicle, ovarian, 9-10, 10i, 67–70
Follicle-stimulating hormone (FSH), 37t, 39t, 40, 41, 42, 45i, 48i, 138, 355
  estrous cycle, 64, 65i-66i, 67
  spermatogenesis, 81
  and superovulation, 250, 251, 251t
Follicular cysts, 370–372, 371i
Follicular dynamics, 67–70, 68i, 69i, 245
Follicular fluid, 46–47
Follicular phase, estrous cycle, 63
Follistatin, 40
Forage, and mycotoxins, 379
Freemartin, 361–362
Fusarium, 380

G

Galactopoiesis, 147
Gametes
  aging of, 105–107
  fertilization, 103–105
  transport, 99-103
Gases, and spermatozoa metabolism, 181
Generation interval, definition, 3
Genetic engineering, 278–282
Genetic improvement, 2–3
Genetic variation, definition, 3
Genetically modified organisms (GMO), restrictions, 282
Genital ridges, 7, 116
Genomics, 287
Germ layers, 113
  organs forming from, 114t
Gestation
  definition, 109
  and heat stress, 340
  length by species, 110t
Gilt. *See* Sow
Glans penis, 33, 34i
Glucocorticoids, 39t, 40, 48
Glycerolation
  frozen embryos, 257–258
  semen processing, 207–208

Glycerylphosphorylcholine (GPC), in seminal plasma, 178

Glycosaminoglycan (GAG), 85

Glycosaminoglycan (GAG)-binding proteins, 177

Glycosaminoglycan (GAG) heparin, 262, 263

Gonadotropin-releasing hormone (GnRH), 37t, 39t, 41, 45i, 48i, 138, 346

in estrus synchronization, 239i, 241

in follicular fluid, 47

in heat stress, 342

in ovulation synchronization, 245

Gonadotropins, 40

during estrous cycle, 64, 65i-66i, 67

intracellular mechanisms, 53, 54i

Gossypol toxicosis, 380–381

Graafian follicle, 9-10, 10i, 12i

Growth factors, 50–51

Growth hormone-releasing hormone (GHRH), 42

Gubernaculum, 22

H

Hearing, and mating behavior, 90

Heat stress, 338–340

Hemocytometer, sperm cell concentration, 186–187, 188i

Hens, delayed fertilization, 107

Herbicides, and endocrine disruption, 384

Heritability, definition, 3

Hermaphrodism, 364–365

Human chorionic gonadotropin (hCG), 37t, 39t, 49, 247

Hymen, 19

H-Y antigen procedure, fetal sexing, 270

Hypothalamus, 39t, 40–42, 41i, 43

Hypotonic diluters, and semen motility, 186

I

Ichiocavernosus muscle, 33, 93

In vitro culture, embryos, 266–268, 267i

In vitro fertilization (IVF), 84, 261–264, 265–266

and embryo development, 268t

In vitro maturation (IVM), 264

Induced parturition, 134–135

Infantile reproductive system, 363

Infectious bovine rhinotracheitis-infections pustular vulvovaginitis (IBR-IPV), 301t, 407

Infertility

age, 377–378

anatomical, 361–369

diseases, 389–411, 390t

nutrition, 348–357, 349t

physiological, 370–377, 371i, 372i, 373i

postpartum rest, 137–140, 139t, 301–303, 302t

psychological, 340–341, 341i, 385–387

seasonal, 338–340, 339i

timing of insemination, 298–301, 299i, 300i

toxicological, 378–385

uterine infections, 402

Infundibulum, 13, 14i

Inhibin, 37t, 39t, 40, 46, 48i

Inorganic ions, in seminal plasma, 177–178

Insemination (cow)

cervical, 223, 224i

equipment, 226–227

problem situations, 226

recto-vaginal, 224, 225i

timing, 298–299, 300t

vaginal, 223

Insemination (doe), 230–231

Insemination (ewe), 230–231, 231i

Insemination (mare), 233, 233i, 301

Insemination (sow), 231–232, 232i

timing, 300t, 300–301

Insulin, in follicular fluid, 47

Interferon *tau* (INFt), 49, 121, 122t

Interferons (INF), 52

Interleukins (IlS), 51

Intersex, 364

Intracytoplasmic sperm injection (ICSI), 268–269, 269i

Intravaginal progestin inserts, 243–244

Iodine, dietary, 353

Isthmus, 13, 14i

J

Jockey Club, and stallion semen preservation, 218–219

K

Karyotyping, and fetal sexing, 270

L

Labia majora/minora, 19
Lactation
 definition, 142
   and estrus, 138
   milk ejection, 149-150
   milk secretion, 147–148
Lactogenesis, 147
Lactose, 151
Laparotomy, embryo transfer, 253, 253i
Lateral suspensory ligaments, 144 144i
Leptospira spp., 396
Leptospirosis, 390t, 395–399, 396i
Leuteinized follicles, 372, 372i
Leydig cells, 27, 40, 75, 76, 78i, 117
Libido, 94
Lifetime record cards, 304, 305i
Light
   and bull sperm, 211
   and spermatozoa metabolism, 181–182
Liquid bull semen, 212–214
Listeria spp. 401
Listeriosis, 390t, 401–402
Live-dead determination, sperm, 192, 193i
Locoweeds (*Astragalus*), 382
Long-day breeders, 72
Lordosis, 90
Lupins, toxins in, 382
Luteal phase, estrous cycle, 63
Luteinizing hormone (LH), 37t, 39t, 40, 41,
        42, 45i, 48i, 138, 355
   estrous cycle 64, 65i-66i, 67
   spermatogenesis, 81, 82i
   and superovulation, 250, 251

M

Male reproductive system, 23i-24i, 25t
   embryonic differentiation, 116–118, 117i
   epididymis, 29-30, 29i
   penis, 33, 34i
   prepuce, 33, 35
   prostate glands, 23i, 24i, 31, 32, 32i, 174t
   puberty, 75–77
   scrotum, 27–29, 28i
   seminiferous tubule, 25, 26i
   spermatic cord, 27–29
   spermatogenesis, 77–81
   steroid hormones, 47–48

   testes, 25–27, 26i
   urethra, 31
   vasa deferentia, 31, 32i
   vesicular glands, 31–32, 32i
Mammary glands
   development, 146–147
   during gestation, 131
   milk ejection, 149-150
   milk secretion, 147–149
   species comparison, 143t
   structure of, 142–146
Managed breeding, 245–246
   females, 292–309
   males, 209-316
Mare
   embryonic development, 112t
   estrous cycle, 62t, 66i
   estrus, 91, 297–298, 301
   estrus synchronization, 246–247
   gestation, 109, 110t
   insemination, 233
   mammary glands, 143t
   maternal recognition of pregnancy, 121
   milk composition, 150t
   parturition stages, 129t
   placentation, 15–16, 16i
   postpartum recovery, 302–303
   pregnancy diagnosis, 331–334, 335i
   seasonal breeding, 72
   twinning, 125
   uterus, 14
Mare reproductive loss syndrome (MRLS),
        383–384
Marker-assisted selection, reproductive traits,
        283, 286
Maternal recognition of pregnancy, 121
Mating behavior
   estrus, 90–91
   hormonal influence, 87–88
   male, 91–95
   senses, 88–90
   social interaction, 90
Median suspensory ligament, 144, 144i
"Medium straw," AI, 158
Medulla, ovaries, 7
Meiosis, spermatocyte, 77, 79i, 80,
   oocyte, 96, 97i, 98
Melatonin, 43
Melengestrol acetate (MGA), 239i, 244

Mesoderm, 113, 114t
Messenger ribonucleic acid (mRNA), 54
Metabolic activity, semen analysis, 196
Metabolism rate, spermatozoa, 179-182
Metestrus, 64
Metritis, 325, 402
Middle uterine artery, 20, 320
Milk
    composition of, 150–151
    as semen diluter, 201, 203, 203t
Milk ejection, 149–150, 149i
Milk progesterone detection kits, estrus
        checking, 296
    pregnancy diagnosis, 326–327
Milk secretion, 147–149
Milk yields, sire proofs, 3i, 3–4
Minerals, nutrition component, 353–354
Mink, delayed implantation, 111
Mitochondrial sheath, 175i, 175–176
Modified Dulbecco's phosphate-buffered
        medium, 255t
Modified live virus (MLV) vaccine, BVD, 406
Mold toxicity, 379, 411–412
Monotocous reproduction, 7
    and twinning, 124
Monozygous twins, 125, 126i
Morula, 110, 111i, 256, 268t
Motility
    photographic determination, 193–194
    semen ejaculate,184–186
    sperm, 192–193
Mount detectors, estrus checking,
        294–295, 295i
Mucous plug, and abortion, 18
Müllerian ducts, 7, 116, 117i, 361, 365
Mummified fetus, cow, 325, 325i
Mycoses, 411–412
Mycotoxins, 379-380, 411–412
Myoepithelial cells, 146
Myometrium, 15, 133

N

Naloxone, 42
National Animal Genome Research Program
        (NAGRP), genomics, 287
National Association of Animal Breeders
        (NAAB), 198
National Center for Biotechnology
        Information (NCBI), genomics, 287

National Research Council (NRC), nutritive
        requirements, 354
Neospora caninum., 405
Neosporosis, 391t, 405–406
Neotyphodium coenophialum (tall fescue), 379
Newborn, care of, 135–136
Nonreturn (NR) rates, reproductive efficiency
        measure, 291–292
Nonreturn rate, bull fertility, 183
Nonspecific uterine infections, 390t, 402
Norgestomet implants, 242–243
Nuclear transfer
    and cloning, 277–278
    and transgenesis, 280
Nutrition
    components, 348–354
    in growth, 354–355
    and reproduction, 348, 349i, 349t

O

Offspring ledger book, 305–306, 306i
Oocytes, 96, 97i, 98i
    and IVF, 264–265
    transport, 99–100, 100t
Oral (feeding) progestins, 244
Organ formation, 114t, 116–118
Organic compounds, in seminal plasma, 178
Osmotic pressure, and spermatozoa
        metabolism, 181
Ovarian arteries, 20, 20i
Ovaries, 7–13, 8i, 11i
    adhesions, 367
Overfeeding, 350
Oviducts (fallopian tubes), 8i, 13, 14i
    incomplete, 363, 364i
Ovigenesis, 82, 96–98, 97i
Ovulation, 63, 64, 67, 69, 98–99
    postpartum, 138–139
    synchronization, 244–245
Ovum, 7, 9, 13
    fertile life, 106t
Oxytocin, 37t, 39t, 40, 42, 46, 131, 133,
        149, 150

P

Palpation
    pregnant cow, 320–329
    pregnant mare, 333

Pampiniform venous plexus, 28i, 29
Paracrine hormone effects, 36
Parturition
  approaching, 128–131
  definition, 109, 128
  hormonal initiation, 131–133, 132i
  induced, 134–135
  physiological events of, 133–134
  rest after, 137–140, 301–303
  stages by species, 129
Parturition rate, reproductive efficiency
        measure, 291
PCB (polychlorinated biphenyls), 384
Pellets, bull semen, 209
Penicillamine hypotaurine epinephrine (PHE),
        IVF preparation, 263
Penile block, 314, 316i
Penis, 33, 34i
Peptide and protein hormones, 36, 37t, 39t, 40
  measurement, 55–57
Percoll gradients, IVF preparation, 263, 263i
Pesticides, and endocrine disruption, 384
"Pharming," 281
Pheromones, and mating behavior, 88–89
Phosphate buffer solution, semen diluter, 200
Phosphorus, dietary, 353
Photoperiod
  and estrus, 340
  in seasonal breeding, 72–73, 73i
Phytoestrogens, 382–383
Pine needle abortion, 381
Pineal gland, 42–43, 43i
Pinus ponderosa (ponderosa pine), 381
Pituitary, gland, 38, 39t, 40–42, 41i
Placenta, 49, 115, 122
  retained, 136–137
Placental lactogen, 49, 124, 147
Placentation, 15–17
  and immune response, 124
Placentome, 15, 323, 324
Polar body, 97i, 98
Polymerase chain reaction (PCR), in
        embryo sex determination, 270–271,
        271i, 273i
Polyspermy, 105
Polytocous reproduction, 7
Porcine reproductive and respiratory
        syndrome (PRRS), 392t, 410–411
Posterior pituitary, 38, 39t, 40, 41, 41i
Postpartum recovery, 137–140, 301–303

Pregnancy
  cow diagnosis, 318–329
  diagnosis value, 318
  ewe and doe diagnosis, 329-331
  immune response in, 124
  maintenance, 121–124
  mare diagnosis, 331–334, 335i
  sow diagnosis, 334, 336–337
Pregnancy-specific protein B
  cow, 328
  ewe and doe, 329-330
Pregnant mare serum gonadotropin (PMSG),
        16, 39t, 49, 123, 247, 251, 333–334
Preovulatory oocytes, and IVF, 264
Prepuce, 33, 35
Prepuce redirection, 316, 316i
Primary follicle, 9, 10
Problem detection, 307–309
Proestrus, 64
Progesterone, 39t, 44, 64, 65, 65i-66i, 67, 133
  and mammary gland development, 147
  and mating behavior, 87
  and pregnancy maintenance, 121, 122, 124
Progesterone assay
  cow, 326–327
  ewe and doe, 329
  mare, 334
Progesterone-Releasing Intravaginal Devices
        (PRIDs), 239i, 243
Progestin method, estrus synchronization,
        241–244
Progestins, 39t, 44t
Prolactin, 37t, 39t, 40, 45i, 65i-66i, 131, 147
Prostaglandin F_{2a} (PGF$_{2a}$), 20, 21, 39t, 50,
        64, 66–67, 99, 121, 131, 132, 247,
        248, 346
  and estrus synchronization, 238–241, 244
  in heat stress, 342
  and induced parturition, 135
  and ovulation synchronization, 245
  and superovulation, 251
Prostaglandin method, estrus synchronization,
        238–241
Prostaglandins, 49-50, 99
Prostate gland, 23i, 24i, 31, 32, 32i, 174t
Protein, nutrition component, 351
Proteomics, 288
Protozoan diseases, 391t, 403–406
Pseudohermaphrodites, 364–365
Pseudorabies, 392t, 409-410

Psychological disturbances, 385–387
Puberty
    environmental factor effects, 62–63,
        76–77
    female age at, 61, 62t
    female weight at, 61–62, 62t
    male age at, 75
Pulse of pregnancy, 320
Pyometra, cow, 325

Q

Quantitative trait loci (QTL), in marker-
    assisted selection, 286
Quiet ovulation, 376–377

R

Radiation shields, heat stress reduction,
    343–344, 344t
Radiational cooling, 345
Radioimmunoassays (RIAs), 55–56
Ram
    accessory glands, 32i
    penis, 34i
    photoperiod, 71
    reproductive system, 23i
    semen collection, 168, 171
    semen composition, 174i
    semen processing, 217–218
    seminiferous epithelial cycle, 84
    sperm cell concentration, 187
    testes, 25
"Ram effect," 89
Range animals, protein in diet, 351
RB 51, brucellosis vaccine, 401
Real-time ultrasonic (RTU) pregnancy
    checking, 328, 329i, 330, 331i,
        336–337
Receptor sites, 36
    regulation, 52–53
Rectal pregnancy palpation
    cow, 318–326
    ewe and doe, 331
    mare, 331–333
Recto-vaginal insemination, 224, 225i, 226
Relaxin, 37t, 39t, 46, 123, 131
Reproduction
    disorders and nutrition, 349t
    and environmental stress, 338–341

genetic manipulation tools, 4
history of, 1–4
hormones regulating, 38, 39t, 40
markers, 282–286
and nutrition, 348, 349t
purposes of, 2
Reproduction management
    efficiency measurements, 291–292
    and environmental stressors, 338–341,
        343–346
    females, 292–303, 356–357
    males, 309-316, 357
    and nutrition, 348, 354–357
    problem detection, 307–309
    record keeping, 303–307
Reproductive efficiency
    maintenance of, 355–357
    measures of, 291–293
Reproductive organ injuries, 366–368
Reproductive toxicology, 378–385
Restraint
    AI facilities, 230
    pregnant cow, 326, 326i
    pregnant mare, 332, 332i
Retained corpus luteum, 373–374
Retractor penis muscle, 33
Rivanol test, brucellosis, 400
Roslin Institute, Scotland, 277, 280
Ruminants, and estrogenic pastures, 383

S

Scrotum, 27–29, 28i
Seasonal breeding, 43, 70
    goats, 70–72
    horses, 72
    and photoperiod, 72–73, 73i
    sheep, 70–72
Second messenger system, 53–54, 53i, 54i
Second polar body, 98
Secondary follicle, 9, 10i
Selenium, dietary, 353
Semen, components, 173. *See also* Seminal
        plasma, Spermatozoa
Semen collection
    artificial vagina, 162–170
    and dilution, 204
    electroejaculator, 170–171
    facilities, 160, 161i
    prior stimulation, 161–162

Semen diluters, 199-200, 202–203, 203t
  buffer solutions, 200–201
  stallions, 220t
Semen ejaculate
  CASA analysis, 195–196
  concentration, 186–189
  gross appearance, 183–184
  motility, 184–186
Semen processing (boar)
  dilution, 214
  freezing, 215–216
  processing, 215
Semen processing (buck), 221
Semen processing (bull), 210–211
  cooling, 206–207
  diluter preparation, 204
  dilution, 204–205
  equilibration, 208
  freezing, 209-210, 210t
  glycerolation, 207–208
  packaging, 208–209
  semen collection, 204
  storage and handling, 211–212
Semen processing (ram)
  freezing, 218
  liquid use, 217–218
Semen processing (stallion)
  freezing, 220
  Jockey Club rules, 218–219
  liquid use, 219
Seminal plasma, 173, 177–178
Seminal vesicles (*See* vesicular glands)
Seminiferous epithelial cycle, 84
Seminiferous tubules, 25, 26i, 77, 78i
Sertoli cells, 25, 40, 76, 77, 78i, 81, 117
Serum agglutination test (SAT)
  brucellosis, 400
  leptospirosis, 398
Services per conception, 291
Sex chromosome abnormalities, 364
Sex determination
  embryos, 269-273
  sperm, 273
Sex hormone-binding globulin (SHBG), 52
Sexual differentiation, embryonic, 116–118, 117i
Sexual exhaustion, 94–95
Sexual satiety, 95
Shades, heat stress reduction, 343
Short-day breeders, 70
Sialomucins, 100

Sight, and mating behavior, 89
Sigmoid flexure, 23i, 33
Silage, and listeriosis, 402
Simple uterus, 15, 15i
Sire proofs, milk yields, 3i, 3–4
Size, and semen production, 309
Size at first insemination, and reproductive
    efficiency, 292t, 292–293
Slide preparation
  sperm morphology, 190–191
  sperm motility examination, 185
Smell, and mating behavior, 88–89
Sow
  embryonic development, 111i, 112t
  estrous cycle, 62t, 66i
  estrus, 91, 297, 300–301
  estrus synchronization, 247
  follicular development, 69
  gestation, 109, 110t
  in vivo capacitation, 84
  insemination, 231–232
  mammary glands, 143t
  maternal recognition of pregnancy, 121
  milk composition, 150t
  organ differentiation, 118t
  ovaries, 7
  parturition stages, 129t
  placentation, 15, 16i,
  pregnancy diagnosis, 334, 336–337
  psychological disturbances, 386
  summer breeding, 339
  superovulation, 252
  uterus, 14
Spectrophotometry, sperm cell concentration,
    189, 189i
Speculum insemination method, cow, 224i
Sperm
  concentration, 186–189
  fertile life, 106t
  freezing and storage, 158. *See also* Semen
    processing
  frozen evaluation, 193–195
  morphology, 190–192
  motility, 192–193
  speed, 192–193
Spermatic cord, 27
Spermatids, 80
Spermatocytogenesis, 77, 79i
Spermatogenesis
  definition, 75

Spermatogenesis (continued)
  epithelial cycle, 82–84, 83i
  hormonal control, 81
  process of, 77–80, 79i
Spermatogenic waves, 84
Spermatozoa, 22, 25, 29, 30. *See also* Semen,
    Sperm
  abnormal morphology, 176i, 176–177
  capacitation, 84–85
  concentration in semen, 173, 174t, 181
  energy metabolism, 178–179
  metabolism rate factors, 179-182
  morphology, 173, 175i, 175–176
  production, 75
  sex preselection, 273–274
  and temperature, 338
  transport, 100–103
Spermiation, 81
Spermiogenesis, 80–81, 87i
Sry gene, 117
Staining slides, 191
Staining techniques, 192
Stallion
  accessory glands, 32i
  penis, 34i
  photoperiod, 72
  reproductive management of, 310–311
  reproductive system, 24i
  secondary sexual characteristics, 76i
  semen collection, 168–169
  semen composition, 174i
  semen processing, 218–220
  seminiferous epithelial cycle, 84
  sperm cell concentration, 187
  testes, 25
Steroid hormones, 36–37, 38i, 39t, 385
  during estrous cycle, 64, 65i-66i, 67
  female, 44–47
  intracellular mechanisms, 55i
  male, 47–48
  measurement, 55–57
Storage livability, semen analysis, 196
Strain 19, brucellosis vaccine, 401
"Straw gun," insemination, 227
Straws, bull semen, 208i, 208–209
Stress
  definition, 338
  disease as, 341
  and endocrine physiology, 341i, 341–343

  and temperature, 338–340
Suburethral diverticulum, 8i, 19
Sulfomucins, 100–101
Summer, and breeding, 339, 343, 344t,
    345–346
Superovulation, 249
  techniques, 250–252
Surface epithelium, ovaries, 7
Syngamy, 105
Synthetic toxins, 384–385

T

Tall fescue (*Neotyphodium coenophialum*), 379
TALP-HEPES, IVF medium, 266
Taylorella equigenitalis, 403
Temperature, and spermatozoa metabolism, 180
Temperature control, testes, 27–29
Teratogenic plant toxins, 382
Tertiary follicle, 9, 10i
Testes, 25–27, 26i
Testosterone, 27, 47, 76. *See also* Androgens
  and mating behavior, 87, 88
  and spermatozoa metabolism, 181
Thawing
  bull semen, 227–228
  straws, 228–229
Theca externa, 9, 12i
Theca interna, 9 12i
Thermoregulation, 343, 344i
Thyroid-stimulating hormone (TSH), 42
Thyrotropin-releasing hormone (TRH), 41
Time-exposure photography, sperm motility,
    193–194, 194i
Touch, and mating behavior, 89
Toxic substances, reproductive effects, 379–385
Toxoplasma gondii, 405
Toxoplasmosis, 391t, 405
Transgenic pharmaceuticals, 280–281, 282
Transgenics, 261, 278–282
Transvaginal ovum pick-up (OPU), 264, 255i
Trichomonas fetus, 403
Tris buffer solution, semen diluter, 200, 203t
Trophoderm, 114
Tumor necrosis factor (TNF), 52
Tunica dartos, 27
Twinning, 124–125
  and freemartin condition, 361
  promotion of, 258–259

U

Udder, 142, 143i
Ultrasonography (pregnancy)
cow, 328–329, 329i
ewe and doe, 330
and fetal sexing, 269-270
mare, 334, 335i
sow, 336–337
Ultrasound-guided follicular aspiration, 264
Underfeeding, 350
Unilateral cryptorchid, 22
Up-regulation, 52, 53
Urethra, 31
Uterine contractions, 133
Uterine deposition AI, 229-230
Utero-ovarian vein, 20, 20i
Uterotubal junction, 13, 14i
Uterus, 8i, 13–17
animal types, 14, 15i
incomplete, 363, 364i
injuries, 366
involution of, 139-140

V

Vagina, 8i,19
injuries, 366
Vaginal biopsy, ewe and doe pregnancy, 330
Vaginal insemination, 223
Variation, definition, 3
Vasa deferentia, 31
Vasectomy, 314

Veratum californicum (false hellebore), 382
Vestibular glands
female,19
Vesicular glands, 23i, 24i, 31, 32i, 174t
Vibriosis, 389, 390t, 393–395
Viral diseases, 391t–392t, 406–411
Vitamins, nutrition component, 352–353
Vitelline membrane, 98, 98i, 105
Vulva, 8i, 19

W

Weight management, dairy cows, 356–357
"Winking," in estrus mare, 91, 297, 298i
Wolffian ducts, 116, 117i, 361, 365

X

X-linked enzyme method, fetal sexing, 270
Xenoestrogens, 384, 385

Y

Yolk-citrate, semen diluter, 202
Yolk-phosphate, semen diluter, 202
Yolk sac, 114, 115i

Z

Zearalenone, estrogenic mycotoxin, 380
Zona pellucida, 96, 97i, 98i, 103
Zona proteins (ZP1, 2, 3), 103
Zona reaction, 104
Zygote, 98